Be Your Own

Doctor

101 Stories

Fifth Edition – Revised & Updated

Natural Remedies for the Health of Your Family

Rachel Weaver, Master Herbalist

Fifth Edition, 2013

For information on distribution contact:

Share-A-Care Publications
240 Mohns Hill Rd.,
Reinholds, PA 17569

To order *Be Your Own Doctor* by phone call: 717-435-4707.

Order online at: www.drmomsherbs.com or

www.share-a-care.com

WARNING - DISCLAIMER

Cover Design by Roger Weaver – son of the author

Illustrations by Carol Weaver, Joyce Hansen and Lisa Strubhar – daughters of the author

ISBN: 978-0-9712669-02

Table of Contents

Foreword

If you read *Be Your Own Doctor* carefully, you will be inspired to realize that God created our bodies to heal when we give them the needed tools. You will be motivated to take back the responsibility of your own health and that of your family. You will find in doing this, the realization that our great grandmothers had much practical wisdom which was not passed on to us. You will, like me, be amazed that helping your family can often be so simple and inexpensive.

Be Your Own Doctor has grown out of thirty-two years of experience with our nine children and twelve grandchildren. It was greatly aided by the countless people who came to my door for help with many things, from small accidents to chest congestion and stomach problems or appendicitis. We always recommended the simplest remedies first and they worked so well that I was usually surprised. These peoples' success stories motivated me to keep on learning. For at least 6 years, people have been begging me to write a book about these remedies so that they would have it on hand to reference it when needed. I also wanted this information to be available to my children and grandchildren, since I will not live here forever. It is too easy for important information to die with a person. Then, too, perhaps my phone will be less busy because this book will be here to refer to.

This book is not about selling herbal products; it is instead, an encouragement to use the things you have on hand in your kitchen to help your family and a tool to help you make your own medicines. Its is also a recommendation to have the things on hand that you need, so that you seldom run into an emergency that you cannot handle. This will be better for your budget and your body.

My first inspiration came from the book *Ten Essential Herbs* by Lalitha Thomas. The next, from *Dr. Mom* by Sandra Ellis. These books brought home-health care to my attention and appreciation. Home health care using herbal remedies, is inexpensive and not harmful to your health. *Be Your Own Doctor* is meant to inspire you to realize that you can care for most of the health problems that arise in your home. I hope that you will continue to study and learn all you can. There is a tremendous amount of information that I did not cover. Many times there are three or more different herbs that could be used to do the job effectively, and I have mentioned only one. Take responsibility for your own health and *"be your own doctor."*

I would like to remind you that no two people are the same and what works for one family may not work for you. Therefore, use common sense, and if a suggested remedy does not make you feel good, do not continue to use it. Be thoughtful, consistent, and temperate in whatever you do. Remember to ask the Lord Jesus for wisdom as you work with your family. He is the Giver of life. He is profoundly interested in you.

Be Your Own Doctor is not a complete list of all the helpful remedies that you can use. It is, rather, a compilation of some of the things that I use the most. As you learn to use herbs, you will create your own list of remedies that your family uses most. You will discover new tinctures to make and other salves and teas that are helpful. You will have your own stories of things that worked and things that didn't.

Treating your family's ailments is a journey, and as time goes on you will feel more and more comfortable with what you know and how to do it. Each success that you have gives you a new level of understanding and appreciation for simple home remedies. You will learn that when one thing is not available, another remedy might take its place just as efficiently. Sometimes the cheapest, simplest remedy will work as good or better than an expensive bottle of pills that you needed to send for.

Be Your Own Doctor is not intended to give you any medical advice. The FDA prohibits me from doing that. I am not a medical doctor and the things that I am presenting here were not scientifically tested at the cost of thousands of dollars. I am only passing on to you common sense information that is the result of common sense living and has been used by many mothers and grandmothers for hundreds of years to heal their families. The proof that these things work, lies in the successes of people, not in the million-dollar tests of the laboratories. But remember that you are responsible for whatever information you choose to use from this book. We, as the authors and publishers, will not be liable for any problems arising from this information.

This information is not meant to keep you from going to your doctor, even though I firmly believe that most doctor visits are not necessary when you are well informed and put that information to work. I know the drugs that they give you are often harmful to your health and should be reserved for REAL emergencies. Doctors are very important for serious traumas and small emergencies like broken bones and they help us in numerous other ways with diagnostic tests and information, when there is a need. But as you listen and read and learn, you will find that you need to use the doctor less and less. God bless you on your journey and give you the courage to be adventurous but wise as you serve your family.

This book is not a complete manual for all the things that you will encounter in your family. I wish it could contain more information on Childhood Diseases, Immunizations, Autism, and Food Allergies. It could cover a whole host of things that it does not. However, three hundred plus pages are enough for one book, so I may need to try to write more later. My main desire is that the information here will help you to gain confidence to do what you need to do to be your own doctor in many situations. If you recognize your story here, thank you for allowing me to learn as I worked with you. Others will be enriched by your story.

I wish to thank my family for their patience, love and support as I wrote endless chapters, for their endurance as I tried out many remedies, and for the fun and love that we share as a family. Life is too short and eternity too long to miss the joy and happiness that we share in Christ Jesus.

Myron, my dear husband, without your support and encouragement this project would never have taken place. Thank you for the strength, love and stability you provide for me.

Roger, Lisa, Joyce and Carol, thank you for the lovely art work on the cover and throughout the pages of this book. Your creativity greatly improves the final results.

Dara and Harold, thank you for the great job you did in proofreading and editing.

LeAnn, your everyday use of these things with your family of boys is an inspiration to me.

James and Grace, thank you for taking on extra chores and doing without me some days while I tried desperately to finish this manuscript. Altogether, without my lovely family this book would not be a reality.

Although I would like to be able to help everyone of you personally, I am seldom available to take phone consultations. My family is my first responsibility. Perhaps this book will do for you what I cannot do in person.

The revised version has a few changes and the addition of a Quick Reference Emergency Chart to post in your kitchen.

One of the reasons that it is so important for me to include the recipes for my tinctures in this book is that many/most companies make tinctures that are really of inferior quality. They are tinctured for only a short time using far less herbs than I recommend. This produces a product that does not work nearly as well. If you cannot make your own, order from American Botanical Pharmacy to get quality products. See Suppliers at the end of the book. Make your own Dental Formula since they do not carry this product.

I would like to thank all of you for the suggestions that I received to make the book better. If you have any significant herbal remedies or personal stories that I could share with others please email me at rachel@shareacarepublications.com.

Or you can snail mail me at:

Rachel Weaver - 240 Mohns Hill Rd., Reinholds, PA 17569

Do NOT expect a personal response to mail or emails.

Rachel Weaver – August 2010

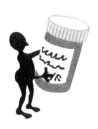

Take Responsibility
for Your Health

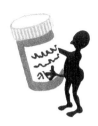

Your Health is Your Responsibility

You may need the help of a doctor, but first you must take responsibility for yourself. Learn all you can about your health problem and do what you can to resolve the issue. It may take some days or even weeks to do this depending on the nature of the problem. If you do what you can and still cannot find the answer that you need, the doctor may be able to help you find a different solution. However, remember that drugs do not usually correct the root problem, they simply put a band-aid on it. To really correct the problem you must go to the root.

Let me tell you one of my own stories from ten years ago.

I was in a dilemma. My blood pressure was high. In fact, it was very high and nothing the doctor had prescribed was working. We had tried this and that for the last year with very little success. The doctor was nonplussed and I was not happy. I did not like to use drugs. They were too expensive, they had dangerous side effects and they were not working. I was ready to try something else. I told the doctor so, and he reluctantly agreed that he was not doing me much good anyway. He was an honest Christian who used some natural things if his clients wanted them. So I went my way and began to research and pray. God gave me the answers in the form of diet and exercise and an inexpensive vitamin. It was not a quick fix, but it benefited my overall health and brought my blood pressure down over a period of time.

Time after time this kind of thing happened to our family and I began to realize that there are alternatives to the expensive, often-dangerous drugs that the doctors use. These alternatives were simple, easy to find and use and worked very well. I began to study and learn. It was an exciting study. I began to understand that the Creator had placed so many wonderful things in this world for the healing of mankind. It made sense to me. God, who created the world, had made what we needed to live in it. That was a wonderful, inspiring thought.. It gave me courage to keep on learning.

God placed plants here for the use of man and animals, and over the many years since then, man has learned much about how to use these plants. Some we use for food, some for clothes, some for medicine, and still others to make a large variety of products that we use every day. In the early days of this country, and today in Germany and England, herbs were and are used for healing. Here, and in many other places, the older women in the country and the villages were the ones who helped folks when they were ill. Folks called for a doctor very rarely. These women learned the information that they knew from their mothers and grandmothers and passed it down over the years. Of course this resulted in some old wives fables and false notions, but often they did have a grip on effective, herbal healing. There are still ladies like this in third-world countries who really understand what the plants of their area can do for folks. Unfortunately they usually get superstition and voodoo mixed into it, so it can be confusing.

We have grown up in a time when herbal wisdom has been largely relegated to the back seat (since about 1945) and allopathic (doctor) medicine has taken the forefront. We do need doctors for emergencies, trauma, and serious difficulties, but we have come to depend on them way too much. This is both hard on our pocketbooks and our health. Why? The first answer is obvious but the second is more obscure. Doctors usually use drugs (*chemicals*) to do their work. They do not go to the root of the problem and advise on diet change, drinking water, and exercise, which will help address most problems. They are taught to use drugs and that is what we have come to expect, "*A pill for every ill!,*" a band-aid for every situation. **Drugs are NOT well tested and this is fast becoming a political problem.** What are the ethics and the motives behind the drug bureaucracy? Today, many conscientious medical doctors are decrying the misuse and overuse of drugs. They are suggesting that the only solution is for us to wake up and take charge of our own health again.

Remember that most doctors do not plan to be negligent or uninformed, but when working with high-powered drugs, the margin for error is slim. Accidents can happen to anyone, but I would rather not be a medical casualty! Doctors may make mistakes because they do not have enough information. That may be your fault. You must take responsibility for your health. They also have been taught to treat the symptom, not the root cause. This is usually counter-productive. If you can learn how to treat the root of the problem you will find that this is far more effective. Doctors often do not spend enough time with you, therefore they often cannot really know the whole of the problem. Finally, they have usually only been taught to use drugs, and EVERY drug has a side affect. Some of the side effects are far more serious than others.

I have discovered a few doctors who do some nutritional counseling and use herbal remedies in conjunction with their other treatments. The number is increasing as concerned physicians look for ways to help their clients. Remember this, part of the original Hippocratic oath that doctors still take is, "First do no harm."

An interesting thing to note is that at times when the hospitals could not function properly, like in wartime, etc., when the death rate should have been the highest, it was the lowest. It appears that when folks need to treat themselves, they often do a good job of it, or else illnesses just resolve themselves if given time. Since many of our illnesses resolve themselves without medical help, that means that they would also resolve often without herbal help, too. But most of us like to do something to help and to shorten distress if possible, and it seems like we should probably learn to help in a drug-free, non-harmful way.

Dr. Mendelson, New York pediatrician and author of *How to Raise A Healthy Child in Spite of your Doctor*, tells us that parents with no medical training are better able than doctors to treat most of the health needs of their children. Why? They have information, time, and love that the doctor does not have. They also know their child very well. Parents can spot subtle changes in their child that will make all the difference in the treatment and outcome of their child's illness.

The question now is, "How can you tell which of the problems are serious and which are not?" The answer is, "You cannot always tell, but really, neither can your doctor." He does the best he can, but often he does not have enough information, and sometimes he has the wrong information.

That is what this book is about. I would like to try to help you understand what is a serious health problem and when you may need to call your doctor. I would like to help you know what to ask your doctor if you do go to him. I would like to help you learn how to check on the medicine doses that he prescribes. This will help you to make sure that there are not more errors than there need to be when an antibiotic or medicine is prescribed.

If you do need to go to the doctor try not to go alone. This will help the doctor to be more careful about what he says to you. Research your problem before you go and know all that you can so that you are able to speak with him about it intelligently.

When he prescribes a drug, ask what the side affects and contraindications of the drug are. Then ask him if there is a less harmful one that could be taken. Finally ask him if there is anything that could be done to resolve your problem without drugs.

Always double check the dosage and the timing to be sure that it is correct for the age and size of the person taking it and make a personal note of what the name of the drug is so that when you get it filled you can be sure the pharmacist could read it.

Here is an interesting personal account of the need to do this. Our nine year old daughter had re-occurring in-grown toenails. Usually I could soak her toe, relieve the inflammation, and then proceed to cut and remove the offending ingrown nail. I had learned how to do this by watching the doctor do it for an in-grown nail that I had. This time, however, I missed it for her. She did not come to me complaining until it was so inflamed that I was afraid to do it for fear of really hurting her. (When this incident happened we did not know how to poultice it with charcoal and flax seed to bring the inflammation down.) We made an appointment with the doctor and he examined the offending toe. "Staph," he pronounced solemnly. "She will need a course of Cipro"

"It is just an ingrown toenail. Can't you cut it out?" I pleaded. He was adamant and busy. He scribbled out a prescription and gave me a sample to start with. I paid the bill, gave the medicine to her to take, and set out for home. On the way home she doubled up with stomach cramps crying that her stomach hurt very badly! When I read the contra-indications on the drug sheet I was alarmed. The drug was doing this!! It cautioned that it could. Hurriedly I dialed the doctor, reminding him that she was a very small nine year old.

"What did I prescribe?" he asked. "Oh, no!" he exclaimed, when I told him what it said on the sample. "That is an adult dose." "Come back in here and I will give you something else." With a sinking feeling in my stomach, I headed the twenty minutes back to the doctor, got the child's dose of medicine, and headed home. When I got home, I found an amazing thing! My little girl no longer had an ingrown nail! After I left she was lying on the couch and her younger brother began to play with her. "Can't get me," he teased. "Oh, yes, I can," she answered forgetting her sore toe and tummy ache. Up she jumped, and after him. The race was on! Mama was gone and there was no one in the room to tell them not to run in the kitchen. Ouch! In her hurry, she collided with the large post that supports our huge room. The impact split her nail and there was the offending corner. With tears, she pulled out the nasty corner and squeezed out the pus. All I had to do was soak it to be sure there was no more infection. Of course we did not give her anymore Cipro. But it made me aware, again, that I had paid an unnecessary $60 for something that we should have done ourselves.

Not too many years later, friends of ours took their 13 year-old son for an appendectomy. All went well and he was discharged and given medicine for pain. For the next week the boy did not really wake up properly. They had to take him to the bathroom, he was so zoned out. Our friends became alarmed and called the doctor. "What did I prescribe" he asked. Once again, there had been an over-prescription. This time it appears that the pharmacist misread the doctor's orders and the boy had been given **four** times the medication that he should have had, a potentially serious mistake that happens far too often.

These kinds of incidents are not isolated ones and they stir me to action. They challenge me to teach folks all I can about being awake and aware of what they can do to help their own families.

Beside this, the cost of medicine, doctor visits, and hospitalization has sky rocketed. America is the most expensive nation in which to be sick. Is it any wonder that people are beginning to seek answers for their many health needs in places other than doctor's offices?

There is a wealth of information to be had and some of it is very exciting and interesting. Some of it is strange and off-the-wall, and some of it has its roots in the spiritual realm of darkness, where one *never* should dabble. Beware of homeopathy. Although it may use some of the herbs that really can heal, the philosophy behind it does not line up with the Bible. Before you decide to use such things, a thorough investigation of it is definitely in order. Stay away from anything that is mystical. Often folks end up getting entangled in other religions' ideas when they dabble in alternative medicine. Stay away from wild advertisements that promise to keep you young, take away your pain and otherwise promise you the moon, money back - guaranteed. These companies are making money on those who are changing their view of doctors and looking for other answers. Research well before you order or you will be scammed like I have been when I returned a doubtful product and never received my money refunded like they had promised.

Discover herbs, the plants God gave us for food, medicine, and enjoyment, and other simple things like charcoal and castor oil. Learn to know what they do and how to use them. The following pages contain exactly that kind of information.

PART 1

Essential
Household Remedies

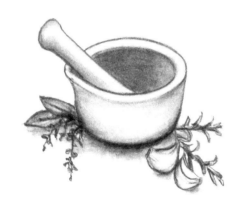

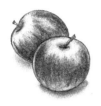

Apple Cider Vinegar

"An All Around Health Aid"

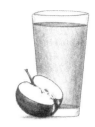

Apple cider vinegar (ACV) is an effective, bacteria-fighting agent that contains many vital minerals and trace elements such as potassium, calcium, magnesium, phosphorous, chlorine, sodium, sulfur, copper, iron, silicon, and fluorine that are vital for a healthy body.

Uses:

- sinus help

- sore throats

- cholesterol

- acne, skin

- food poisoning

- allergies

- immune aid

- stamina

- weight loss

- digestive aid

- constipation

- arthritis

- urinary tract
  health

Natural apple cider vinegar is made by crushing fresh apples and allowing them to mature in wooden barrels. This boosts the natural qualities of the fermented crushed apples, which differs from the refined and distilled vinegars found in supermarkets. When the vinegar is mature, it contains a dark, cloudy, web-like bacterial foam called the *mother*, which becomes visible when the liquid is held to the light. The mother can be used to add to other vinegar to hasten maturity for making more apple cider vinegar.

Natural vinegars that contain the mother have enzymes and minerals that other vinegars in grocery stores do not have, due to processing, over-heating, and filtration.

For this reason, I recommended that you purchase only natural apple cider vinegar when you want to use it for healing purposes.

Benefits of Apple Cider Vinegar

Apple cider vinegar is a helpful natural remedy for a number of ailments which often require antibiotics and other medications.

Pectin in the vinegar is a fiber which helps reduce bad cholesterol and regulate blood pressure. Vinegar also helps extract calcium from the fruits, vegetables, and meat you eat, assisting in the process of maintaining strong bones. Apple cider vinegar is loaded with potassium. Potassium deficiency causes a variety of ailments including hair loss, weak finger nails, brittle teeth, sinusitis, and a permanently running nose. Many ailments can be avoided with the intake of apple cider vinegar. The potassium aids in eliminating toxic waste from the body. The beta-carotene helps in countering damage caused by free radicals. Apple cider vinegar is good for weight loss because it helps in breaking down fat deposits.

Apple cider vinegar contains malic acid which is very helpful in fighting fungal and bacterial infections. It's malic acid dissolves uric acid deposits that form around joints, helping relieve joint pains. This dissolved uric acid is gradually eliminated from the body.

Take your apple cider vinegar the first thing in the morning and with your meals for the best results.

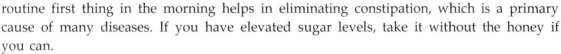

Mix two teaspoons each of apple cider vinegar and honey in a glass of water and drink it. (If you have a problem with sugar levels skip the honey.)

This solution may taste slightly acidic and may not seem to be the best way to start your morning, but once you know of the immense benefits that follow, it will not feel all that bad. You will likely find that following this routine first thing in the morning helps in eliminating constipation, which is a primary cause of many diseases. If you have elevated sugar levels, take it without the honey if you can.

Vinegar and Acid Reflux

An effective remedy to help reduce or eliminate acid reflux is to take the following apple cider vinegar tonic:

Apple Cider Vinegar Tonic

2 teaspoons of apple cider (10-15 ml) in an 8 ounce glass of water (with a teaspoon of honey if desired) before meals or whenever heartburn is experienced.

It appears that the lower esophageal sphincter (LES) is a pH sensitive valve. When there is food in the stomach with insufficient acid present, the LES valve can periodically flop open, causing acid reflux. Too little acid in the stomach may be caused by different factors, but one of the most common one is that as we grow older, our body does not produce as much stomach acid. As a result, the LES valve, sensing less acid, periodically flops open causing acid reflux. Drinking apple cider vinegar supplies the LES valve with the acidity it needs to function properly and the heart burn is resolved.

Trouble with the Flavor?

Here is a recipe that tastes a little like lemonade and makes it easier for some folks to take their ACV.

One cup water   2 tablespoons ACV   2 packets lemon powder

This is ground up, powdered lemon in a box of 18 packets. Grocery stores carry it in orange and lime, too! This tastes like lemonade with a kick!

Detox with Apple Cider Vinegar

To detox:

Use 2 **tablespoon** *of organic ACV in a one or two liter water bottle.*

2 tablespoon = 1/8th cup.

You can add more vinegar than this amount, however, make sure you dilute it with plenty of water. Do not add a sweetener. Drink this solution throughout the day. The solution will be cleansing your system and kidneys all day long.

There are several things you will notice within a week or two of drinking apple cider vinegar· your allergies should begin to disappear, your face should have a more healthy look, you should have more energy, better elimination, and you will more easily digest your food. Apple cider vinegar is an effective, cheap detoxifier for the body.   However do not overdo this. Follow the directions or you may detox too quickly and feel bad.

I have an interesting note to add here. When I began to add ACV to my daily water, I noticed something interesting. The scaly, patchy redness that I had been developing over the months when I was taking heart medication began to leave. In its place my skin became softer and smoother.

Vinegar for Acne

Another lady tells us, "I've suffered from acne for six years now. It developed in my teen years. I've tried everything, from prescription antibiotics, to salicylic acid, change in diet, and drinking liters of water...but to no avail! I decided to give ACV a try. After taking two teaspoon. of vinegar mixed in warm water three times daily, and also applying it topically each night with a cotton swab, I found my skin was clearing. My skin did flare up again after a week and the vinegar was very drying to my skin. I applied the ACV to my face every few days while moisturizing with oil in between, and continued drinking ACV three times a day. After about half a month my skin was clear, with only a few spots every now and then." Apple cider vinegar probably helped her digestion thus eliminating her acne.

For Eczema

One mother says that apple cider vinegar is the only thing that has cleared her youngest son's eczema 100%. They put lots of money into soaps, lotions, and special dietary consideration over the last three years for him. He now drinks ½ cup of tonic three times daily before his meals (see tonic recipe in the beginning of chapter) and she puts a cup of ACV in his bath water. Before he started ACV they had to bathe him twice a day, once with soap, and the other just a water bath. Then they lathered him down with lotions and prescription creams. Taking ACV has leveled him out and his skin is clear for the first time since birth. I suspect that the reason the ACV helped, is that it normalized his digestion. Faulty digestion is one of the main reasons for eczema. When the root problem, digestion and absorption, is aided, the body can begin to heal and the eczema goes away.

For Arthritis

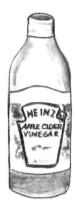

Use the vinegar and honey treatment internally for arthritis and also apply cider vinegar externally to painful joints.(perhaps with cayenne-see cayenne chapter) This entails soaking the arthritic hand, or foot in a strong, comfortably hot solution of cider vinegar for ten minutes, two or three times a day – Use a quarter of a cup of cider vinegar to one and a half cups of water. Arthritic knees can be attended to by making a poultice - soak the cloth in a mixture of cider vinegar and water, (as per above mixture) wring out and wrap it around the joint, then secure with a dry cloth to retain heat. When the wet cloth cools, it should be wrung out in the hot solution and applied again. Repeat several times daily. To speed up the healing benefits add a bit of cayenne to the soaking solution. (a big pinch to ¼ cup of vinegar) See the Cayenne chapter for a story of how apple cider vinegar and cayenne together, helped clear up arthritis pain in my friend's knee.

Sharon writes: "In the mid to late 1980's I was working in an Extended Care Unit in a hospital as a Care Aide. Throughout this time I had been seeing my doctor because of constant pain due to arthritis. My back and knees hurt so badly sometimes it was nearly unbearable. X-rays were taken of my knees, showing spurs under the knee cap itself. The doctor said he'd never seen arthritis so bad in someone so young; even my fingers were beginning to twist. He tried me on different arthritis pills to see which would work the best, and one finally just eased the pain slightly. The pills the doctor had me on cost $60 a month. He said I would have to take them the rest of my life. One day (no longer working at the hospital), I ran out of pills and out of money and remembered what my chiropractor had once said. "Take two teaspoons ACV, two teaspoons of honey in water." I thought there would be a transition period for the ACV to work, I prepared myself for a whole lot of unbearable pain. I started the drink that night and every night for 1 week. Besides flushing my kidneys out, there was no transition at all. There was no pain, absolutely nothing... and still there is no pain. To this day I have not taken any pills from the doctor for arthritis. It has now been sixteen years. If you read the instructions on how to clean a drip coffee machine, it says to use vinegar. Vinegar dissolves calcium build in the machine and I've found it dissolved the build up in my body, too." An interesting response to a simple thing. I think that if I had arthritis I would surely try ACV.

Shingles

Cider vinegar relieves the pain arising from shingles, if applied, undiluted, six times daily to the area of distress. It also promotes the healing. Take internally as well, in a three times daily ACV drink. Try this simple remedy for at least a month and see if it makes a difference in your life.

"ACV has helped with a recent bout of shingles. I applied a solution of 1 tsp. ACV with 1/4 cup of water with some cotton balls. I also made a foot-bath with 1/4 cup of ACV and 1 gallon of warm water, twice a day for three days. The sores were healed within a few days and gone was the pain." Usually this pain lasts much longer than three days. Apple cider vinegar is definitely anti-viral and it must have worked against the virus effectively.

ACV for Wart and Mole Removal

For this simple procedure, you need just three things:

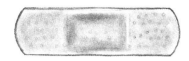

    ☒ *apple cider vinegar*

    ☒ *cotton balls (end of a Q-tip will do)*

    ☒ *band-aid*

Each night before going to bed soak a cotton ball in apple cider vinegar, apply it to the wart/mole and then hold it in place with a band-aid. Leave it on all night, or if you like, twenty-four hours a day, but change the soaked cotton and band-aid each evening for a week. The wart/mole will swell and redden and it may throb or sting as it reacts with the vinegar and then start to turn black within the first two days and after a week or two it should be completely gone. ***It is important to continue the treatment for a few days to a week after the wart has fallen off to help ensure that it does not come back since they tend to have roots or "seeds" that make them grow.***

We had a friend who had quite a few uncomfortable moles on her back that her clothes were irritating. She decided to try the apple cider vinegar cure and followed the directions carefully. This young lady experienced stinging and some redness at the site of the mole she was treating, but she persisted and the mole began to change color and dry up and in a few more days it fell off. Thus encouraged, she treated all of them and rid herself of the annoyance she had been having. She had no doctor bills and very little pain involved, and they were gone.

High Blood Pressure

Charles has had high blood pressure for the last ten years or so and its been getting progressively worse. His doctors had put him on a wide variety of pills, but nothing they had done was of any real benefit to his health. Nothing. Recently he went to the emergency room because his pressure was reading 210/160. He was experiencing pain in his head, neck, back, and eyes. The pain was unbearable. He left the emergency after five and a half hours without being seen by anyone other than the intake nurse because they were so busy and that's when he decided to take his health into his own hands. He began a regime of two tablespoons of ACV in water three times a day. After two weeks he was tempted to give up because he didn't see any results but he remembered that results sometimes take time, so he kept on with the ACV and after his third week there was a breakthrough. His pressure came down significantly. Though this does not help everyone, here is what he takes.

3 tablespoons ACV
1 teaspoon cinnamon
½ teaspoon cayenne pepper
1 glass of water

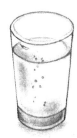

Vinegar for Burns

One lady tells us the following account. "I have always known ACV is good for sunburn, one cup in a tub of water and the sunburn is gone! So, when I was at work alone and severely burned my hand, I put ACV in a sink of water with ice cubes. I had to wait until someone else came into work before I could go to the hospital. On and off for about an hour I kept soaking my burnt hand in the ACV solution. When I arrived at the hospital my hand was bandaged and treated and I was told to return the next day to have this treatment repeated. The next day I went back to the hospital and as the bandages were removed, the doctor was shocked! The deep red welt, the blister, and all signs of a burn were gone. I had only a pink line. I can thank my mother for this. She used apple cider vinegar when I was growing up."

Vinegar for Blood Sugar

Research suggests that vinegar has a beneficial effect on blood sugar levels. In the study, ingesting a couple tablespoons of apple cider vinegar before a high-carbohydrate meal was found to help dampen expected spikes in blood sugar levels from the meal.

Vinegar is no substitute for healthy eating habits or proven methods of blood sugar control. But in a recent study, Carol Johnston, a professor of nutrition at Arizona State University East, proves that taking two tablespoons of apple cider vinegar before eating a high-carbohydrate meal improved insulin resistance.

Study participants who experienced the blood sugar control benefits from vinegar were either diabetic or had insulin resistance syndrome. They followed the twenty grams of apple cider vinegar with a high-carbohydrate meal consisting of a white bagel, butter, and orange juice. After the high-carbohydrate meal, the acetic acid from the earlier serving of vinegar reduced blood sugar levels by nineteen percent in people with diabetes and by thirty-four percent in people with insulin resistance.

Acetic acid may help lower blood sugar levels by suppressing enzymes required to break down sugars, resulting in slower absorption.

Canker Sores

Shirley tells us that she decided to try home remedies for her canker sores. First she tried hydrogen peroxide and that didn't work, then she rubbed salt on it and it hurt so badly, but it didn't work. A few hours later, she couldn't take the pain anymore, so she decided to try apple cider vinegar. She put some on a Q-tip and it really hurt, but a few minutes later the pain was basically gone. She says she went from not being able to talk, to eating dinner within a matter of an hour. She was so amazed! She repeated the procedure a couple more times that day and it did not hurt as much second time around. She was just amazed as how fast the ACV worked." The antiviral effects of apple cider were working for this lady.

Vinegar Tincture for Calcium

This old fashioned remedy is a simply made form of calcium, easily digested and absorbed. It is beneficial to the hair, nails and bones.

Collect eggshells from one dozen free-range eggs, dry them, and remove the membranes if you like. Powder the shells, using a blender or mortar and pestle, and add to a pint of pure apple cider vinegar. Use a quart or larger glass jar or bottle as the mixture will bubble. Immediately cap the jar.

Take a tablespoon of this tincture three times a day.

This does not taste much different than the ACV that you have been drinking and it is a very cost-effective remedy that will supply you with good calcium. I would use free-range eggs so that you have a product that is not damaged by chemicals.

Kidneys and the Bladder

Due to the eliminative nature of cider vinegar, the kidneys and bladder can benefit tremendously by the 'flushing' which they receive when the following cider vinegar therapy is undertaken: two teaspoons of cider vinegar in a glass of water six times a day. It is beneficial to drink a couple of glasses of water in the morning, taking one teaspoonful of cider vinegar in each drink. Inflammation of the kidneys, called pyelitis, in which pus cells are present in the urine, will generally clear up with the above treatment.

Hay Fever

This ailment is marked by watery eyes, sneezing, and running nose. In other words, there is an excess of fluid which the body is drastically trying to offload. For an effective relief, honey and cider vinegar should be taken.

The ordinary dosage of cider vinegar and honey should be:

2 teaspoons of cider vinegar and 2 teaspoons of honey

Take in a glass of water, three times a day. This dosage should be maintained during the entire hay-fever season. This may help to bring relief when other things have not worked.

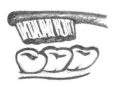
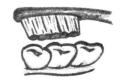

Black Walnut

"The Household Dentist"

The active ingredient of black walnut hulls is nucin or juglone. Iodine is present in all usable parts of the black walnut, but the highest concentration is in the outer hulls of the nuts. As a rich source of organic iodine, black walnut has gained much popularity as nourishment for the thyroid, especially where sea vegetables were hard to come by. Black walnut is a significant source of potassium, magnesium, manganese, sulfur, copper, and silica. Black walnut tones and helps heal inflamed tissues. It is also effective in enhancing the elimination of various microbes and parasites from the bowel. This interesting herb strengthens and builds tooth enamel. It contains organic, assimilable fluoride. Dr. Christopher writes,". . . it is a muscle and nerve food, and a food for the hair, nails, skin and nerves." Never mind that he does not mention the teeth. He still added black walnut to his tooth powder.

For Cavities and Tooth Repair

I read it again, and again. "You can fill in your children's cavities," the ad promised. This was not some "fly by night" firm. I was reading the catalog of a reputable family-based business that I often ordered from. I kept promising myself that I would order their product to check it out since our one daughter had trouble with cavities, but it was a rather expensive kit and I did not get around to it.

Uses:

- antibacterial

- rebuild enamel

- take away toothache

- kill parasites

- cure impetigo

- rich source of iodine

Then I enrolled in the "School of Natural Healing" to get my Master Herbalist Certification, and somewhere in the course, Doctor Christopher talked about using black walnut to heal tooth enamel. It was just a mention and that was all, but I was intrigued. I purchased his tooth powder and gave it to my married daughter to try. She used it faithfully and said that it took away the pain in her teeth, but that it was not enough. It did not seem to fill in the cavities that she always dealt with. Her diet was good, but she had been a premature baby, and I did NOT understand nutrition when she was little. She was missing some necessary mineral or something. I kept searching. One day, a friend who knew that I worked with lots of people's health problems, gave me six or seven bottles of black walnut tincture from the food co-op that her husband worked for. They had just gone out of date and she thought that maybe I could use them for someone. Interestingly enough, I had read again that week, that black walnut helps with cavities. Here was my chance to try it. I was having tooth pain from some cavities that I had. I dislike going to dentists so I immediately went to work swishing black walnut in my mouth and presto, my toothache was gone. If it would return, I would swish a few times a day and it would be gone for awhile. Then it went away and did not return. Interesting!

I began to give the black walnut to my children when they got toothaches and if we were faithful and swished two droppers three or four times a day for a week or two, the small cavity filled in. I was impressed! I could not find much information anywhere on my idea, but it seemed to be working. What I needed was a few others to try this experiment.

One day I got a call from a friend. "Can you come over quickly? Our son was in a bike accident and his face is all messed up. We'd like your help." I went as quickly as I could. His face was messed up - way too messed up for me to deal with! One glance told me that he would need extensive stitching to repair his mouth and chin area. There was a huge split above his lip and the skin on his lower jaw hung slack. I sent them in to the hospital for repair, wishing that I could have helped them. The next morning the mother called and asked if I had anything to repair teeth. The doctors had put in about 40 stitches and told them to go to the dentist since her son's front teeth were all cracked and would need extensive work. The X-rays agreed, and the dentist told them to come back in two weeks when his mouth was healed and she would begin to work on the teeth. We all knew that would be expensive. Dental work always is these days. I thought of black walnut tincture and gave her a free bottle with these instructions:

Use 2 droppers of black walnut glyceride in a small bit of water. Swish it around in the mouth and swallow it. Repeat at each meal time and just before bed.

Of course that was just a good guess and I had no idea what the results would be. But I was confident that it would do some good.

Imagine my surprise and delight when she phoned me after his next visit to the dentist two weeks later. "His teeth are fine."

The dentist got him into the chair and took a look at his teeth and said, "There must be a mistake. He does not need any work on his teeth." "Get the x-ray," requested my friend. Ms. Dentist obeyed and behold, the x-ray showed very cracked teeth.

"How did the teeth heal?" she asked.

"We used black walnut tincture," replied my friend.

"Never heard of it." said the dentist. "But his teeth are fine." That is all she said.

This incident gave me the courage to really begin to introduce people to the healing benefits of black walnut. I have found that children's teeth heal far more quickly than adults. In adults it takes the pain away and sometimes it heals their teeth. Other times it is only a pain reliever. I suspect the reason lies in the fact that the potassium actually aids in the enamel repair in young, healthy children and younger adults. Older adults who heal less quickly and have greater mineral deficiencies may need to work at it longer than a child to heal the problem. Finally, in elderly people total repair may be impossible for the same reason. Another reason that I suspect that this works is that black walnut is highly antibacterial, thus eliminating much of the bacteria in your mouth and allowing the enzymatic saliva to do it's job of rebuilding your enamel.

Since that time quite a few folks have taken this tincture and really feel that it helps. Some of these folks are in their 50's. They feel that it has helped them keep their own teeth longer, without so much work at the dentist. Most of them are younger people with families and they tell me that it has helped them avoid many fillings and dentist visits. Many times with children, the amount used to heal a cavity is 3 droppers a day or less over a period of a few weeks. If the child is small you must use half that amount or less.

For toothache and for cavities:

Put 2 droppers of tincture in about 1/8th glass of water, swish well and swallow. Repeat as needed, 3 or 4 times daily. Note - if you do not have black walnut, try making a warm rinse with 2 teaspoons of salt in a ½ cup of very warm water. Swish the water around well and hold a bit in the side that hurts. Repeat in 5 minutes if needed. Repeat as often as needed. Some folks say that this is very helpful in relieving the immediate pain of a cavity. It will kill any bacteria that is giving you a problem as well. Do the black walnut to rebuild the tooth but the salt might be helpful immediately, for pain. For a child of 5 – 7 it may only take a dropper a day. Do not use if pregnant or nursing. If nursing, it may dry up your milk supply. Use Calc Tea - see p. 30

One day I read this little comment. "A lady told me that she took her son to the dentist and he had a cavity. They scheduled to get it filled two weeks later. She had him brushing with black walnut powder and when they went back to the dentist, the cavity was not there." I was encouraged. Black walnut powder does work, but it is messy. I like the glycerite best, myself. It is less messy to swish and swallow.

Black Walnut Powder

Here is a story to reinforce the benefit of black walnut for teeth.

Susan had not been to the dentist in two years. Only two weeks before her dental appointment she began using the black walnut as a tooth polish after brushing. (She just emptied a capsule into a jar cover and applied it with a damp toothbrush.) The dental hygienist couldn't believe how clean and white her teeth were, especially since she had not seen the dentist for so long! Black walnut powder to the rescue!

Make Your Own Black Walnut Tincture

Collect freshly, fallen black walnuts that still have the husks on them. You can also pick them from the tree when you know they are ready. This is usually in September or October, and you will notice that the nuts have begun to fall off the tree. Use a few of the nicest <u>black</u> husks, crushed. Do not use the green husks since they *may* be somewhat toxic. **Never use the powder for a tincture. It simply does not strain out nicely.**

> *3 parts black walnut hull – dried (not green and not powdered)*

> *2 parts comfrey leaf –* FDA does not approve of comfrey for internal use

> *1 part white oak bark cut and sifted*

> *1 part marshmallow root cut and sifted*

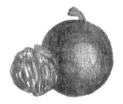

> *1 part peppermint leaf*

> *1 part horsetail herb*

> Fill the jar with a mixture of glycerine and vodka. Use ½ glycerine and ½ vodka. Cover the jar and store in a cool dark area.Let set for two to four weeks and then strain off the liquid and bottle it.

> Pacific Botanicals (see suppliers) is one of the only places to get hulls. You will need a 1 pound order.

I recommend that you do not use this when pregnant or nursing and not for more than 6 – 8 weeks at a time. Switch to Calcium tea for about 2 months before using the Dental Formula again. See Calcium Tea recipe on page 30.

Black Walnut Tea

You can make a nice tasting tea that may do the same thing as the black walnut tincture. In fact, for some people it seems that the tea actually works better than the tincture.

Mix together:
1 part marshmallow root powder
1 part comfrey root powder
1/3 part black walnut powder
¼ part anise seed ground or powdered

Use three to four teaspoons per quart of boiling water. A drip coffee maker with a filter simplifies this greatly. Use the tea mix in the place of coffee. Adults -drink at least 3 cups daily.

Tea for Toothache

My husband recently had a toothache, which was unusual for him. Up to that time he had only one filling in his mouth and he was fifty-four. He began to use black walnut tincture like our children do, but, although it helped it did not completely clear up the problem. Finally, he went to the dentist, who found a tiny cavity and filled it. The sad part of the story is: the hundred dollar filling did not fix the problem. When he went back to the dentist again, they could not find the problem and offered to do a root canal which he declined. He came home and began experimenting with black walnut tea. Drinking a cup of it daily helped him far more than using the tincture did. Then he discovered that he actually enjoyed the tea, so he has been drinking the tea regularly as a deterrent to more cavities and his tooth pain.

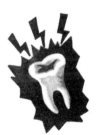

Re-mineralization of Tooth Enamel

Here are a few things you can do to effectively create a favorable body chemistry for re-mineralization of tooth enamel and possibly bone re-mineralization.

1. Sea weed capsules or super food tablets (American Botanical Pharmacy).
   Dose: Take up to twelve capsules a day, three or four with each meal.

2. Black walnut tincture – take two droppers in a bit of water with meals and at bed time. Swish and swallow.

3. Drink black walnut tea, two to four cups daily. Recipe on previous page.

4. Make a powder mixture to use with the oils in #5. (Directions below #5)

   ½ cup sea salt

   3 tablespoon white oak bark powder

   3 tablespoon black walnut hull powder

   2 tablespoon marshmallow root powder

   2 tablespoon comfrey root powder

5. Mix Tooth Oil.

   Use 1 part each of thyme and oregano oils, and four parts each of peppermint and wintergreen oils. These oils are antibacterial and contribute to general oral health. Store in an air-tight glass container.

Directions: To maintain an alkaline environment in your mouth, use the following procedure: *Place ½ a teaspoon or more of tooth powder in a cup. Add three or more drops of tooth oil. Add water to liquefy. Use this mixture as a mouthwash, swish it in your mouth for ½ - 1 minute daily. Repeat this at least four or more times a day if you need an intensive treatment to avoid an upcoming dentist visit.*

Parasites

Taking black walnut for your teeth will likely have another effect on your body. It may effectively rid your body of other parasites like pin worms and round worms that live in your intestines. Everyone has these critters living in their gut and black walnut is a reliable worm remover. Black walnut glycerin is easy to take and may be more effective than over-the-counter pin worm medicine. You will have the benefit of knowing that it is good for your child's teeth as well.

Black Walnut for an Itchy Red Rash - permission of The Bulk Herb Store

One mother writes: "We used black walnut for my daughter's problem several years ago! She had an itchy red, dry rash on her hands. We decided that the rash was caused by a yeast infection or a parasite. We treated her (after getting no help from a doctor) with black walnut. We used the leaves and hulls in a tea, and they both work. She drank the tea twice a day for about 2 weeks. She had immediate results after drinking the first batch of tea. I made black walnut tincture and treated her again a month later because of a recurrence. I rather think it was a parasite. We never had another problem. This was a very painful rash that responded to an easy remedy. It made me a believer in herbs. I hope this remedy is helpful to many mothers out there in the trenches fighting for their children's health."

Black Walnut Tincture for Impetigo

The late Dr. Christopher, told this story of the time he cured a serious case of impetigo with black walnut tincture. The fellow that he was treating had been hospitalized nine times and nothing had worked. He had a huge scab over his whole scalp. Dr. Christopher made a gallon of black walnut tincture. He tinctured it only two days instead of fourteen because he was dealing with an emergency. He made a cap of layer after layer of gauze, and he taped it to hold it down. At the places where the tape didn't cover, there was room to insert a syringe filled with the tincture. He inserted tincture a number of times a day to keep the area moist with black walnut. The man spent four days with this fomentation on his head. The fifth morning came, and Dr. Christopher loosened the adhesive tape that was holding the headpiece down and took it off. Inside the cap was ¾ an inch of scar tissue and scab. The man's head was clean as a baby's, with no sign of impetigo at all. The secondary infection where the scalp had bled was healing. Taken From Dr. Christopher's writings

Use black walnut tincture to heal impetigo. Take it internally and apply a bandage soaked in it to the affected area. You should see results in a few days. Keep on with the treatment until the area is clear.

Fungus

Black Walnut tincture is one of the best known remedies for any fungus. Use externally and apply frequently. This includes ring worm, athlete's foot, and others. You could add it to a soak, use it in a bandage, or rub it into the affected area a few times a day. For quicker healing you can also drink the tea or take the tincture while working on the skin.

Energy

Low thyroid levels usually mean low energy and reduced resistance to disease. We are noticing that folks that take black walnut regularly for a few weeks often notice an increase in energy. This may be due to the fact that black walnut is high in natural iodine and iodine encourages thyroid health.mAmericans, across the board, have low thyroid functions. When the thyroid is functioning normally your body fights infection more effectively, you sleep better and your energy level is improved. Maybe black walnut will do more than one thing at a time for us.

Herbal Calcium - for rebuilding teeth, hair and fingernails, and for osteoporosis -

6 parts horsetail herb

2 parts nettle leaf

2 parts red raspberry leaf

3 parts oat straw

1 part lobelia herb

1 part peppermint leaf (optional for flavor)

Do not use powdered herb - use cut herb. Mix these herbs and store in a glass jar ready to use. If you desire to you can add 4 parts comfrey leaf for more healing (optional: if you think of comfrey as I do – the FDA says not to take it internally.) **Do not take herbal calcium with comfrey in it for longer than 4 weeks at a time.** Without comfrey you can take it indefinitely. Adults: two cups daily. Small children – ½ cup or less

Herbal Calcium Tea or Syrup

*Make a **strong** tea with ½ cup of the mixed herbs for 2 quarts of water. Bring water to a boil, turn off heat and add the herbs. Cover and let set for 30 minutes. This is the tea. Strain, sweeten and drink in three days.*

For Syrup, Using 2 quarts of tea, heat and simmer until the two quarts are simmered down to 1 quart of liquid. Add 1 pint of honey and 1 pint of apple cider vinegar and refrigerate indefinitely. Use by the spoonful as often as desired for ages two and up. Good for nursing and pregnant mothers.

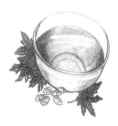

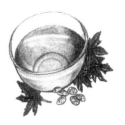

Castor Oil

"The Healing Oil"

Castor oil is extracted from castor beans. The oil has a long history of use as a healing agent in medicine around the world. Castor oil, known for its emollient and lubricating properties, is unique in that ricinoleic acid, an unsaturated hydroxy fatty acid, makes up 90% of its composition. Doctors from the early 1900's taught that castor oil packs help rebuild and increase the effectiveness of the lymph system and the mucous membrane of the small intestine.

Castor oil packs over the abdomen and liver enhance liver function, stimulate the gallbladder, increase elimination, and promote relaxation. A double-blind study, described by Harvey Grady in a report entitled *Immunomodulation through Castor Oil Packs* published in a recent issue of the *Journal of Naturopathic Medicine,* examined lymphocyte values of 36 healthy subjects before and after topical castor oil application.

Uses:

- pain relief

- drain abscesses

- increase milk

- for sore nipples

- inflammation

- abscesses

- headaches

- appendicitis

- constipation

- intestinal obstructions

This study identified castor oil as an anti-toxin, and as having impact on the lymphatic system, enhancing immunological function. The study found that castor oil pack therapy of a minimal two-hour duration produced an increase in the number of T-11 cells within a 24-hour period following treatment, with an increase in the number of total lymphocytes.

This T-11 cell increase represents a general boost in the body's specific defense status, since lymphocytes actively defend the health of the body by forming antibodies against pathogens and their toxins. T-cells identify and kill viruses, fungi, bacteria, and cancer cells.

Castor oil packs are a simple therapy which often produces amazing results in boosting the immune system, relieving pain, and in healing disease.

Castor Oil Internally

Castor oil should not be applied to broken skin, or used internally during pregnancy, breastfeeding, or during menstrual flow. Always seek advice before using it internally. Castor oil may induce labor if taken internally since it causes spasms of the colon which tend to irritate the uterus for some ladies causing them to go into labor. For some ladies, all it does is give them the "diarrhea". Castor oil should not usually be taken internally.

Castor Oil Packs

"Modern uses for an old folk remedy"

By Simone Gabbay, RNCP excerpt used by permission from simonegabbay.com

My first encounter with the amazing healing powers of castor oil took place during a business trip to Amsterdam, Holland, some 25 years ago. As I got off the plane from Toronto, I felt a sharp pain in my lower back, radiating down into my leg. Whether it was triggered by the long hours of sitting crunched up in an uncomfortable airplane seat or by the heavy suitcase I was carrying, I'll never know. By the time I got to my hotel room, I was in agony, barely able to stand up straight. Even lying down on the bed was painful.

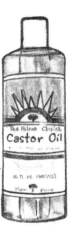

What was I to do? I didn't know anyone in the city, and I was scheduled to attend some important meetings the following day. The staff at the hotel reception desk couldn't tell me how to locate a chiropractor. I wasn't interested in going to a doctor for a prescription painkiller or muscle-relaxant. I remembered that Edward Cayce frequently suggested castor oil packs for various aches and pains, and I remembered having read of this remedy's effectiveness in cases of sciatica.

I managed to take a cab to a nearby drugstore, where I purchased a bottle of castor oil. No doubt the pharmacist thought that I was bent over because of constipation.

Back at the hotel, I soaked a towel in the oil and wrapped it around my lower back. In a proper castor oil pack, a cloth of wool or cotton flannel is folded in several layers, then saturated with warm castor oil and placed on the affected area. But I had to make do with a hotel towel and oil at room temperature. I also didn't have access to a heating pad or hot water bottle to add the prescribed warmth to the pack. The idea is that heat allows the oil to penetrate the skin and work its way deep into the tissues. I figured that the heat generated by my body would have to do. Finally, I cut open some plastic bags and spread them on the bed before lying down, to avoid getting oil on the sheets.

Tired from the overnight flight and exhausted from the pain, I drifted off into a deep sleep. When I woke up a few hours later, I was drowsy with jet lag, but the pain was gone! It had completely disappeared, and I was able to sit, stand, and walk normally. An impressive result for a clumsy first attempt with makeshift tools!

My family and I have successfully used castor oil packs and rubs for various kinds of abdominal complaints, headaches, inflammatory conditions, muscle pains, and skin eruptions and lesions. Castor oil is a staple item in our medicine cabinet at home, and whenever we travel, we pack a small bottle of the oil.

Instructions for Castor Oil Pack

You will need: flannel   plastic sheet   electric heating pad   towel

- ☒ *Pour castor oil into a pan and soak the cloth in the oil.*

- ☒ *Wring out the cloth so that it is wet but not drippy with the castor oil (or simply pour castor oil onto the pack so it is soaked).*

- ☒ *Apply the four layers of wool flannel to the area of the body that needs treatment.*

- ☒ *Cover the flannel with a plastic sheet, or large plastic bag. Then place the heating pad on top of the plastic sheet and keep the heat on low at first, gradually turning it up to medium.*

- ☒ *Do not have the heat so high that it will burn the skin.*

- ☒ *Finally wrap a towel over the treated area to keep the heat in.*

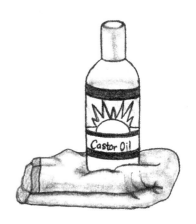

The pack can stay in place from 45 minutes to two hours, and the skin can then be cleansed with a solution of baking soda and water. The amount used is two teaspoons to a quart of warm water. The flannel pack can be used up to 30 times. Each person should have their own pack. Keep in a plastic container in the fridge. The pack should be warmed up before application. So, relax and enjoy.

Note: Always use a high-quality, cold-pressed castor oil, available in health food stores if you can.

Abdominal Pack

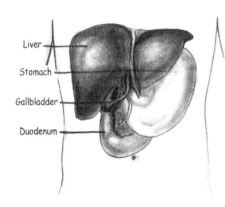

Liver
Stomach
Gallbladder
Duodenum

Prepare a flannel cloth which is two or three thicknesses when folded and which measures about eight inches in width and ten to twelve inches in length after it is folded. This is the size needed for abdominal application - other areas may need a different size pack. Most often, the pack should be placed so it covers the area of the liver.

When I was detoxing as I was loosing weight, my kidneys became sensitive. I had been reading about castor oil packs and how they actually help with detoxing, so I made the choice to aid my kidneys by using a pack over the liver to eliminate some of the waste that way, taking the stress off my kidneys. The pack felt warm and cozy and I fell asleep for the night with it on. I awoke later and took it off, noting a relaxed feeling in the liver area. Because of how good it felt I repeated the process for a few nights and it noticeably relieved the strain on my kidneys and reduced swelling over my liver area.

Pain Relief

One writer recalls the time when her mother had fractured her back due to severe osteoporosis. She was prescribed very strong painkillers during her ten day stay in the hospital. The writer remembered the information she had read about castor oil packs. On her mother's return home she proceeded, with her mother's permission, to very gently apply castor oil packs to her back. After the very first application the mother no longer required the painkillers and after using the packs for three consecutive days per week for several weeks, they changed to a maintenance program of once a week. This kept her spine more flexible and supple. In fact the mother actually looked forward to her *castor oil day* and found it extremely relaxing.

Varicose Veins

Apply castor oil packs at night for the relief of pain and swelling associated with varicose veins. The castor oil soothes the inflammation and increases the circulation which begins to heal and tighten the veins. Repeated applications will be necessary.

Fertility

When it comes to fertility, castor oil packs are great for women who are experiencing:

- Ovarian and uterine cysts
- Blocked tubes
- Uterine Fibroids
- Ovarian Cysts
- Endometriosis
- Detoxifying before conception

Castor oil therapy consists of using a warm castor oil wrap over the abdomen in order to stimulate blood flow to the uterus and ovaries. Castor oil treatments are recommended to treat many gynecological disorders. This type of treatment is helpful to resolve infertility in many cases, because the castor oil pack relieves congestion and inflammation of the uterus, ovaries, and fallopian tubes.

Castor oil therapy increases circulation to the reproductive organs and helps detoxify the liver improving the metabolism of hormones. In these cases, castor oil is used by employing packs over the abdomen (see castor oil abdominal packs) covering both the uterus and liver. Castor oil is absorbed easily into the body through the skin and its healing components are delivered directly into the body tissues.

Concussion

A child (six years old) took a nasty spill on his bike. This story is an excellent report on what happened:

"He had a 'goose egg' over his right temple and surrounding area. I checked his eyes, and they seemed to focus alright. I asked him if he wanted to go to church or stay home. He opted to go to church... but instead of going to his class, he stayed with me, head in my lap. When we got home he complained of not feeling well, and vomited. In talking to him, I discovered he couldn't remember what had happened from the time he fell off his bike until sometime on the way to church. I was very concerned by this time and felt he must have had a minor concussion. I put a castor oil pack on the bruise and around his head, and asked him to lie down and remain comparatively quiet. In about an hour and a half he was asking for something to eat, playing a game on the bed with his sister, and when I checked the swelling, it was all gone. I removed the pack and he got up. That night I put it back on until morning. We had no further repercussions that I could see."

Hyperactive Children

There have been many positive reports on the use of warm castor oil packs for hyperactive children. In each case the mother placed a warm pack on abdomen of the child for 20 minutes to a half hour at nap times and bedtimes. The packs seem to help a bit immediately but it does take some while before the treatment can be discontinued. This simple treatment might be an answer to prayer for many a weary mother whose child cannot sit still and does not sleep well. The children that were treated actually seemed to enjoy the treatment and that was probably because it noticeably relaxed them and they felt better.

Lower Back Pain

If you suffer from lower back pain, you are not alone. Lower back pain is a common condition that affects most individuals at some point in their life. While there are a number of causes for this condition, in most cases identifying the culprit of your lower back pain can be difficult.

Kidney problems are one cause of lower back pain and using a castor oil pack will be extremely helpful if that is the reason for your pain. Castor oil packs relieve tight muscles and pull out toxins. This treatment can be a very relaxing, soothing treatment, especially if you have had a lot of pain. Castor oil packs can often take the place of pain medication and do healing at the same time.

For lower back pain, follow the treatment as outlined for castor oil packs. Leave the pack on for at least thirty minutes, longer if desired. The pack can be stored in the refrigerator for future use. Heat to desired temperature and reuse. After about three days of using this treatment, you should see a significant improvement in your condition, if not before.

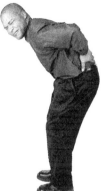

I experienced the benefit of a castor oil poultice when I was having a fair amount of kidney pain and nothing that I used seemed to be helping. I tried my normal kidney herbs, I drank more water, I soaked in an herbal bath designed to address the kidneys, but when I used a castor oil pack two times in one day, the annoying ache simply disappeared.

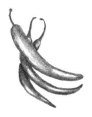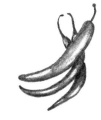

Cayenne

"The Remarkable Healer"

Cayenne is one of the best all-around herbs to use and have on hand. Its name comes from the Greek "to bite." The highly stimulating properties of cayenne aid in increasing circulation, stopping bleeding, and healing things quickly. It is an inexpensive, effective herb to use. Keep a small bottle of the powder and one of tincture in each car and in your medicine cabinet and you will always be prepared for an emergency like shock, heart attack or bleeding. It can be given with complete safety.

Cayenne – a Blood Stopper

"My foot is bleeding, and I am all alone with 5 young children. What can I do to stop it?" asked a distressed young mother. " I cut it and the blood keeps running unless I put my foot up and pinch it tightly."

"What happened?" I asked.

"It was a foolish thing. I dropped a jar and broke it. Then I accidentally stepped on a piece of the broken glass. I tried to brush it off with my foot and accidentally cut my other foot rather deeply."

Uses:
- bleeding
- ulcers
- anemia
- energy
- heart attacks & strokes
- shock
- flu and virus
- circulation

"Do you have any cayenne?"

"Yes," she replied a bit hesitantly. "But won't it burn?"

"It shouldn't. Pack it into the cut and hold it tightly for a bit. Wait for a bit. If that does not stop the bleeding, do it again. Call me back if it does not work for you and I will take you for stitches." In about ten minutes my phone rang again. "It worked!" she said happily. "There was only a slight sting and the bleeding stopped almost at once. I added a bit more just to be safe and then I bandaged my foot and I can even walk on it."

"Good," was my response. "That is usually how it works. And it works very quickly." Time and again I have found this to be the case, even in more serious situations.

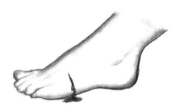

More Cayenne Stories

We were away on a trip giving lectures about herbs and I was ready to give my lecture on First Aid and Emergencies in just ten minutes. Suddenly there at my elbow was my sixteen year-old son. He looked distressed and was holding his hand tightly. "I need People's Paste, Mom," he said. "But I do not have any. I just sold it all at the last meeting."

"But Mom, I need it. I have a deep cut." Even as he spoke the blood was seeping through his fingers and dripping to the ground. "Let me see it," I responded with concern. "

"I can't take my fingers off or it will really bleed," he responded with a worried look. What could I do? I was not at home and I did not have my usual supplies. Then I remembered cayenne. Perhaps the lady where we were staying would have cayenne in her cupboard. She was not at home at that minute, but I could check. We hurried over to her house and a quick search disclosed the cayenne.

"Please mom, don't. It will burn like fire." he begged, remembering a story I had told them one day.

"Let me try just a pinch and if that is too bad we will think of something else." I responded. I took a tiny pinch and placed it at the beginning of that gaping wound. A tiny sting and that was all. Maintaining pressure on his hand to keep the flow staunched we added more cayenne until the wound was packed with it. In just a minute, the bleeding stopped. I hurriedly bandaged the fingers and got back to my seminar just a few minutes late. What a good illustration I had for my first aid class that day!

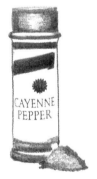

My next surprise came the following morning when I re-bandaged it. Never had I seen a cut healing so quickly and neatly. In just a few days the deep cut across two fingers was healed without a scar. Why? Cayenne increases the circulation so much that it speeds the healing and the powder mixed with the blood forms a nice, tight bandage that holds the wound shut. Seldom, if ever, do I need to apply more cayenne after the first five minutes. When the wound is packed with the powder it does it's job neatly. Remember to use pressure on the area around the wound to help slow the bleeding, too.

Occasionally I have to add a bit more powder if the wound is bleeding very quickly. In that case drink a glass of water with ½ - 1 teaspoon of cayenne mixed into it. This also helps to stop the bleeding from the inside out. It is hot but drink a glass of milk when you are done and you will be fine. This is cheaper than a trip to the emergency room.

"Fire Water"

Cold and Flu Fighter

Mix together:

½ cup boiling water   ½ cup apple cider vinegar   1 teaspoon cayenne powder   1 teaspoon salt

Stir until the salt is dissolved. Add ½ cup apple cider vinegar (not white vinegar) Take 1 tablespoon every 15 - 20 minutes until the flu is gone.

My first experience with "fire water" was a favorable one. I am a skeptic that needs to prove things before I am sure that they work, so I had to try this one before I would tell others that it really did the job. I came down with a bad case of the flu, fever, body aches and all. Since I was lying there unable to do anything else, I decided to try "fire water" and see if it did what the book said it would. My taste buds did not tend to the really "HOT" spectrum, so I kept a piece of bread in a bag by my side and a cup of water. Every 15 minutes I took a big spoonful of fire water and then a bite of bread to cool my tongue, followed by a half glass of water. By lunch my fever had broken and the aches had gone away. (fever usually rises as the day progresses) I took it every half hour for the next hour or two and then every hour for the rest of the day and the flu was over! I was happy because I seldom get the flu, but when I do, it is usually stubborn and I ache and have fever for more than one day.

40

Now I needed another test case. This came from a lady, a distance away, who needed immediate help and wanted me to Fed-Ex her an overnight package of some Echinacea Plus tincture and Throat and Tonsil tincture for her daughter's strep throat. The girl had had re-occurring strep infections and doctor visits. She was desperate. I told her about this remedy and 1000 mg. of Vitamin C hourly, and mailed the package overnight. She called me in the morning, jubilant. The "fire water" had worked so well that the girl was already 75% better. If she had known, she could have saved herself an overnight charge and the cost of my tinctures. But she was still very happy and so was I! Another experiment had worked! I do think, however, that one must be diligent and take "fire water" every 15 minutes for it to really work. I think that water is also a key factor and that starting the treatment immediately makes it more effective. So the next time you feel a case of the "bug" coming on, pull out the "fire water" and "get" the bug before it "gets" you.

Quick Energy Blast

Here is a recipe for a quick "pick-me-up" using cayenne.

Mix together: ¼ - ½ teaspoon of cayenne powder in ½ glass of grape juice.

Energy Blast will provide you with an alert mind and energy for at least an hour. It will give you a pick up that does not give you the jitters that caffeine does and will also allow you to sleep if you do not take it within an hour of going to bed. It also seems to be helpful in bringing up the hemoglobin if you need to build red blood cells in your blood. Drink one-half a glass 2 - 3 times a day until your hemoglobin is where it should be.

During a phone call from a young mother in another state I recommended this tonic. She called, 35 weeks pregnant, complaining of fainting spells. Her midwife was not available and she wanted help NOW. She had had a few black-outs that had not been serious, then, when she was taking a walk along the road, she suddenly felt woozy and blacked out right there along the road. We discussed blood sugar issues and she was familiar with that and did not think that was what she was facing. I told her to get someone to take her blood pressure a few times that day and call me back. The next morning she called me to tell me that her blood pressure was very low. I told her about this tonic and asked her to try it for few days, *drinking a half cup, at least 4 times a day*. I received a call from her a few days later and she was very pleased. The tonic had done it's job.

Her father tried the same thing because of his low energy and was also, very pleased with how it helped him feel "up to the job."

This tonic works because it dramatically increases the circulation and this helps the body and the brain to do the work at hand. When you take Energy Blast, think ahead.

Our oldest son decided to try this tonic out since he would often come home from work weary and would have no energy to do anything in the evening. He took his drink, felt the pick-up it gave, and went off for an evening of shopping with his wife. To his dismay, an hour and a half later, in the middle of the mall, his energy was gone. "Mom, you did not tell me that would happen," he complained. I had not known it either, but have noticed the same thing, since then, when I have taken just one dose. If you do not want that to happen, mix a larger quantity and sip it from a thermos now and then. You will stay wide awake and alert. It is especially useful when driving for a long period of time, to replace caffeine.

Cayenne for Shock

This is one thing about cayenne that I really like! Anytime anyone feels faint, or begins to go into shock, cayenne will help to pull them out of it.

Stir ½ – 1 teaspoon of cayenne powder into a glass of warm water and have the person drink it down.

The increased circulation that this brings helps to stabilize the person for a bit until you get the help that is needed.

I have used cayenne quite successfully a number of times even when the person was not conscious. If they are not conscious, either rub cayenne into their gums or drop a few drops of cayenne tincture into their mouth taking care to do it slowly so that they do not choke.

One day I was called to help a lady who was having a miscarriage. She had lost a lot of blood and they felt like they wanted someone to come and check things out. When I got there, she indeed had lost a lot of blood. I proceeded to check things out and then when I had gotten her comfortable and stable, we visited a bit so that I could observe her. Everything was stable and the mother seemed fine. Finally I got her up to use the bathroom before I left, and while there, she went into a grand-mal seizure. The blood began to pour, and I knew that I had to do something to bring her out of the seizure immediately. I reached for the cayenne powder, rubbed it into her clenched mouth, and prayed. The lady relaxed, the bleeding stopped, the color came back into her face and she opened her eyes. We got her onto the bed and she was able to talk to us coherently. God answered our prayers. The cayenne increased the circulation so much that it snapped her right out of the seizure and did not leave her with the after effects that such seizures usually bring. She wondered what I had done and said she never felt the sting of the cayenne in her mouth. We called 911 and transported her to the hospital immediately. NOTE: For midwifery-type bleeding always transport even though the bleeding has stopped unless you have addressed the root problem, like delivering the placenta, etc, because the bleeding will often begin again in 15 – 20 minutes. The cayenne is helpful because it will buy you time.

Cayenne for Heart Attack or Stroke

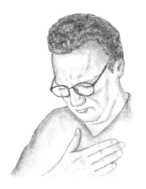

If you are dealing with someone whom you think has had a heart attack or a stroke, call 911, and then while you are waiting for the ambulance, give them a glass of cayenne water, ½ – 1 teaspoon of powder in a glass of warm water if they are awake and alert. If not, rub the powder onto their gums or give them cayenne tincture drop by drop into their mouth, taking care not to choke them. Repeat the dose in a few minutes, especially if the person is not responding. When you administer cayenne orally you will likely increase the circulation enough to bring the needed oxygen to the brain. This will greatly improve his chance of living. When you have him awake and alert, keep giving small doses until you have medical help. This procedure has saved lives! Cayenne is a powerful stimulant and greatly increases circulation to the brain. This may help to keep your loved one alive, and if you are careful not to choke them, you will do no damage. It almost always takes at least 9 minutes for the ambulance to get there and in that time your loved one could be gone. One nurse that we know of kept a small packet of cayenne powder with her and used it whenever one of her elderly patients had a heart attack or a stroke. She says it worked miracles quite a few times.

The effect of cayenne powder on a heart attack is quite amazing. A widow friend of ours experienced increasing heart pain. She is the kind that does not call the doctor easily. The pressure increased and she says it felt like an elephant was sitting on her chest. Her shoulder hurt and her arm ached and it got worse. Concerned, she called her neighbor lady, who told her to stir a teaspoon of cayenne into a glass of warm water and drink it. She did this and immediately the symptoms began to recede. She repeated the procedure until she felt better. Her doctor agrees that she probably had a heart attack, and he wanted her to go for tests. Instead she opted to take therapeutic doses of the high quality heart tonic from American Botanicals, change her diet and begin walking. Her follow-up blood work has improved and her heart pains are nearly a thing of the past. She still takes cayenne in water if she gets chest pain, and she says the pain goes away immediately.

Heart pain is not something that you can play with. Take your cayenne and head for the doctor unless you are really serious about changing your life style. This, of course, will do far more for you than any pill ever could do. But you cannot ignore your body's signals. If you do, you may not live to talk about it.

Cayenne Warms Cold Feet

If you struggle with cold feet or hands in the winter when skating, hunting, or anytime at all, sprinkle 1/8 teaspoon of cayenne in your shoes/gloves before you put them on. The cayenne acts to help the body generate heat. If you do it too liberally, your feet will get so **HOT** that you will not be able to keep your shoes on. Water-soluble components in cayenne dilate capillaries in the skin surface, producing an immediate sensation of heat. Within 15 minutes, oil-soluble compounds reach deeper tissues, generating warmth for hours. This will also work if you just feel chilly or have a hard time staying warm. Take a glass of water or juice with ½ one teaspoon of cayenne in it and you will be warm. Why? As we learned before, cayenne dramatically increases circulation which warms you up.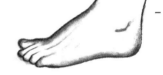

Cayenne for Aching Muscles and Joints

Mix one heaping teaspoon of cayenne powder into ½ cup of apple cider vinegar and shake it well.

Let it set a few days and shake often.

After a few days it is ready for use as a liniment for arthritis or rheumatism. (You can use it immediately though it is not as strong then.) Rub it on wherever there is an ache or a pain. Try it on a small spot first and if it is too strong for your skin, dilute it with a bit more vinegar.

As I was writing this, a lady from South Dakota called for help with severe rheumatism.

She asked me to send her a bottle of Deep Tissue Oil to use and I wrote her order down, but suggested that she try this recipe until her order arrived. She called back a day later and canceled the order. This is what she said. "I don't need the oil. The cayenne in vinegar worked immediately. I had been hurting for three days and now my knees feel better **in just one day**." She did not even let the vinegar set a few days. She just mixed it up and used it immediately.

People report back to me again and again that they have been able to get off their pain medicine and begin to function using this liniment. Not everyone sees the results in one day but usually it is helpful in a few days.

Varicose Veins

Cayenne mixed into some lotion will help with the pain of varicose veins. I would rub a small amount of cayenne cream and into my legs morning and evening, or you could use the vinegar base like you would for arthritis.

How Cayenne Works

Cayenne works because it contains an amazing compound called capsicum. Capsicum relieves many types and sources of pain, and is used to temporarily help relieve the pain from osteoarthritis and rheumatoid arthritis. It lowers the level of Decapeptide Substance P (DSP) in the joint fluids that provide cushioning between the bones. It also breaks down the DSP, which can destroy cartilage and also magnify the sensation of pain. It is unique compared to other "spicy" substances such as mustard oil, black pepper, and ginger, in that it causes a long-lasting desensitization to the irritant pain. Many pain killing salves and creams use capsicum as the active ingredient, but you can use the red pepper in your kitchen to make this helpful remedy.

Cayenne for Arthritis

Peter from New York wrote: "I read that cayenne pepper could alleviate the excruciating pain of arthritis that I had in two fingers on my left hand. I'd awaken daily in pain to find my pinky and ring finger locked in a bent position and it would hurt very much to straighten them. I would run hot water over them but they got worse as weeks went on.

I had been playing the piano several hours daily, and this was most likely the cause of this painful arthritis, a common piano-players ailment. If left unchecked it would surely end my piano playing and the use of two fingers. I met several ex-piano players who had exactly the same symptoms and quit playing because of the pain. After reading about the topical use of castor oil I thought it would be good to mix the cayenne pepper with castor oil so the mixture would stick to my fingers. So before bedtime, I took a paper towel and cut it to about 10x6 inches. Then I folded it to 10x2 (triple thick). Next, I mixed some cayenne into castor oil until orangey/red and smeared it onto the first four inches (to cover both sides of fingers) of the paper towel and also onto my fingers.

I wrapped my fingers with this bandage and excess paper, and finally used a rubber band to hold it all together. Every night I did this and I took it off in the morning. There was a noticeable reduction in pain immediately the first day and more use of my fingers. After three months I was 80% normal and within nine months I was completely healed."

This remarkable story exemplifies how increased circulation helps to bring healing. This could be done in many other areas where there is pain and stiffness.

Cayenne for Ulcers

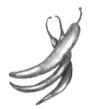

If you suffer from a peptic or duodenal ulcer, the last thing you might consider taking is hot cayenne pepper. This goes against everything you've ever heard about what aggravates an ulcer; the facts are that most "spicy" foods do just the opposite.

Cayenne can reduce pain and serve as a local anesthetic to ulcerated tissue in the stomach. It can even help to control bleeding in the stomach. Some individuals may be bothered by eating red pepper or spicy foods, but these foods do not cause the formation of gastric ulcers in normal people. People suffering from ulcers usually avoid cayenne pepper, but those people would actually benefit from its therapeutic action. Taking capsicum may significantly reduce the risk of ever developing a peptic ulcer. A Chinese study published in 1995 stated, "Our data supports the hypothesis that the chile used has a protective effect against peptic ulcer disease."J. Y. Kang, "The effect of chile ingestion of gastrointestinal mucosal proliferation. Researchers have concluded after experimenting with human volunteers, that capsicum has a definite gastro-protective effect on the mucous membranes of the stomach. However hot sauce will do the opposite and irritate the stomach.

Cayenne has the ability to rebuild stomach tissue. It also has the ability to bring blood to regions of tissue at a faster rate, boosting the assimilation of foods that are consumed with it. Several clinical studies support this phenomenon. Capsicum stimulates the release of substances which increase secretions in the stomach and intestines, and can increase an abundance of blood to the stomach and intestines. Cayenne increases the flow of digestive secretions from the salivary, gastric, and intestinal glands. This makes cayenne an excellent choice when working on healing the stomach and digestive system.

"But," you say, "I cannot tolerate spicy foods." *Begin with one-eighth teaspoon in one half cup of juice 4 times a day.* As you tolerate that amount, take one-fourth teaspoon in a half glass of juice or water. Keep increasing the amount that you can tolerate until you reach ½ – 1 teaspoon 3- 4 times daily. If you take this with slippery elm powder (see Slippery Elm chapter), you should notice significant healing in a few weeks.

An Ulcer Story

I had been working with a young man who had been having stomach ache after eating. He did not call until it was really hurting him so much that he was unable to work. At that point, he was also unable to eat without severe pain and he was a miserable boy.

We tried the simple things like slippery elm powder and a bland diet, but that was not enough to take away the pain. We started him on lots of water, 2 cups an hour (to dilute the stomach acids) and ½ teaspoon of cayenne in ½ glass of water every other hour. That is a hot dose, but he was desperate to feel better. He went off all food but a little yogurt during this time. When he drank the cayenne water he would feel a very hot burning area in his stomach but it would subside leaving him more comfortable than he had been for the last few days. As the day wore on, the extra water and the cayenne drinks made him more and more comfortable. He slept much better that night and the next day he was able to be up and around with much less pain. We switched the cayenne to every 3 hours and continued the bland diet and the 2 cups of water every hour. He continued to make good progress. In another day he was back to cayenne every four hours with lots of water every hour. His ulcer improved to the point that he had little or no pain. He took slippery elm and aloe vera for another week to give his stomach the nourishment that it needed to heal completely. He was very happy for the help that cayenne gave him on a weekend when the doctor was not in.

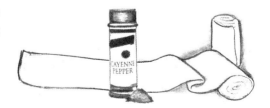

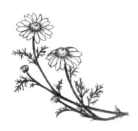
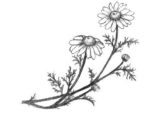

Chamomile

"The Quieting Herb"

Chamomile is an old stand-by for relaxation and digestion. It is a cure-all for many every-day problems. It reduces inflammation, relaxes nerves, and promotes tissue repair. Studies indicate that it is active against E. coli, strep, and staph bacteria. It helps restore exhausted nervous systems. Topically it is often used in salves to soften skin, treat inflammation, and heal wounds. It has a relaxing and calming scent. People use the dried flowers to stuff into pillows as a sleep-aid. A wash of the tea sprayed onto the skin will repel insects. People who are sensitive to ragweed should be careful about their use of chamomile. Use it with caution. It may not bother you.

Tea for Colic or Tummy Ache

Give this tea to your infant to relax his intestinal muscles and calm him down. Make it very warm to increase the relaxing effect.

Uses:
- Stomach Ache
- Cramps
- Gas
- Menstruation
  Difficulties
- Insomnia
- Fever
- Infection
- Inflamed Eyes
- Urinary
Problems

Steep one teaspoon of flower heads, or one tea bag, in a cup of boiling water for four to five minutes, cool to room temperature. Give 1-2 ounces.

This is great help in easing a baby's tummy ache, or anyone's tummy ache for that matter. We tried this with baby number eight who cried a lot with tummy aches. I mean, she screamed a lot, slept a little, and was always spitting up. I had read about chamomile, so I asked the children to make a bottle of tea and bring it to me to try. She drank one ounce and fell asleep immediately, after a large burp. In fact, she zonked out! The bottle was really warm. It was warmer than I would have made for a baby but it did the trick. I think the warmth and the chamomile made a great

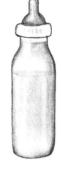

combination. Adults and children alike will find their stomachs calmed and the gas dissipated when drinking a hot cup of chamomile tea. Use it after a meal that has been too heavy, or whenever you struggle with a tummy ache. One mother told me that the cost of this book was really worth it for this bit of information.

For Sleep

Chamomile is a gentle sleep-induction aid. If you have a child that has a difficult time going to sleep, it is just the thing. Make him a warm, mildly sweet cup of tea before bedtime. It will calm his jitters and send him to dreamland. It is soothing and sedative, and works for adults as well.

Infusion:

Add 1 heaping teaspoon of flowers to 1 cup of boiling water. Let steep for at least 5 minutes. Strain and sweeten. We often add a little bit of milk to make it taste even better.

Chamomile Oil for Aches and Pains

You can make a nice chamomile oil to use in massage for aching limbs and even for paralyzed limbs. With time and care, this massage may bring back movement if the nerves are not severed.

Fill a small bottle full of fresh flower heads. Cover the flowers with olive oil and keep the jar in a warm dark place for two weeks. Do not put a lid on the jar so that the moisture can evaporate. Otherwise you may have a problem with mold. Strain and store in the fridge. Warm the oil to use for a massage or to make it into a salve.

For Infection

If you have an infected wound, grind chamomile blossoms into a powder and wet them with boiling water to make a paste. Apply the paste to the sore. It will clear the infection and ease the pain.

Chamomile Salve

This salve is very nice for diaper rash or other skin disorders. Use it liberally.

Heat 1 cup of lard or coconut oil

Add 2 handfuls of fresh chamomile flowers

When it foams, stir it well.

Remove it from heat and place the lard or coconut oil in a cool place overnight.

In the morning, warm it and strain it through a cloth.

Squeeze out the last bit by twisting the cloth.

Bottle in small baby food jars.

Chamomile Bath for Relaxation and Soothing Sore Muscles

To end the day in a relaxing bath or to soothe your sore muscles, take a long, warm chamomile bath.

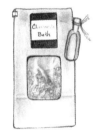

Add 2 double handfuls of fresh or dried flowers, or 10 - 16 teabags to a gallon of boiling water.

Turn off the heat and steep for 20 minutes.

Strain and add to a tub of hot water.

Soak and enjoy.

This bath works well to relax a fussy baby or a hyper child.

Try it and enjoy the results.

Chamomile Steam

For clogged sinuses, pour one quart of boiling water over 2 tablespoons of chamomile and inhale the steam under a towel. This will open up the sinuses so that you will feel able to breathe easily again. When you are finished with the steam make sure that you stay very warm for a few hours. Do not do this if you have ragweed allergies.

Chamomile Implants for Fevers

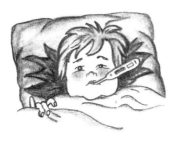

If your child has a high fever and you feel you need to bring it down, do it without drugs and use chamomile. Make a chamomile infusion like you were taught to under "chamomile for sleep." Cool it till it is comfortable to your underarm. Put it in a bulb syringe. Lubricate the tip of the bulb syringe with Vaseline. Lay your child on its tummy, on a towel. Depress the syringe while it is upright before inserting to remove air and then insert it slowly and gently into the rectum. Inject the contents of the syringe very slowly so that the child will not expel the contents. This is not an enema. This is an implant. You are injecting liquid into the body that you want to stay in the body.

Here is an unusual story about my journey with chamomile. I was teaching a class about how to deal with fever and flu and I opened it up for discussion at the end.

"Do any of you have a way to deal with fevers that I have not discussed?" I asked.

"Yes," said a mother. "I have found chamomile to really bring down fevers. My children tend to spike fevers of 105 and that is hard for me. So when I have a child with a fever, I use chamomile to bring it down."

"That is interesting." I responded. "How do you use it? And where did you learn about it?"

"From you," she responded, smilingly. "I called you about what to do with fevers and you told me to use a chamomile implant. It really works!"

I do a lot of reading and one day I must have read about using this herb to bring down a fever. That mother called me at just the right moment and I passed the information on to her. I did not need it myself and had never used this information, so I soon forgot it. Now here it was, called to my attention again. God has a way of doing that. Often I find that He brings things to my attention over and over again. So, instead of being frustrated when things continue to happen, I try to remember that I am in school, and I am learning valuable lessons.

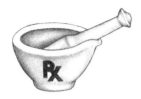

Charcoal

"What the Doctor Ordered"

Powdered charcoal has been in use for at least 200 years in America. It was eliminated from general medicine in 1950 when the drug industry began to mushroom and all the drug companies wanted to sell their drugs. It is still in use in hospital emergency rooms for poisoning.

Activated charcoal is a light, fluffy, black powder. It contains certain electrostatic properties that favor the binding of most poisons to itself. Lancet Medical Journal says that when they apply charcoal superficially somehow it pulls the toxins from deep tissues and organs. Every home should have charcoal on hand for an antidote in poisoning and as a treatment in diarrhea, nausea, vomiting, and any intestinal infections.

Charcoal is harmless and can be ingested in large amounts. Most types of viral infections can be helped with drinking charcoal slurry, especially if taken within a few hours of onset, particularly for a histamine reaction to some sort of allergen, which causes sneezing, weeping eyes, coughing, sore throat, or hives.

Uses:
- drug overdose
- reaction to drugs
- counteract poison
- diarrhea
- intestinal gas
- bad breath
- bites and stings
- jaundice
- infections
- draining wounds
- Filtering water
- Lyme disease
- Vomiting

Here is an acronym that I like which applies to charcoal. Using charcoal is: **SAFE!**

Simple

Affordable

Feasible

Easy to use.

Reasons to Use Charcoal

Why would you use charcoal instead of going to the hospital? **First,** you can treat yourself immediately. We know that this is usually more effective than waiting until you can get care in the emergency room. **Secondly,** there are no side effects. Our body does not digest it and so it is not assimilated and it passes through. **Thirdly,** organisms are not charcoal resistant and many organisms are antibiotic resistant. **Lastly,** it is so inexpensive and has a very long shelf life. This way every family can have it on hand to use it. When you are looking for charcoal it should say activated, or USP which means that it has been washed before sale. It may also say food supplement although it is not really a food supplement. Charcoal does not seem to adsorb food or take away nutrients.

Charcoal Slurry

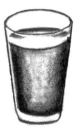

The usual dose of charcoal powder is:

1 tablespoon of charcoal in 1 glass of water

Stir and drink immediately. Repeat in 30 minutes Follow the cup of slurry with another cup or two of water to avoid constipation.

When Poison Has Been Taken

Use this treatment when you need help <u>immediately.</u>

Increase the charcoal to 4-10 tablespoons in a glass and a half of water. (Adult dose)

Drink quickly and follow with 2 more glasses of water. Repeat in 30 minutes.

On an empty stomach, the amount of charcoal should be twice the amount of the poison the child has swallowed. (Use 2 heaping tablespoons if the amount is unknown.) It is important to do this promptly. Do not use a large amount of water for a child. Preferably put the slurry in a bulb syringe or something that you can use to get it down the child's throat. Give it to him, head tipped back, until he has swallowed it all. The benefit of this is that you can get it into him **immediately** whereas it would take time until you got to the hospital and more time until they treated him. Give fresh water after the dose to assist the body in clearing out the charcoal. If the child vomits, repeat the dose, until it is kept down. Then repeat it in an hour if he exhibits signs of poisoning like paleness and lethargy(slowness to respond).

Another advantage to doing it yourself is that your child will probably respond better to you than a stranger.

The slurry is somewhat sandy in texture but does not have a bad flavor. If you have a problem with the texture, use a straw to drink it and it will not be a problem. We often use this treatment with a few droppers of digestive tonic added to give it a nice flavor and aid in treating the stomach.

In 1831, Professor Touery drank a lethal dose of strychnine in front of his distinguished colleagues at the French Academy of Medicine, and lived to tell the tale. He had combined the deadly poison with activated charcoal. He caused a medical sensation that has not been forgotten.

One of the families from church had a two year old that got into the rat poison in the barn. No one knew how much he ate and when they called me I recommended that they go to the emergency room for treatment because I was unsure of what the treatment of choice would be. Guess what the ER did! They tried to make him drink charcoal water! He did not cooperate well and it went everywhere. Imagine how much cheaper it would have been if my advice had been to stay home and force him to drink a half cup of charcoal water over the period of a half hour and to repeat that process in another hour to be sure.

Read the book Rx Charcoal by Agatha & Calvin Thrash for more specific tables on types of poisons, how to identify them, and what to do for each. The book Charcoal Remedies.com by John Dinsley is also very helpful. **It is a must have for your library.**

Have it On Hand

If you place 4 tablespoon of activated charcoal in a quart jar of water, and put it in your cupboard, it will always be there for an emergency. When you need it, shake it up to mix well, and use it immediately. Give lots of charcoal with lots of fluid. If you give enough you will resolve the problem more quickly.

My husband came down with a bit of food poisoning and lay groaning on the couch feeling really badly. I suggested charcoal and he was slow to take my suggestion. But after a few glasses of charcoal water from the jar I keep in the pantry, his ailment subsided and he slept well, waking without the symptoms he had before he went to bed.

This even works for animals. You can treat their illnesses with charcoal too. One lady who heard about the benefits of charcoal did not want to try it on herself. She decided to do it on her dog. Her elderly dog had a softball-sized growth on his abdomen. She gave him a capsule of charcoal every day for a few weeks and the growth reduced dramatically. (We would have used a lot more than that!) She then began to add it to his food for further healing. The results astounded her. Now she uses charcoal for herself and her family.

Charcoal in the Sears Catalog

Back in 1908 the Sears catalog actually carried charcoal. They said it was good for gas, indigestion, nausea, etc. Somehow it disappeared off the screen until recently. It is now coming into use again. Even medical personnel are recognizing that it is a great remedy to help with eliminating problems, especially at the very first sign of the symptoms. They use charcoal patches on wounds, and charcoal filters. Charcoal also is used to relieve itching related to kidney dialysis treatment, and to treat poisoning or drug overdose.

Charcoal Slurry for Dysentery

You will find that the slurry works well for dysentery. Our daughter was in Haiti on a mission assignment. She contracted the dysentery, probably from bad food. Everything was running straight through, even water, and they needed to take a trip out to the city. It was a 5 hour trip with almost no restroom accommodations available. She took a charcoal slurry immediately upon rising, and then one every time she had to run to the bathroom. By 10 AM when they were due to leave, the problem was over, and the trip uneventful. People going on trips to third-world countries do well to carry a cup of powdered charcoal in their possession. Capsules are fine for some things but not for dysentery. They tend to go straight through and never open.

Charcoal deals well with severe diarrhea from many sicknesses including cholera. Taken when needed, it could save your life. You are the gate keeper of your health. Use charcoal!

Charcoal to the Rescue

Our first exposure to charcoal was nine or ten years ago when our oldest daughter was preparing to go to Africa on a mission trip. She was due to take her anti-malaria medication 2 weeks before she flew. She was to take one pill one week, and another pill the next week. When she took the 2nd dose she started with a blinding headache immediately. It progressed quickly to include extreme light sensitivity, inability to sit or stand, and excruciating pain.

I called the doctor, but he had not prescribed the medicine. The mission board had gotten it from Africa. He definitely did not want to be involved. I began to pray in earnest. Then I remembered that just a few weeks before, someone, knowing my interest, had given me a book on charcoal and a can of the powder. "Just in case someone needs it," they said. God had provided.

The drug that she had taken was listed in the book along with how to take the charcoal. I mixed the stuff up and took it to her with a straw and the instructions to drink it down. In 10 minutes she reported to me that she was feeling a bit better. I immediately repeated the dose, and within a half hour she was able to converse with us and the pain had gone down considerably. I gave her another dose on the hour which gave us even more improvement. An hour later I gave her the last dose and we were able to pull up the blinds. She sat up in the chair although she was very weak.

My next step was to call the mission board and tell them what had happened, and request that she would not need to take that kind of medicine when in Africa. I began to research to see what she had reacted to. I discovered that one of the main components of the medicine was chlorine. We knew that she could not use any chlorine when cleaning or washing, but we did not think about her ingesting it. That chemical is in many drugs as a preservative. Now whenever she might need to take some drug, she always checks out the chemical composition of it, especially the preservative that was used.

Activated charcoal is estimated to reduce absorption of poisonous substances up to 60% so it is wise to have it on hand for any poison emergency that you might face.

Charcoal Water

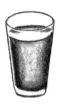

Put ¼ cup of charcoal powder in a 2 quart jar.
Slowly fill the jar with water (the powder will puff and float around).
Cap the jar and shake well. Set on the counter to settle for about ½ hour.

Now you have charcoal water and you can drink it all day. When the jar begins to get empty, fill it up and shake it again. You can refill the jar as often as you wish until the charcoal is all used up.

I like to use the charcoal water when I feel like I am "coming down with something." If I start it immediately, I often get ahead of whatever is giving me the "uh-oh" feeling and it does not develop into a flu or cold. This is especially helpful for intestinal upsets. The water is not difficult to drink and does not have an unpleasant taste although it is gray. This is a very good way to purify water if you are not sure that your source is pure. I would much rather drink "gray water" than get seriously sick with food poisoning or bad water. These are the two most common reasons that visitors get sick when they visit third-world countries. Activated charcoal does not irritate the mucous membranes of the GI system. The American Journal of Gastroenterology also did a double blind study which showed that charcoal decreased intestinal gas and nausea.

Charcoal for Lyme Disease "Die-Off"

Here is an account used by permission from charcoalremedies.com:

"I have Lyme Disease. My body's response to Lyme Disease treatment is worse than the disease itself. As the Lyme is killed, it creates a die-off of Lyme toxins. My Lyme doctor recommended activated charcoal to absorb the "die off" (which turns to ammonia and creates pain). I have NEVER in my life seen anything like this substance- what a miracle! I am recommending activated charcoal at forums to Lyme patients who suffer and need detoxing that is safe. I was skeptical, but I have been made a believer. My son, also with Lyme Disease, was so sick from "die off" that I was going to take him to the hospital. I gave him activated charcoal water and within hours he started to return to "normal". In 4 days he was completely himself again. . . . ."

We have Lyme sufferers in our own family, and we have also found charcoal water to be very helpful in dealing with die-off. We take it in-between our herbal or medical treatment.

Chronic Ear Infections

One lady wrote that she had an ear infection for over a month and no antibiotic from the doctor helped it. She finally mixed a bit of charcoal in a bit of water and let it set. Later she strained out the sediment and put a few drops of the "gray water" in her ears. The next day she applied a bit more and that was all it took to clear up the pain and the infection. *Put a few drops of warm charcoal water in your ear at the **first** sign of infection. Do it 2 – 4 times a day to get quick relief. Or, make a charcoal poultice and place it over the problem ear with heat on it, for extra help.*

Breast Infections

After reading more about charcoal I determined not to forget how well it worked in stubborn infections. I soon had another chance to try it on a friend who was having a re-occurring breast infection. She did the normal hot showers, massage, and cabbage leaf treatments that usually bring swift relief, but to no avail. Her infection would get a bit better and then it would flare back up. In desperation she went for an antibiotic, thinking that that would be the answer. But 2 days later the infection was even worse. It was then that I remembered charcoal. I made her a flax seed/charcoal poultice and she applied that overnight and drank about a quart of charcoal "gray water". In the morning the pain was gone and she felt so much better. She continued the treatment for another day and her infection was gone. Now whenever she feels an infection coming on she drinks charcoal water and massages the area and she usually can stay on top of it. NOTE: Do not use the poultice on the breast too long, since it seems to start to dry up the milk.

Make a Charcoal Poultice

Grind a cup of flax seed in the blender. Mix it with an equal amount of charcoal. Moisten it with olive oil/castor oil or hot water to a pie dough consistency. Spread it out about ¼" thick on a sheet of plastic wrap. Heat it in the microwave or oven. (Make it nice and warm, but not too hot.) Oil the painful area and flip the poultice onto it, leaving the plastic wrap on. Bandage it onto the area and apply heat if you wish. The poultice can stay on for an hour or overnight.

When you are finished with the poultice, peel it off and roll it up again. It can be stored in a plastic bag in the fridge for future use, unless you were using it over an infected area.

Charcoal Poultice for Pain

A charcoal poultice is helpful for almost any kind of pain. Make it very warm. Oil the area and apply it. Top it with a towel and a warm rice sock or heating pad for the best effect. This works for gall bladder pain, appendicitis pain, painful joints, chest pain, and any place where there is infection, abscess, or inflammation. If the spot of infection is an open one, do not reuse the poultice.

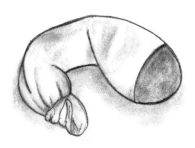

I came down with some pretty bad kidney pain one day. I took my kidney/bladder tincture and lots of water, but I still had a lot of tenderness. I finally made myself a poultice and applied it very warm over my kidney area. I topped it with a warm rice sock and left it on for about 30 minutes. It felt really good and took the pain away immediately. Sometimes the poultice does not work that fast and you will need to do a few applications. If you want to keep the poultice on longer you can reheat it and apply again, or cover it with a heating pad instead of a rice sock.

Rice socks can be made easily by filling a clean sock half to two-thirds full of rice. Knot it or sew it shut. Heat this in the microwave or oven until it is really warm before you use it. Do not scorch it! If you make it too hot, lay a towel between your poultice and the sock. Heat it as often as needed to keep the poultice warm and cozy. We use these socks for cold feet in a cold bed, for ear aches, and monthly cramps. We try to keep at least two on hand to use when we need them.

Charcoal for Infection

Another interesting case was the young man who developed a very sore hand. His hand was too sore to use at work. They called me to find out what they could do for him.

"What had happened to make the hand sore?" I inquired.

They did not know. Perhaps he had gotten a sliver in it but he did not remember. I suggested drawing salve and they tried that but it did not do any good. Then I thought of charcoal. I told them how to make a charcoal poultice and apply it.

They made the poultice and applied it before going to bed. In the morning the swelling, the redness, and the pain were gone. They could not believe how simple it was and how well it had worked. He had had a painfully sore hand for a week and in one night, with one application of charcoal, it was over. The only problem that they had was that she had made the poultice too thin and there was charcoal all over the sheets. You can hardly wash out charcoal! But they were so impressed that they ordered a pound to take with them to the mission field when they went. This is just one example of what charcoal can do in a poultice. Try it yourself and write your own story.

Charcoal for an Infected Finger

One day at work John got a wood splinter in his middle finger close to the middle joint. He pulled it out and didn't think much of it. Within a day or two his finger swelled almost double in size. Thinking there might still be a tiny piece left in there, he casually poked around at it every evening for about a week. Some pus came out, so there must have been some infection happening. He thought that was all that needed to be done since he had done this procedure dozens of times over the years.

The swelling slowly went down and by the end of the second week his finger felt normal. Then, a month after the initial splinter incident, his finger suddenly began to throb badly at night, keeping him from sleeping. After the second night of it, he took his stiff, throbbing fingers (by now more fingers were stiff and swollen) to the doctor.

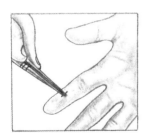

The doctor listened to his story and decided that he was either dealing with a present joint infection or arthritis of the joint because of the injury. His response was - antibiotics for the possible infection and if it did not respond to that, an arthritis shot in the joint every year or two. John casually mentioned that he should have let his wife treat his finger earlier. Doctor said, "I know your wife uses home remedies but trust me, there is no home remedy out there to treat a joint infection. Patients need 6 weeks of antibiotics to clear up joint infections."

When John went home and immediately soaked his finger in strong, hot salt water with some ginger powder. He reasoned that salt would address the infection and ginger would increase the circulation to speed healing.

This immediately helped with the pain and the mobility his fingers. He took a good dose of Super Duper Tonic (natural antibiotic), stuck the bottle in his work jacket and went to work taking 4 droppers every two hours for the rest of the day. Still worried, he contacted me and asked what else he should do. I suggested a charcoal poultice overnight, every night, until the fingers were normal again. He applied a poultice that evening and left it on until the next morning. His finger felt perfectly normal in the morning, but he took doses of Super Duper Tonic and did the charcoal poultice one more night to be safe. He is very happy that *"home remedies"* actually worked on a "serious joint infection" in less than six weeks. If a problem should re-occur they know exactly how to deal with it.

I often see healing like this taking place with this kind of poultice. When it does I never cease to be amazed and grateful that God has given us what we need to do the job.

For an Inflamed Colon

As I was writing, I had yet another opportunity to see the value of a charcoal poultice. I was called out to see if I could help a young man with appendicitis. On arrival I did the usual rebound tenderness test to see if we were likely dealing with appendicitis. The test did not point to appendicitis, neither did his answers when I asked him about life style, fluid intake, and bowel habits. The location of the pain was in the lower center of his abdomen, too. We decided that he was probably dealing with gastro-enteritis, another problem which closely mimics appendicitis. We made sure his colon was not full, gave him very warm chamomile tea, and slippery elm to soothe his insides. We rubbed his abdomen with lobelia to relax it and then applied a charcoal/flax seed poultice. He did not have the poultice on long before he visibly relaxed and then fell asleep. He had slept almost none the night before because of his pain. When he relaxed I went home with the instructions to keep a warm poultice on him part of every hour or continually if need be. They were to use lobelia as needed for the pain and give frequent doses of garlic for infection. Other than having some toast with the garlic (to keep his stomach happy) he was to have only liquids for a day or two to give him a chance to recuperate. When I called back that night to check on him, he had slept most of the day and the pain was completely gone. In two days he was working with no sign of the pain that had kept him up all night! We are not sure what his problem was but does it matter What matters is that the treatment worked!!

Charcoal Poultice for Poisonous Bites and Stings

Charcoal has amazing abilities to neutralize the poison of stings and bites. One of our daughters had an encounter with a spider. We did not see the spider, but the way the bite progressed, it appeared to be a brown recluse. The venom from these bites causes serious damage to tissues and the medical field does not have a good way to combat it. Often it results in amputation of the finger or toe, and sometimes a whole leg.

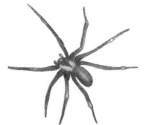

As the bite progressed to a huge, dark-red area the size of a man's hand, I began to give her natural remedies by mouth (now I would use charcoal water and my freshly made Echinacea Plus and apply charcoal poultices.) She ran a fever and felt very ill. We used natural remedies and gradually the bite receded and the leg healed.

Here are incidents where charcoal helped with a poisonous bite. Reprinted by permission from the amazing book *CharcoalRemedies.com*.

"While teaching a course in Scottsdale, I noticed a small ulceration on my friend's leg. Maxine had not noticed it, but by the next morning it had gone from less than dime-size to quarter-size and had become angry and inflamed. A large, open ulcer had developed, and she had enlarged lymph nodes in the groin. I immediately prepared a poultice, and placed it over the open ulcer. The poultice was replaced several times daily over the course of a week. Maxine also took a couple of herbal supplements and charcoal internally. By the second week there was no evidence of a bite at all.

We've used activated charcoal many times for our family and friends for the brown recluse spider bite. (These friends are from the south.) Even a couple of doctors here were amazed at what it did! We would make up a paste and change it the first day about every 2 hours and then the next day just a few times and would keep watching it. Usually the bite was shrunk and just a little scab after a few days. Usually we would also drink some charcoal water so that we would have any poison from the bite eliminated from our system."

Wasp Sting

"My three year old was stung by a yellow jacket on his little hand.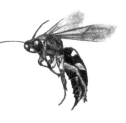
Amid his hysterical screams, I dumped some charcoal powder into
a large bowl and added water. I plunged his hand into the black
water and, instantly, his screams stopped. We swished his hand
around in it for a few minutes while looking at a book. Then he
took his hand out and said it didn't hurt any more. That was truly the end of the sting."

Allergies, Anaphylactic Shock and Dialysis

JMA and the medical magazine, "The Lancet", have picked up on the medicinal ability of
charcoal to counteract mushroom poisoning and insect bites. They report that sometimes
charcoal can stop anaphylactic shock (the constriction of the throat which obstructs
breathing)when people have been stung by bee or hornet. One of the foremost allergists
on peanut allergies from Canada writes that it has been clinically proven that charcoal
can adsorb the peanut protein in 30 seconds. Clinically there is a lot of research to back
up why it can be used in the home. If my child responded badly to a food that he was
sensitive to, I would use charcoal to help with his reaction. Dr. Hillabrand - La Loma, CA
has developed a liver dialysis machine that uses charcoal to clean up the liver. Kidney
dialysis machines use a bed of charcoal to filter the blood for the kidney patient.

Charcoal for Abscesses

Here is another story from the CharcoalRemedies.com website. Jeremy, a Physician
Assistant, but also trained for several years in natural medicine, writes of a recent
experience he and his wife had. "My wife had what appeared to be a small cyst in her left
auxiliary (armpit) region for several days and it kept getting bigger, more painful, and
more red and inflamed. She had no fevers, chills, malaise or night sweats, and no
streaking was seen radiating out from what we thought to be a cyst. The pain increased
and was to the point of not allowing her left arm to comfortably rest by her side - I could
not even lightly touch it without causing her a lot of pain. It grew to the size of a golf ball
and looked as if it was coming to a head. By this time I began to think we might be
dealing with an abscess.

Activated charcoal was the first thing that came to my mind in the form of a poultice that might bring this through the skin more effectively and allow it to drain.

I mixed activated charcoal with ground flax seed in no 'special' ratio, but simply made a paste with it that would stay on the gauze and not be runny. I taped the poultice down over top of the abscess and left it on overnight.

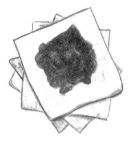

The next morning when the poultice was taken off, the abscess appeared to have a thinner wall in one area. The erythema (redness and inflammation) was virtually gone and the pain was completely gone. My wife very gently squeezed the lump and it burst open and released large amounts of pus. She continued to expel the material until nothing more came out. We cleaned the area well and dressed it with gauze. She could rest her arm by her side and had no pain. By the next morning the swelling had decreased to about ¼ inch in diameter and finally disappeared several days later.

Without question, a poultice of activated charcoal holds tremendous value for post-surgical patients as well."

All said – charcoal is one of the most inexpensive and effective remedies that a home can have. We always keep at least a pound on hand (about 2 quarts) and use it for all kinds of things. You can buy your charcoal at buyactivatedcharcoal.com if you wish. The address and the phone number are also listed in the medicine making chapter.

Charcoal for Throat Cancer

A wonderful testimony from charcoalremedies.com tells how charcoal helped a couple in distress. "I just had to let you know how charcoal has helped our friends. . . . .Our friend, George, had throat cancer that the doctors said was well advanced, and my husband told his wife about charcoal. They immediately got some and began using it. We saw them a few weeks later, and you could hear George coughing up that junk in his throat. Today, some several months later, George is cancer free. And imagine this, his doctors can't figure out why!   This procedure may not always work but it is surely worth a try.

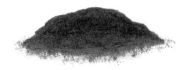

Brighten and Whiten Teeth

Nothing whitens teeth better than activated charcoal. Though a tasteless black substance, this stuff whitens teeth and removes plaque at the same time. The substance is very powerful and also helps to maintain a healthy mouth pH balance.

Charcoal is a better, more effective, and cheaper alternative to laser cleansing of the teeth as well. Our dentist actually admits that using a dental cleaning tool on your teeth actually harms the enamel a small amount. Hmm – always thought it did!!

One herbalist knew a Native American woman who had the whitest teeth he ever seen. He thought she was crazy when she told him what she did to have her pearly white teeth. She told him that as a little girl her father used to make charcoal from burning plant matter and their family brushed their teeth with charcoal (carbon), using their fingers to brush their teeth. He said that he, too, learned of the valuable benefits of activated charcoal and has been using the substance for his teeth ever since. I want to try this one since I have stains on my teeth from the braces that I wore.

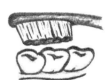

A Few Charcoal Notes

It should be noted that while charcoal has many benefits, there are some minor precautions to keep in mind. It may cause constipation if you do not drink enough. You must drink plenty of water when using it. Also important to note, milk products may decrease the ability of the charcoal to work. Don't eat or drink dairy products when taking it. And usually do not take it for long periods of time. Remember, charcoal does not discriminate when it is taking things out of your body. It will take out prescription medicines while it is taking out other things. Take it one and a half to two hours away from your other meds. You can order charcoal and books at this address from John & Kimberly Dinsley. Their prices are right and their service is prompt and friendly.

Ordering Information

Email: customersupport@buyactivatedcharcoal.com   Phone: 308-665-1566

BuyActivatedCharcoal.com PO Box 261 Crawford, NE 69339

website: charcoalremedies.com

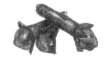

Cloves

"The Pain Relieving Herb"

Clove is an important herb to have on hand just for pain! Reach into your spice cupboard and you have what you need. The oil in the clove bud provides a numbing effect when rubbed on locally and a relaxing effect when taken internally.

Clove Oil for Toothache

Clove oil is a great pain reliever, especially for toothaches, abscesses and mouth difficulties. It can be applied with a q-tip. A drop will do. Remember it is very potent; you may even want to consider diluting it for this purpose.

A whole clove can be crushed slightly and placed on the gum where the toothache is located, or place a small amount of ground cloves into a piece of coffee filter, wrap, wet and place between gum and lip. Using any of these applications will alleviate the pain, the higher the potency, the quicker the relief. Using clove oil will not only alleviate the pain, it will also draw out any infection from an abscess so you will likely not need antibiotics for your problem.

Uses:
- pain relief
- toothache
- sleep aid
- burns
- scabies
- fights flu

Clove Tea for Pain

Make a tea from the clove buds.

Use 1 tablespoon of whole cloves to 2-3 cups of water.

Boil the whole cloves in the water for about 15 - 20 minutes.

Strain out the cloves and sweeten the tea.

We like to add a bit of milk for taste. Swish the tea in the mouth and swallow and it will gently numb it and take the pain away. It is helpful for pain anywhere. The pain of a broken bone responds well to clove tea. This is probably because it relaxes the muscles that are spasming from the break. Sip on it and feel the difference. Or you can take a few drops of clove oil and rub them into your gums when you have pain in your mouth. Almost all tooth and gum medications have oil of clove in them. Go for the plain clove oil and you will find cheaper, quick relief.

Sleep like a Baby with Clove Tea

This tea is also very helpful to some people as a sleep aid. Make it hot and take it just before going to sleep. It works for a lot of sleep problems but not all. (It does not seem to work for sleep problems when they are hormonally related.) After I read about clove tea for sleeping, we had a relative visiting who was not sleeping well. He was complaining about it and I felt sorry for him since I had had some problems with sleeping, myself. I mentioned the tea to him and he laughed at me and we dropped the subject. However, just before he went to bed I made him a sweet cup of clove tea. He drank it, laughing, and went to bed. In the morning when I was preparing breakfast for everyone he was the first to come down. "Your tea worked like a charm," he said with a smirk. He is such a joker that I did not take him seriously. "No, really," he said. "I went to sleep promptly and did not wake up until now." I was happy to hear it and add this to my list of herbs that work for some folks.

Fight Off the Flu

To fight bacteria, colds, and flu this season try this homemade tea. It also helps to fight allergies and asthma. It is soothing and battles stress too. In one cup of water brew together the following natural ingredients:

1 whole clove   *½ teaspoon of sage*

½ teaspoon of thyme   *½ cinnamon stick*

¼ teaspoon of cayenne pepper   *juice from half a lemon*

1 teaspoon of honey

Let steep for several minutes and drink for good health.

This wonderful recipe will help you to retain your health and wellness in the midst of stressful circumstances. When you are surrounded with flu and you drink a few cups of this tea daily you will likely not come down with any of the flu symptoms. Getting enough sleep is important, too. When you loose one or more hours of needed sleep it lowers your immune system and makes you much more vulnerable to the flu.

Scabies

To treat the rash from scabies apply this mixture generously to the affected area before bedtime every night.

Mix together well:

  ☒ *½ cup of vegetable oil*

     ¼ cup water and ¼ cup of honey.

  ☒ *5 drops of clove oil*

Clove oil can be very irritating to skin, so do a test patch before applying to a wide area.

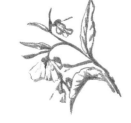

Comfrey

"The Knit-bone Herb"

Comfrey knits broken bones back together and doubles the rate of cell growth, rapidly speeding up healing rates. It is my favorite herb. Comfrey is a sweet, cooling herb with expectorant, astringent, soothing, and healing effects. It reduces inflammation and controls bleeding. Comfrey contains a special substance called allantoin, which is a cell proliferative. In other words, it makes cells grow faster. This is one of the reasons why comfrey-treated bones knit so fast, wounds mend so quickly, and burns heal with such little scarring. Comfrey is often called knit-bone or healing herb.

My first experience with comfrey happened about 30 years ago. It was before the advent of car seat laws, and I was driving our two-door sedan around a curve in a nearby countryside. My seven year-old was seated on the right side, and had fallen asleep against the door. As I rounded the corner, the door, which sometimes did not latch properly, swung open, and she rolled out onto the road and into the ditch. As you can imagine, my mother heart almost stood still, aghast at what I thought I would see as I stopped. To my relief, she stood up, so I knew that she hadn't broken a leg, or rolled under the wheel. But she HAD gotten severe road rash. The skin and flesh was rubbed away to the bone several places on her face, knuckles, and hip. Other areas were severely brush-burned. My husband's mother came to the rescue, introducing me to comfrey and recommending that I make a tea of it to soak the wounds. After cleaning the wounds we soaked them in a strong, comfrey leaf tea. Since some of the worst wounds were on her face and hip where we could not soak them, we dipped clean rags in the comfrey tea and laid the wet cloths over them (a comfrey poultice). We soaked her hands in the tea, too. She cried when we put her hands into the soak because of the open wounds. To help her keep her mind off the immediate pain we read her some of her favorite stories. The pain would subside and we would soak her

Uses:
- abscess
- breaks
- bruises
- burns
- cuts
- IBS
- pain
- pneumonia
- sprains
- ulcers
- varicose veins

brush burns for 20 minutes twice daily. Then we would wrap the wounds to keep them clean and dry. Within one week, fresh, pink skin had formed over most of the brush burns and she could use her fingers to write again. In 2 weeks the deepest wounds were almost completely healed.

Not only that, but there was so little scarring that today the only noticeable scarring is a ¼ inch scar on one knuckle of her right hand, and a bit of scarring on her hip where we did not do the comfrey soaks. We were favorably impressed, to say the least. This was the first, but not the last time, we have used comfrey to help with healing. If we were to repeat the process today we would probably use a comfrey poultice since it would not cause the pain that the soak did, and then we would apply comfrey salve when we wrapped the wounds to keep them moist and further speed the healing. But the interesting thing to note is that the herbs worked when we used them, even if there might have been a better way to do the process.

Comfrey Root Poultice

For a stronger healing aid use the fresh root. Dig the root, and peel it. Blend it to pulp in your blender with a bit of olive oil. Mix just enough slippery elm powder to the root to hold it together. Apply over the wound for quick wound healing. Bandage the area. It will often bring pain relief and will facilitate healing. This is called a poultice. Repeat this 2 or 3 times daily.

You can use the fresh or dried leaf if you want to and it will also speed the healing, but the root is more powerful than the leaf. The fresh root is best, but powdered dry root mixed with castor oil or olive oil will also do the trick.

*Do **NOT** use comfrey on any wound that may have any infection in it. Comfrey will heal the area so quickly that it can heal over the infection and then you will have a problem. This has happened before.*

Clean the wound, deal with any existing infection and then use comfrey!

You can use blanched burdock leaves over a dirty wound to draw out dirt and infection. Bring water to a boil. Dip the fresh or dried burdock leaf into the boiling water just long enough to soften the leaf.

Some time ago, a friend was holding a router between his knees as he changed the bit.

Then his grip slipped and his knee hit the switch. Before he could turn the machine off, it made several deep cuts on his hand. As he ran to the house, he grabbed a leaf of a comfrey plant, stuck it in his mouth, and started to chew. Once inside, he grabbed a jar of cayenne and threw some cayenne down into the cuts to stop the bleeding. He then put the pieces of comfrey leaf he had chewed up over the wound. The cayenne stopped the bleeding and he bound up the cuts with a cloth.

Two weeks later, he told us about the accident. Everyone crowded around to see his hand. It had healed so well you couldn't see a scar.

Comfrey Mint Drink

This is simple-to-make, pleasant-to-drink shake.

Pick several leaves of comfrey, and 2-3 sprigs of fresh mint. If the leaves are large, cut the spine off and chop a bit, before putting them in the blender. The spines of large leaves add toothbrush-like fibers in your shake even after blending. Add to blender:

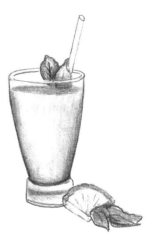

> 2-3 comfrey leaves, *spined and chopped*
>
> *2-3 sprigs of mint*
>
> *1-2 cups of pineapple juice (canned or fresh)*

Whiz till smooth and thick. Thoroughly blend the comfrey leaves. It isn't nice if there are still leafy pieces in it. Add ice to thicken as much as you wish. Enjoy! It has a nice minty flavor and a lovely green color. Refreshing on a hot day and healthy and healing as well. Use frozen cubes of pineapple juice to thicken, and make a more flavorful shake. Children enjoy this shake just because it is good.

Comfrey is very rich in chlorophyll. That is why it is so useful. After all, the only difference between chlorophyll and our blood is that our blood molecule is built around an iron atom and the chlorophyll molecule is built around a magnesium atom.

NOTE: The FDA considers comfrey a dangerous herb to ingest, but I feel that this is misinformation based on a study that they did with rats. This study (The Carcinogenic Activity of Symphytum Officinale by Hirono, Mori, and Hago - Japan, 1978, which sparked the U.S. legislation regarding the use of comfrey.) focused on injecting newborn rats with PAs (pyrrolizidine alkaloids) which is unrealistic. We never inject that compound into our bodies. They also fed the rats extremely larges amounts of comfrey daily. I propose that this is a biased study. If you were to feed anyone Tylenol or Pepto Bismol in such large quantities, or inject it into their bodies, these medicines would quickly cause liver cancer and be pulled off the market. Furthermore, they used only isolated PA's and not the whole plant for that experiment. None of us take comfrey that way. When the whole plant is taken, you cannot ingest enough PA's to damage you.

Because of this study though, I must advise you to do your own research before accepting my opinion that comfrey is safe for internal use when taken in normal amounts, using the leaf and not the root.

Malignant Ulcer

Dr. H.E. Kirschner, M.D., author of Nature's Healing Grasses (H.C. White Publications, 1975), describes one of his most interesting cases involving comfrey: "A middle-aged woman came to me with a large malignant ulcer below the eye and close to the nose. I prescribed a comfrey poultice and a "green drink" containing comfrey leaves. Soon after the application of the comfrey leaf poultice, the painful swelling subsided and rapid improvement was noted. Only a few months after the initial treatment there was complete healing over the infected area and the malignant ulcer had disappeared."

Comfrey Salve

Comfrey salve is so easy to make that you really should take the time to do it. The cuttings from one plant will make at least one quart of comfrey oil that can be turned into salve. Then you will have all you need and some to spare. This salve is good for brush burns, chapped lips, cold sores, burns, diaper rash, varicose veins, psoriasis, excema, and anywhere you need healing to take place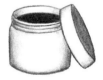

Cut the comfrey leaves and shake them clean. Chop the leaves (and at least 6 inches of root) like you were going to make salad. Put them loosely into a wide-mouth quart jar. Cover with olive oil (or a mix of olive and almond oil). Heat to 100 degrees in your oven for one hour. Turn off heat and let set, covered with a cloth, on your counter for one to two weeks. Strain and squeeze out the leaves and you have a lovely, green oil.

Make your salve with this recipe.

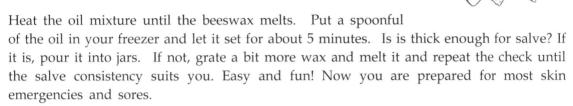

2 cups of comfrey oil

1 ounce grated beeswax

1 tablespoon vitamin E oil

15 drops of lavender essential oil

Heat the oil mixture until the beeswax melts.   Put a spoonful
of the oil in your freezer and let it set for about 5 minutes. Is is thick enough for salve? If
it is, pour it into jars. If not, grate a bit more wax and melt it and repeat the check until
the salve consistency suits you. Easy and fun! Now you are prepared for most skin
emergencies and sores.

Comfrey for Varicose Veins

Deborah had deep, burning pain and discomfort in her legs from her varicose veins.
Someone told her to use comfrey salve. At first when she rubbed it on it was very
painful. But Deborah persisted and after 2 weeks there was very little pain. Soon there
was none. The burst veins and red areas disappeared gradually over the next few weeks!

More Comfrey Stories

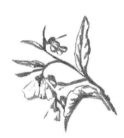

Thomas had bouts of trouble with his digestive system and he decided to try green
drinks. He drank a green shake at least once or twice a day and he liked them. His
stomach troubles cleared up in no time at all. But there was an unusual twist to this
story. After about two weeks of drinking his comfrey faithfully, Thomas reported that
his ankle which had given him trouble from a long past injury was not bothering him
anymore when he ran and played with his children. Comfrey is like that. It heals old
scars and helps repair damage to any cells and muscle and bone that we have.

My husband heard that story and began to do his own experiment. He had a large scar on his wrist from an accident as a child. What do you know! After about two weeks of drinking the green drink, his scar had softened noticeably and was definitely smaller. He also experienced an unexpected side effect. His bad breath was much improved. The comfrey's excellent healing ability had aided his digestion, too.

I have had psoriasis since I was thirteen. No medications and creams had given any lasting help. I decided to test the effectiveness of comfrey salve on my stubborn skin inflammation. To my surprise a twice daily application of comfrey salve did more to ease it than any prescription drug ever did.

Comfrey Tincture

This is a simple tincture that you can make from the root of your prolific comfrey that will be very helpful. You can use it for sprains and bruises and any goose egg your child gets.

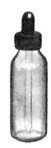

> *Dig a comfrey root.*
> *Use the leaves for green drink and wash the root.*
> *Peel the root and chop it finely like you would for a salad.*
> *Fill a pint jar loosely with chopped root.*
> *Cover it with 80 proof vodka.*
> *(You can use vinegar but the tincture will not keep as long.)*
> *Let it stand for 2 – 6 weeks, shaking often.*
> *When you are ready, strain and bottle the liquid in a dark jar.*
> *Use for sprains, bruises and aches. This liquid is called a tincture.*

To show you the effectiveness of this simple, comfrey tincture, I'll tell you a story.

John dropped a very heavy table on his toe. He yelled in pain and began hopping around on one foot. His wife immediately brought him pan of water to soak his toe in. She added a few droppers of comfrey tincture to the water. He soaked his toe and soon the toe felt better and he went on with his work.

That night she rubbed the toe with comfrey tincture again and they went to bed. In the morning a friend was helping him move the table and he mentioned his accident. "How in the world are you walking?" asked his friend. "I dropped a rock on my toe in the same area and I could not walk for a week."

They looked at his toe together and other than a slight discoloration, the toe was doing well and it was not painful. In a few days the nail did come off and there was a new nail growing beneath it. The toe had obviously sustained trauma, but the wonderfully healing comfrey had come to the rescue again. This kind of story could be repeated over and over.

Another Tincture Story

"I fractured my right fifth metacarpal the beginning of this month. I saw the orthopedist and he set it with a cast. I used a tincture of comfrey acquired from the local health food store. I applied it with a q-tip under the cast at the site of the fracture once or twice a day. I went back to the doc for my followup visit two weeks and two days after the injury. The doc asked three times, "When did this injury occur?" He could not believe how fast it had healed. He left the cast off and I have a soft splint. Now I apply the comfrey tincture on a bandage and leave it on overnight. I hope to be splint free when I go for my next two week checkup. Not bad for a 58 year old lady!"

I have used comfrey tincture myself for a badly bruised area and it took away the pain and the bruising disappeared more quickly. I try not to be without this tincture because I can use it when my huge comfrey bed is frozen in the winter. I just add some tincture to water to make a healing foot soak or saturate a gauze pad with it and apply directly over a wound. You can change it often and there is no mess or fuss.

Comfrey Burn Paste

How to Make Burn Paste

½ cup wheat germ oil

½ cup honey

Add only enough comfrey root or root powder to thicken it nicely.

Keep tightly covered in fridge when not in use. It will last a while. Use this mixture to heal burns. I make it when I need it, or make it ahead and freeze it in small amounts in a Ziploc bag ready for emergencies. **If you are covering a large area make sure that you use plenty of oil and change it at least every 8 hours to keep it from drying out and sticking to the burned area.**

When the comfrey is growing – from May to October, I use the fresh leaf and root to make the burn paste. Use 3 fresh, chopped comfrey leave and root. Add the wheat germ oil and the honey. Blend to a fine pulp. Thicken to spreadable consistency with comfrey root powder or slippery elm powder if needed. Use plenty of wheat germ oil!

Deep 2nd Degree Burns

5:00 PM – my phone was ringing again. A busy 2 year-old had climbed up by the stove just as his sister pulled the kettle off the stove. You guessed it! Both little palms laid flat on a burner that was on high! I went flying over with a large bottle of aloe that was in my fridge while she held his hands in cold water to take out the heat. These were deep 2nd degree burns. His dad beat me there by 5 minutes and he was holding him, screaming, both hands in the water. I poured the cold aloe juice in a bowl and stuck his hands in – hiccup, sob and the boy was quiet!

It never ceases to amaze me what cold aloe does for a burn and I intend never to be without it. This is the 5th time that I made a run like this and it always works. Over the next few hours we had to keep trading the warm juice for some that was chilled to keep his pain at bay. But by 9:30 he was falling asleep and by ten we wrapped his hands with comfrey burn paste and bandaged them and he slept all night.

In the morning, though his hands were badly blistered, he had no severe pain. We definitely had deep burns, but by hydrating the tissues in the aloe, healing had already begun.

Each day we unwrapped his hands, gently patted off the loose paste, added new burn paste in a thick layer, and re-bandaged them. The burns were severe enough that the little one ate almost nothing for the first three days. He ran a fever which is normal for this severe a burn, His parents gave him hi-protein drinks and good juices (without added sugar) to hydrate him and soon he was up and around playing.

By the fourth day he was out riding his tricycle with his bandaged hands and playing happily. It took a few weeks until his hands were healed but we bandaged them morning and night until the new skin had formed and he did so well.

If you have a burn like that and bandaging does not take care of the pain, there is something else you can do. Find a burdock leaf in the field (use plantain if you do not have burdock), and blanch it in boiling water. Pat out the water and lay it over the burn paste before you bandage it. Believe it or not, there is something about the plant that will actually help to take away the pain of the burn.

For more information on burns and how to care for them see the burn chapter. We have detailed information there on how to care for burns and where to get supplies when needed. There is also another story there of how to heal burns using B&W salve. Study these accounts and you will be prepared to care for most burns that your family receives.

Bleeding Hemorrhoids

Colitis and IBS

Drink three cups of comfrey tea daily along with lots of water. Take a teaspoon of prepared, powdered slippery elm before each meal and at bedtime, and with each loose bowel movement. Usually this brings relief for most people. If not see *cayenne chapter.

A Fissure

My email held yet another question. The lady had a fissure, or tear that was giving her pain and bleeding when she moved her bowels. She had been doctoring this thing for three months with no success. What could she do for it

I pondered the problem and decided that comfrey might help and recommended that she make a strong solution of comfrey leaf, calendula flower and plantain leaf and use it as a sitz bath. *see sitz bath p. 261 I suggested that she do this two or three times daily until she experienced healing.

To my surprise, she emailed me and reported that one sitz bath corrected the problem . One sitz bath corrected a problem that had been ongoing for three months! The healing abilities of comfrey and the simplicity of its use never cease to amaze me.

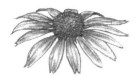
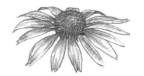

Echinacea

"The Immune Builder"

Echinacea (Purple Cone Flower) is not only a beautiful flower, but also a potent medicine. This plant works with the body's defense mechanisms against the spread of pathogens and reduces inflammation. The American Botanical Council tells us that echinacea may be of value for any infection, chronic or acute, but especially where there is not long-term immune deficiency or dysfunction.

Echinacea improves immune function by increasing the chemical recognition of an invading pathogen. The speed at which the immune cells migrate to the site of infection and destroy the invader is markedly increased. Herbalist Jeanine Pollak, of Santa Cruz, California, explains this process in layman's terms: "The immune cells devour things that are bad for your body before they can develop and make you sick. "

Uses:

- sinus help

- sore throats

- acne, skin

- food poisoning

- allergies

- immune aid

- stamina

- weight loss

- digestive aid

- constipation

- for arthritis

- urinary tract

Echinacea helps to prevent colds and flu when everyone around you is getting sick. **If you take it at the first sign of an illness it will work a lot better than if you take it later**. But even if you don't start taking echinacea at the first sign of illness, it can shorten the severity and duration of many common illnesses. I have found that it helps a lot to keep infections from settling into the lungs and sinuses.

Take Echinacea as Fresh as Possible

Freshness is important. This seems especially true with echinacea. Dried roots and powdered herbs in capsules can be old, minimizing their effectiveness, so look for **"fresh root"** when you are buying it or make your own fresh root tincture.

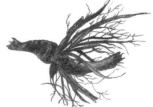

If you go to buy dried root - check for freshness by tasting a piece: It should have a "tingly" feeling on your tongue and cause you to salivate. If not, it will not be effective. You can get around this difficulty by buying four, 3 year-old echinacea plants at your local green house in the spring. Plant them by your house, or any place in the sun where you have room. In early August, harvest one plant with flowers and stems for tincture. Allow the others to stay to scatter their seeds so that you can start new plants in the spring. Harvest by cutting the stems at least 6 inches off the ground. Strip the leaves off the stem and discard the stem. Chop up the leaves, the petals and the seed head. Now you are ready to make your tincture. Fill your jar with a mixture of leaf, flower and seed head and cover it with either the glycerin mix (see Making Medicine for Your Family) or with vodka. If you are making the Tasty Echinacea formula, you will add about ¼ chopped fresh peppermint leaf. *See recipe in Making Medicine.

When the plant dies down, then you are ready to get your root. You really need to have a 3 year plant for sufficient root "strength" to be worth anything. Dig the root of one plant. This way you will leave 3 mature roots for you next year.

Wash your root. Chop it up with a very sharp knife or put it in a good quality blender and shred it. Fill a jar with the shredded root and cover it with alcohol to tincture. The root tinctures best with alcohol.

Your flower and leaf tincture will be ready before your root tincture is, so strain it and put it in a dark place, labeled well, to wait for the root tincture. When the root is ready, strain it and add it to the flower tincture. I usually use a ½ root and ½ flower/leaf/seed mix. This stores well and is nice to use. You could use less root if you want to.

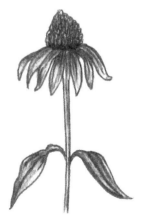

If you want to have a no-alcohol tincture for babies you can tincture a bit of root in glycerin, but glycerin does not extract as well from the root as alcohol does.

If you want an all-alcohol tincture you can use alcohol to tincture the flower/leaf/seed mixture as well. This is all up to you. Remember to be sure to label all your jars well since it is very hard to tell tincturing herbs apart. Alcohol makes the strongest tincture.

The reason for making tinctures of echinacea is that the plant is usually dormant when we need it the most in the fall and winter. You can make a tea out of echinacea root or herb to do the same thing and it works well, too. I would mix it with another herb that has a pleasant flavor, like peppermint, so that folks would want to drink it. In my opinion, the fresh root/herb tincture is the strongest way to take it. Here is an interesting story in our herbal journey.

The Effectiveness of Fresh Echinacea

We have never used the doctor often, and as time went on and our family grew, I began to experiment with herbs. I would read that this herb was good for colds and flu and then go to the health food store and get a bottle of capsules or a tincture, but I was rather disappointed when they did not perform as well as I had expected that they would. After I began serving as a midwife, I needed herbs that would help with difficulties that I encountered during and after the delivery, and I needed them to work well. I was directed to a producer of herbal tinctures that were supposedly stronger. She sent me a little flyer in which she advertised her other tinctures. She made one that she called "Immune Awake". That tincture was the turning point in my herbal journey. It worked for the cold and flu, and it worked well. As I asked her questions I learned that she used fresh plant instead of dried plant to make many of her tinctures and that is why they were stronger. See Wish Garden Herbs.

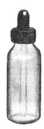

Then I found American Botanical Pharmacy and their products worked even better. Finally I began to make fresh tinctures of echinacea myself. Folks tell me that they are ten times stronger than any they have ever used. I expect that it is because of the fresh products that I use and because I fill my jars full with the herb. Many herb companies fill their jars less than half full with herb and they use dried herb, so the resulting product is definitely inferior though it may still work. You get out of it what you put into it!

How to Fight off a Cold

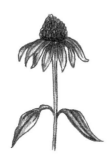

Barb writes, "Last night, my throat felt a little sore, and I took a couple of zinc tablets and irrigated my sinuses. This morning when I woke up, my throat was *really* sore, and I had the generally yucky feeling that goes with a cold. I used to get very, very sick with colds -- the initial viral infection would almost always be followed by a secondary bacterial infection. I'd be sick for at least two weeks. For the last few years, I've been able to cut the process short by taking zinc tablets at the first sign of a cold and irrigating my sinuses every 3 or 4 hours with a neti pot, and eating citrus. Taking vitamin C tablets doesn't help me, nor does frozen orange juice; it has to be fresh citrus.

This cold that started last night was one virulent infection. For a while, I was sure it was going to lay me low. Still, it was worth trying to fight it. I added a 30 second gargle with Listerine to the routine every time I used the neti pot, but I kept getting worse. About noon, I went out to the garden and dug up an echinacea root. . . . One thing I can say for sure -- it works to ease sore throat pain. The inside of the root is brownish gray with dark brown rings. What I do is slice off little bits of the root and chew it, holding it in my mouth for a while. The taste isn't 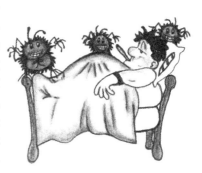 bad at all, a bit like a radish. At first, it makes the tongue feel prickly, then the prickles spread to the nasal sinuses and throat. Then the pain just goes away. It's similar to the way aloe vera leaves stop the pain of minor burns. I've eaten a slice of echinacea root every couple of hours for about six hours. For a while, my throat felt better, but the rest of me kept feeling worse, but around 6:00 I started feeling better all over. I now feel almost normal, but I've continued the treatment. I'm a little worried that the virus will get the upper hand again during the night, since I won't be doing the treatment as often. But I feel so good, perhaps my immune system has things under control." She wrote again the next day to say she had the flu licked and she was happy.

Dosages of Echinacea Tincture

You need to take enough to make a difference.

If you have a fresh root/herb tincture and you begin to feel a scratchy throat or a sniffle coming on – take four droppers (one tsp.) every three hours for a day or so.

If you are already sick with sore throat and fever you will probably need to take that much every 2 hours.

And if you have a bad case of the flu you can take twice that much every hour for a day, or until the symptoms break.

If you want to add extra protection take Super Duper Tonic with the fresh echinacea tincture in equal doses. When I do this, I find that the symptoms disappear and seldom develop into anything serious. In fact, I seldom have even a serious head cold if I start my Hot Echinacea and Super Duper Tonic at the first sign of the sniffles and sore throat.

I also take it as a preventive if I am nursing a bunch of people who have come down with the flu. I know that I do not have the time nor the desire to go to bed with the flu so I reach for my bottles of echinacea and Super Duper Tonic and usually I stay flu-free.

A number of researchers feel that you reach the maximum immune stimulation after five days of use, after which its helpfulness begins to decline. Some think that the maximum is two weeks and a few say it does not matter at all. I am not able to comment on this except to say that the body does gradually accommodate itself to most things and this is probably true for echinacea, too. In that case, it would be helpful to take echinacea for a week or two, and then take two or more weeks off before taking it again.

I usually only take it until I feel better which is at the most three days and then I set it aside until I need it another time.

For Sore Throat

Mix 4 droppers of echinacea in a small amount of warm water. Gargle and swallow every 2 hours or as needed (every hour is OK). If you use the Tasty Echinacea. See *Medicine Making section. It does not even taste bad.

Tasty Echinacea

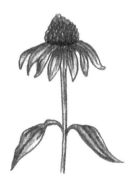

   2 parts fresh echinacea herb, chopped

   1 part fresh echinacea root chopped. (dried will work but it is much

   weaker in strength)

   1 part peppermint leaf chopped (for flavor)

Make a mix of 75% glycerin and 25% water. Cover the herbs. Let stand two to four weeks shaking daily. Strain and bottle. Use liberally for children and adults alike.

Hot Echinacea

2 parts fresh echinacea herb, chopped

1 part fresh echinacea root chopped

1 part fresh garlic cloves

1 part cayenne (this one is hot and it is much more effective than Tasty Echinacea.)

Some folks put it in capsules to take since it is hot. This will not work quite as well, but it does keep your mouth from burning. Three capsules equal about 1 dropper. Cover the herbs with vodka. Let stand two to four weeks shaking daily. Strain and bottle.

Tasty Echinacea Tea

Combine these ingredients and put 4 tablespoons in a non-metal 1 quart pot:

- *Echinacea root*
- *Grated ginger root*
- *Fennel seed*

Add 1 tablespoon of these ingredients:

- *Licorice root (if you do not have high blood pressure)*
- *Orange peel or slices*

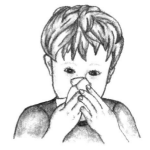

Fill the pot almost to the top with water, cover, and simmer for 20 minutes. Pour it through a strainer before you drink it.

Drink 3 hot cups of this yummy concoction per day until your symptoms improve.

If you must use dried root, then order it from Mountain Rose Herbs and use this recipe. The extra ingredients make this tea taste good, plus they have added effects: ginger is an expectorant; licorice soothes your throat; fennel moistens your throat and lungs and helps to settle your stomach; the citrus is antiseptic, antibacterial, and rich in bio-flavonoids.

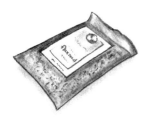

Flax

"A Healing Seed"

Flax seeds contain high levels of lignans and Omega-3 fatty acids. Lignans may benefit the heart, may possess anti-cancer properties, and studies performed on mice found reduced growth in specific types of tumors. Flax seed may also lower cholesterol levels, especially in women. Studies suggest that flax seed taken in the diet may benefit individuals with certain types of cancers.

Flax may also lessen the severity of diabetes by stabilizing blood-sugar levels. Due to its fiber content it can help to remedy constipation. Because of this, flax seed is one staple that I try to keep on hand all the time. It is useful for so many things.

Uses:

- poultices
- foreign
  objects in the eye
- infection
- arthritis
- women's
  health
- cancer
- bowel aid
- kidney disease
- weight loss
- skin aid

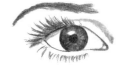

Remove Foreign Material

from your Eye

My first exposure to the lowly flax seed was when someone got a particle of something in his eye. A friend was here when I got the call asking what they could do to get it out. My friend is a construction worker and has trouble with getting foreign material in his eyes from time to time. This is what he does, and it has worked for everyone that has used it like I recommended.

Take one flax seed and place it in the eye in the lower corner by the tear duct. Do this just before you go to bed. In the morning the foreign material will be right there for you to wipe out.

What a simple, simple remedy. It works and I have used it again and again.

Flax Seed Poultice

Flax seed used as a poultice is very healing, takes pain away, and helps with infection.

Making a flax seed poultice is very simple.

Grind 1 cup of flax seed (depending how large a poultice you need) to a coarse powder in your blender or coffee grinder. Dump the ground flax into a bowl and mix it with a little olive or castor oil. . Add hot water a bit at a time, stirring well, until you have a thick, smooth paste that will spread but not be runny.

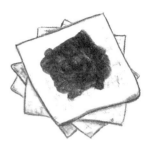

Lay out a piece of plastic wrap, the size that you need to liberally cover your sore area. Spread the poultice material over the plastic wrap about ¼ inch thick. Oil the sore area and flip the poultice onto the area, plastic side up. Cover with a towel and a heating pad or warm rice sock. Keep the warm poultice on for at least a half hour. It may stay on as long as you desire. If it was not against any infection, you can roll it up, refrigerate, and reuse it again. Unroll, sprinkle with water and reheat in the microwave or oven, or use hot water to heat it.

Poultice for Appendicitis

I have found the flax poultice to be an invaluable help when dealing with pain and infection. The following is an account of how we used a flax/charcoal (*See charcoal chapter) application to bring relief for appendicitis.

One Sunday morning, just as we were ready to leave for church, a lady called and asked if we could help her husband who was suffering from abdominal pain. I had her do the rebound tenderness test and it indeed confirmed the likelihood of appendicitis. I got the man on the phone and asked him a lot of questions.

Yes, he had been working in the hot sun the last week. No, he had not been drinking much water. It was too inconvenient on the job. Yes, he had been having pain and bouts of soreness off and on the last two weeks, but today it was very intense and he was running a fever. Yes, he would do whatever I said. "OK. Put on the tea kettle and make and drink a cup or two of hot tea while I drive over." I put a bunch of things in my basket and headed out.

When I got there we immediately gave him a number of herbal laxative capsules, and another cup of hot tea. Then I prepared a flax/charcoal poultice. She rubbed lobelia tincture on his sore tummy and then applied the very warm poultice. We covered that with a towel and a warm rice sock. His pain noticeably lessoned and he became more comfortable. I chatted with them about what I was doing, and why, and how it had helped others in the same situation. In 45 minutes I gave him another bunch of herbal laxative capsules and another cup of hot tea. I was really trying to get his bowels moving because I knew that if we could, we could calm down his inflamed appendix and avert an operation. She rubbed more lobelia on him and I reheated the poultice. By now he was much more comfortable.

It took an hour and a half and lots of laxative capsules and about a quart of tea. Finally he headed for the bathroom and really emptied out. He was now very sore but not having the waves of pain that he had had. I put the poultice on him again and gave him slippery elm gruel by mouth. This serves to soothe the irritated colon. I urged them to use vitamin C and hot echinacea to deal with any infection that might still be there and to stay on a liquid diet for 2 days. He was to use lots of fresh juice and herbal teas and water to give his colon a rest. After that he was to eat a soft diet for 2 days and stay away from meat and eggs and hard to digest foods. I left them and went to enjoy the rest of my church service.

A week or two later I received a card and a gift with a note of thanks for helping them to stay out of the emergency room. He was feeling so much better and he had learned a lot about how things work and why he got that way. I believe that he got an education that will help him for the rest of his life, and the cost was minimal.

Flax to Soothe Eye Irritations

Empty a tea bag and fill it with ground flax seed and staple it shut. Moisten it with hot water and lay it in place over your sore or inflamed eyes to soothe them and take away the irritations.

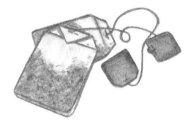

This procedure will often relieve sore eyes, or eyes that have been over-strained from computer usage.

Our daughter received a scratch on her eye that caused her tremendous pain for nearly a week. It had nearly healed and she was doing computer work again. Suddenly she came down with severe eye pain again. We tried quite a few things but nothing was successful until we did flax tea bags moistened with eye bright tincture (you could also use eyebright tea). These slowly brought about relief and healing.

Flax for an Abscessed Cyst

It was Sunday and Susan was in pain from an abscessed cyst in a sensitive area. A few months earlier she had had the same problem and the doctor sent her to the hospital to have it lanced and drained. Susan said she had spent the next week laid up with quite a bit of pain. Here she was again, with the same problem. Was there any thing that she could do to avoid another costly hospital bill and all the time in bed?

I was definitely not sure, but I recommended the old stand-by, a flax/charcoal poultice mixed with castor oil. Susan and her husband came over immediately to pick up the supplies (see why it is important to keep these things on hand) and set to work to follow my instructions. She kept a poultice on all night and the cyst swelled and became more painful. (This is a normal response) In concern she called the doctor and asked for an antibiotic. Her husband went to get it early in the afternoon and she took a sitz bath to the area to try and relieve the pain.

As she checked the area she thought that she saw a bit of pus coming from the abscess so she began to work with it. She was able to drain the cyst completely before her husband got home with the medicine. She never did take the antibiotics, but she put another poultice on overnight simply to be sure that the infection was all gone.

Susan called me to let me know that the abscess was resolved and she was so thankful. The cost was only a few dollars and the pain was minimal compared to what she had gone through the other time.

This treatment is not invasive, expensive, or painful. There is no recuperation involved and it works so well. I have been glad for it many times.

Flax/Charcoal Poultice for Infection

By permission from John Dinsley from CharcoalRemedies.com, I have included the following example of a flax seed/charcoal poultice that did a beautiful job of healing infection.

"My husband had toe surgery to correct his hammertoes on both feet (8 of them!). He picked up a Staph infection in the hospital and almost lost one of his toes due to infection. The toe looked like ground burger. The surgeon prescribed a powerful antibiotic, but it did not do anything for him. He was then prescribed another, more powerful antibiotic. Again. Nothing!

I have used charcoal drinks and poultices over the years, but never for anything this serious. It has always worked well and efficiently for stomach ailments and wound infections. This was going to be a test. We trusted in God, and with prayer we placed his toes in the sunlight for sun treatments. We also placed some charcoal poultices on several times throughout the day. His toe healed wonderfully. After a while, his other foot began to swell and turn dark. Apparently the staph infection had gone throughout his body. He had a terrible skin reaction in his groin area, too. I treated this with a garlic poultice and sun baths. But the foot was the worst.

I called the doctor and she told me to take him immediately to the emergency room. We knew what emergency rooms can be like and didn't want the long hours and hassles-- and more drugs that didn't work! We prayed to God for guidance. I told the Lord that if we didn't see any results by next morning, we would then go to the ER.

It was 6 p.m. when I applied the first poultice. I used flax seed powder and mixed it with the charcoal. This produced a flexible poultice that wrapped completely around his foot and then covered it with plastic. I covered this with a heating pad set to LOW. We pleaded with God to allow us to glorify His name and to vindicate the use of this natural, harmless treatment. At midnight, I woke to change the dressing. The foot was remarkably lighter in color and the swelling had gone down.

I placed another poultice on, and while praising God, I went back to sleeping peacefully. At 6 a.m. I woke and took off the dressing. The foot looked like new! No swelling. No darkness. There was, however, a red mark on the top of his foot. I continued to place a smaller poultice on this red mark and in a few days, the redness burst open and produced a discharge. I continued the poultices and in the next day or so, the wound began to show signs of healing. I exposed it to a little sunlight during the day with a poultice change once or twice throughout the day--then a poultice at night.

Within the next few days, it was dried and healed. Praise the Lord! Apparently there was a deep infection in his foot that was being drawn to the surface by the poultice. The antibiotics did not work, but God sure did!"

This happens time and again when charcoal and flax are used together. It is amazing how powerfully a poultice like this can work. You need to be consistent and work with the infection carefully. But I believe that it is a wonderful way to get healing. The hospitals are having more and more difficulty healing staph infections. These bugs are becoming antibiotic resistant and it is a source of great concern in the medical world. Why not learn all you can now and then if you get an infection, treat it yourself and gave God the glory. He is the one that made all these things for us to use.

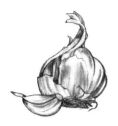
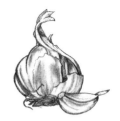

Garlic

"The Natural Antibiotic"

If garlic were not so cheap and did not smell so bad, we would treasure it more. As it is, most people do not really know how effective garlic is. They do not know that until 1942 when penicillin was manufactured, doctors routinely used garlic to kill virus, bacterias and fungus. They used garlic to fight infections on the battlefields in World War I. Garlic still works well for an antibiotic although it tastes worse and needs to be taken more often. It works well for the common cold, combats hypertension, quiets the body, and gets rid of parasites. Simply put, garlic is fantastic!

Uses:

- antibiotic

- relaxant

- high blood

pressure

- coughs & colds

- pneumonia

- abscesses

- fungal infections

- high blood sugar

- bacterial

 infections

- stops bruising

- immune system

The Medicinal Qualities of Garlic

There are two main medicinal ingredients which produce garlic health benefits: allicin and diallyl sulphides. Allicin does not occur in "ordinary" garlic, it is produced when garlic is finely chopped or crushed. The finer the chopping and the more intensive the crushing, the more allicin is generated and the stronger the medicinal effect.

Until 1942 when penicillin was made, doctors routinely used garlic to kill virus, bacteria and fungus. Garlic formed the principal ingredient in the 'Four Thieves Vinegar,' which was used so successfully in Marseilles for protection against the plague when it prevailed there in 1722.

The active properties of garlic depend on a pungent, volatile, essential oil, which may readily be obtained by distillation with water. It is a sulphide of the radical allyl, present in all the onion family. This oil is rich in sulfur, but contains no oxygen. The peculiar penetrating odor of garlic is due to this intensely smelling sulphate of allyl, and is so diffusive that even when the bulb is applied to the soles of the feet, its odor is exhaled by the lungs.

Studies by competent multi-degreed scientists have shown beyond any reasonable doubt that consuming garlic generally has the following physical effects:

- *Garlic lowers blood pressure a little. (9% to 15 % with 1 or 2 medium cloves per day).*

- *Garlic lowers LDL Cholesterol a little (9% to 15 % with 1 or 2 medium cloves per day).*

- *Garlic helps reduce plaque buildup within the arterial system. One recent study shows this effect to be greater in women than men.*

- *Garlic lowers or helps to regulate blood sugar.*

- *Garlic helps to prevent blood clots from forming, thus reducing the possibility of strokes and thromboses (blood clots) (Hemophiliacs shouldn't use garlic).*

- *Garlic helps to prevent cancer, especially of the digestive system, prevents certain tumors from growing larger, and reduces the size of certain tumors.*

- *Garlic may help to remove heavy metals such as lead and mercury from the body.*

- *Raw garlic is a potent natural antibiotic that works differently than modern antibiotics and kills some strains of bacteria, like staph, that have become immune or resistant to modern antibiotics.*

- *Garlic has anti-fungal and anti-viral properties.*

Let's take a simple overview of how garlic works. A bulb of garlic has from four to sixteen or more cloves. In each of these cloves are cells containing the main compound of garlic, an amino acid called allicin. In separate cells an enzyme called allinase resides. Whenever the cellular walls separating them are damaged, some of the enzyme comes into contact with the amino acid and this sets off a chemical reaction that causes sulfenic acid to form instantly. But sulfenic acid is unstable and reacts with itself and breaks down at a steady rate into another unstable compound called allicin, which has a strong antibiotic property.

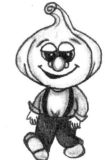

Allicin is the "magic bullet" in garlic from which its many benefits are derived. Because garlic forms the active compound allicin steadily and in regular spurts, rather than all at once, it is better to chop it fine and to let it set for 15 minutes to an hour before using it in order to build up a greater amount of allicin.

One of the simplest ways to use garlic as an antibiotic is to chop it or grate it finely and let it set for about 10 minutes. This gives the allicin time to activate in the air before you use it. Then swallow it without chewing, if you wish to eliminate the problem of garlic breath. Or, if you find the taste of garlic too distasteful, drizzle it with honey before swallowing. Do this for all kinds of infections.

Consistent doses are important. Garlic is not a drug; it must be taken often and faithfully to do the same job as one antibiotic pill a day. However, you need to know that instead of lowering your immune system like antibiotics do, garlic actually enhances your immune system.

Did you ever notice that when you take antibiotics they usually work, but often in a few weeks or months you need to go for another one? This is because antibiotics lower the immune system, making you susceptible to the next infection.

I find that you must take garlic every 2 hours or oftener for serious problems like abscesses or bacterial infections. If you find it difficult to take chopped raw garlic you can take Super Duper Tonic instead. You can purchase it or make it yourself. Variations of this recipe have became widely known through the teachings of Dr. Richard Schultz.

Super Duper Tonic - An Inexpensive Antibiotic Formula

Chop finely equal amounts of :

raw onions, garlic horseradish ginger root cayenne (use less if you do not want it too hot)

Use equal parts of all of them and fill a quart jar full to the brim.

Fill the jar up to the neck with raw,apple cider vinegar, (preferably from the health food store; this kind has not been pasteurized.) Let it set for 2 - 4 weeks, shaking every day. (You can use it as soon as you wish, but it is stronger if you let it set longer.) Now strain it through a cloth and bottle in dark bottles.

When you need to take it, take 1 spoonful in water or juice. This is hot. Take it hourly if you wish, or 4 times a day. If you take it hourly you will notice improvement more quickly.

Super Duper Tonic to the Rescue

We use natural medicine for nearly all our ailments and the children are not always grateful for the medicines. But as they grow older and leave home and are responsible for their own health and their own bills, they appreciate these simple remedies more than before.

Our sons-in-law had not been accustomed to Super Duper Tonic and it's powerful effects before they were married. In fact one of them was quite skeptical about whether these things worked at all. His folks had always used the doctor. One day, he was sick in bed, groaning with the aches of flu and fever, and his wife persuaded him to try the tonic. He did try it every hour, like I recommend, and he was back to work the next day. He could hardly believe how simple and inexpensive it really was, but it worked! Now when he feels the slightest hint of the flu coming on, he reaches for his Super Duper Tonic bottle and he soon feels better.

This remedy is so simple that your children can make it if they are careful with cutting up the hot peppers. The oil of these peppers can really burn. Some folks wear gloves, and if you are making a large amount you should. You can figure on getting about 2 cups of tincture from a quart of the chopped mixture. If you are sick and take it every hour or two, you will need about ¼ to ½ a cup to get over your flu. For a family, it will usually take a quart or more for a flu season. If you make more you will have some to share. You will want to make it fresh every year. Try to make it in the late summer when you can get jalapenos and horseradish at your local grocery, or at roadside stands. You can usually get ginger root at a grocery store anytime.

Quite a few families around us are making and using this tonic. They find that it saves them many doctor visits. When I begin to get the sniffles or feel like I am coming down with the flu, I get my own two ounce bottle and set it where I am working.
I take a spoonful of it every hour and usually that is the end of the bug.

Garlic Salve – the Antibiotic Salve!

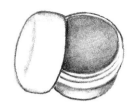

Here is an all-purpose antibiotic salve that you can use for babies, children and adults alike. I first read about it in Debbi Pearl's articles. Garlic salve can be made in a few minutes and stored in the fridge to be readily available whenever you need it. When I read about this simple salve I really questioned whether it could do all they said. But I have no more questions about its ability. It is a valuable, inexpensive home remedy that no mother of little ones should be without. Once again I wish it did not smell like garlic, but the results are worth the smell. Apply directly to sores inside the mouth. Rub it on athlete's foot or use it for jock itch, or yeast and other related infections. Apply on rashes any place. If you have a sensitive place where you want to apply it, try a small amount first to be sure that it does not burn too badly. However, if you follow the recipe you will have a salve that usually does not burn. Place it on a cotton swab for ear infections. Garlic salve kills candida, parasites, bad bacteria, and virus by direct application. In addition, it treats systemic infections by absorption through the skin into the blood supply and it travels throughout the body. After two weeks, make a new batch of garlic salve.

Garlic Salve Recipe

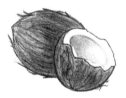

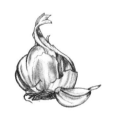

Put in blender:

1/3 cup coconut oil

2 Tablespoons olive oil

8 cloves peeled garlic

5 or so drops of lavender oil

*Blend at high speed until liquified. Strain through a fine sieve to catch any pieces. Pour into a wide mouth, small jar and **refrigerate.***

Note: **If the salve causes a rash, dilute with more coconut and olive oil.** Your child may have sensitive skin and this should help. There is an occasional baby who cannot tolerate the salve anywhere but on the soles of his feet.

Garlic Salve Stories

My first exposure to garlic salve was when a young mother near here used the salve to keep her 3 month old baby out of the hospital. The baby contracted pneumonia and the doctor wanted to hospitalize it, but she begged for 3 days to try home remedies... She faithfully applied garlic salve liberally on the chest, the back, and the soles of its feet, 4 times a day, and the pneumonia cleared up quickly!

I was favorably impressed and began to recommend it to other mothers with little ones who had coughs, colds, and RSV. My recommendation was to rub it liberally on the back over the lung area, on the chest, and up to and around the throat and ears, and on the soles of the feet. I tell the mothers with tiny babies to do it every time they nurse the baby. Older ones should have the treatment at least 4 times a day, oftener if they are sicker. Whenever a mother calls and says it is not helping, I always ask, "How often are you doing the treatment?" Her reply is usually, "Once or twice a day." That might work for small infections, but if you have RSV or pneumonia or croup, it will not work fast enough to keep your baby out of danger. *See Respiratory Illness to determine danger signs.

Recently I worked with a 3 week old baby who sounded and looked bad. The hospital was full of RSV and the doctor had hoped that this baby would be alright if the mother worked with it, but the baby was sounding worse and worse. I was dressing the 3rd degree burns that his two-year old brother had, so I got to see that baby every day. The mother knew about garlic salve and was using it, she said. "Use it more," was my advice. "Use it every time you nurse." This worked, and though the baby smelled like garlic, the RSV slowly but surely cleared up. The mother was very diligent and determined to get her baby well because she did not want to be in the hospital with it.

Remember this – begin with the salve as soon as your baby begins to cough or sniffle and you will clear the problem up very quickly. Most of my experience has been with the salve working after a week or more of the problem because that is when mothers call me. "My baby has had a cough for a week and it will not clear up." Salve to the rescue. It helps noticeably in a day and in a few days the problem is usually gone. Though it may smell, germs do not become resistant to garlic salve. So, no matter whether virus or bacteria, garlic works! Did you know that viruses do not respond to antibiotics? NOTE: This will not clear up whooping cough. *See chapter on coughs. This salve will also work on an infected cut. Rub it anywhere there is bacteria and the bacteria will have to go. There are scientific studies out there which show this fact.

Garlic Oil

This is a mild oil that you can make for your family.

Chop 2 bulbs of garlic coarsely

Fill baby food or other small jar 2/3 full of chopped garlic

Now fill the jar full with olive oil

Let the jar set for at least 2 weeks and shake it daily

Finally strain out the garlic through a cotton cloth and bottle your oil.

Use this warm oil in the ear for any earache or ear infection. Warm a teaspoon of the oil slightly. Test it on your inner arm by dropping a drop there. The ear is very sensitive. Drop a few drops into the painful ear with a spoon or dropper. Keep the head tilted up for five minutes, then place a cotton ball in the ear. This can be done up to four times a day. It may be helpful for a yeast rash in the diaper area, too.

Garlic for Earaches

Children are usually the most at risk for earaches, but people of all ages can be affected. Earaches can result from swimming, getting water in the ear during a shower, pollen in the air getting trapped in the Eustachian tubes of the ear, or even excessive wax buildup or more often because the child has had overmuch dairy in his diet.

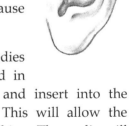

Since garlic is a natural antibiotic, there are some garlic-based remedies that can be administered at home. Fresh garlic cloves can be used in several ways. Dip a peeled, *unnicked* clove of garlic in olive oil and insert into the opening of the ear canal. Cover the ear with a warm rice sock. This will allow the bacteria-fighting garlic to penetrate the ear, and the heat will be soothing. The garlic will fight the infection and should reduce the pain.

Eating a whole clove of garlic several times a day will aid earaches as well. Ingesting raw garlic is easier for adults than children. Do not forget that you can chop garlic and cover it with honey. Put it on a spoon and take it quickly. This makes it more palatable. Garlic salve rubbed around the ear a few times a day will also help.

Garlic for Abscesses

Garlic cloves did the job when our twelve- year old daughter came down with a bad tooth abscess on a weekend of church meetings. We were working in the dining room serving one thousand people. She kept complaining of an ache in her mouth and, sad to say, I wrote it off as her cutting a molar. But on Friday night, she came to me looking very pale and said, "Mom, I feel really bad and my whole face hurts." I groaned.

The girl was visibly ill. Now it was Saturday night. Our dentist was not in, and we would need to pay a lot to fix the problem on the weekend. We packed up and went home. All the while I was thinking about what I could do. This child hates my bad tasting potions, so I fixed her up with a drink of strong clove tea (* see clove chapter), and gave her garlic capsules and vitamin C, and she relaxed and fell asleep. In the night I needed to repeat the process because her pain got too bad. In the morning our guests suggested that we use fresh raw garlic instead of the pills. I, too, knew this would be better, but the taste had been the deterrent. What could I do?

We came up with an idea that I have often used since then. I toasted a slice of bread, spread it lightly with cream cheese, and topped it with two cloves of chopped, fresh garlic. We folded it over and she ate it. She kept drinking her clove tea and taking 1000 mg. of vitamin C. We gave her another slice of toast and more vitamin C in an hour. The pain really improved. She had more toast and vitamin C every two hours for about 3 more bread slices, and the pain was gone, and the abscess was nearly gone. We went back to church in the evening and did our job and repeated the toast when she came home. The next day the abscess was gone, and though I had expected to need the dentist on Monday, we never needed to go. This was especially helpful since we do NOT do root canals and hate to extract teeth if not absolutely necessary.

NOTE. "Often" is the key, if you want to do something like this. **Never make your child take something that you have not tasted yourself.**

If you cannot make yourself take raw garlic, try **Nutrimedical.com**. It is a great place to order processed garlic called Allimax, that is stronger and more cost effective than most processed garlic. This company has a great reputation for helpful products. Order online if you can- if not call them at 888-212-8871 9:00 A.M. to 4:00 P.M. Pacific Time, Monday to Friday,

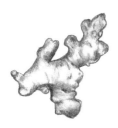
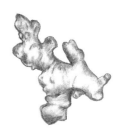

Ginger

"A Circulatory Herb"

Ginger increases circulation and is a carrier herb. This means that if taken with other herbs, ginger will increase their effectiveness. Similar to cayenne pepper, ginger reduces the pain of arthritis. It also reduces the pain and swelling caused by rheumatoid arthritis and osteoarthritis. The healing powers of ginger help prevent the nausea and vomiting associated with motion sickness and pregnancy, enhance digestion and circulation, and ease intestinal gas.

There have been clinical studies to prove that ginger has the healing powers to prevent and treat various illnesses. This research showed that ginger relieved pain and or swelling in seventy five percent of arthritis patients. Natural healers already knew this for many years. People who took it for their health attested to its benefits.

Uses:

- cold feet

- nausea

- flu

- circulation

- aches & pains

- indigestion

- morning

 sickness

- migraine

 headaches

- intestinal gas

One side effect of taking ginger is blood thinning, so use caution if you are on blood thinning medicine.

Ginger Bath for Colds & Flu

A hot ginger bath really speeds up the circulation. This, in turn brings sweating and moves the toxins out of the body. Actually, it produces a bit of a fever. Contrary to what most folks think, this fever is good for you. It increases the action of the macrophages (the critters that eat up the bacteria and virus in your blood). To take a ginger bath there are a few things that you should know.

Fill the tub with very warm water. Add 2 - 4 tablespoons of ginger powder to a full tub of water. Before you get in the tub, drink two cups of hot peppermint or ginger tea .

Have a cup of cold water close by in case you get too hot and feel faint. If you do, drink some cold water, and dip your wash rag in the cold water and put it on your head or back of your neck for a bit. Soak in the hot tub for at least 10 – 20 minutes.

When you feel your heart begin to race and you get flushed, get out of the tub, dry off quickly, and get into a really warm bed. Drink another cup of hot tea, curl up, sweat it out and go to sleep. When you wake up you will usually feel much better.

Our second oldest daughter battled Lyme disease, and often ran a low grade fever and felt ill. She learned that if she would do a ginger bath when this happened, she would wake up the next morning feeling very much better. Because of this I always keep at least a quarter pound of ginger on hand. It is ready when we need it.

This bath, with only 2 tablespoons of ginger powder, will also help for aches and pains that one gets from sore muscles. It will increase the circulation and relax the body all over. Relax in a steaming tub of ginger water and let your aches and pains float away. You will get out relaxed and refreshed, and you will sleep very well. **Caution – If you have heart disease or high blood pressure it is not wise to do this. Also <u>be careful bathing children</u>..** use **half** the ginger, be sure they are **well hydrated**, and their baths must be of **shorter duration. It can be done for a baby but I seldom do it unless it is an emergency since a baby cannot tell you how it feels.**

Ginger for Nausea, Indigestion & Morning Sickness

A cup of hot ginger tea often is "just what the doctor ordered."

Make a cup of boiling water.

Stir in ½ teaspoon of ginger powder.

Sweeten (add milk if desired) and sip first thing in the morning or when ever you need it.

You can repeat as often as needed in a day. For some mothers, this is the thing that helps them over the nausea of morning sickness.

One young lady called me rather desperate for an idea of how to stop throwing up. Sipping ginger tea did the trick for her. I wish that I could say that it works for everyone, but unfortunately this is not the case.

Another young lady needed to take ½ teaspoon in water, every hour for 3 or 4 hours before her nausea went away. She found that some days she only needed 1 or 2 doses and other days she had to be more persistent. As the days went on, she found that she needed less and less. If the ginger does not do it, try taking 1 drop of peppermint oil in a ½ glass of water. Perhaps that will make a difference.

Morning Sickness Testimony

Rosalyn was dealing with serious morning sickness. At your suggestion she took chromium, ginger tea, and dandelion tincture. At first the ginger tea was almost overwhelming but when it had a few minutes it quieted down her stomach and she was able to work on her second cup of tea. After that she got up, showered and ate!! Today she is pretty excited to feel so much better.

I am happier than you can know to tell you I am already feeling MUCH better! Today I feel like I am living again, instead of barely surviving. Thank you for your wisdom. I am doing all you told me to do, and it works! I do mix the ginger tea with chai, simply because I couldn't handle the taste. (no milk or sweetener)

Migraine Headache

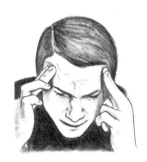

If you have one of those awful headaches that nothing will shake, try a ginger foot bath for it. This not only feels good, but it often helps the headache.

Make a very hot foot bath.

Add 2 tablespoons of ginger to the water.

Soak your feet and sip a cup of ginger tea.

This will increase the circulation to the brain so that, hopefully, the headache should soon be gone.

Ginger for Constipation

Ginger is stimulating to the bowel. So drink a cup of ginger tea if you are having trouble with constipation. That might be all it takes to get you moving!

Delayed Period

Ginger tea is also great for helping to bring on that late period when you are just plain down uncomfortable, and a day or two late. Sip a cup of good, warm tea and get ready! Or take a hot ginger bath or have a cup of hot ginger tea and see what happens!

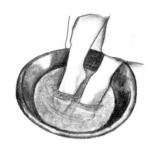

Arthritis Remedy - Ginger/Mint Tea

I have found that making tea out of ginger root and mint is more helpful than any capsules. Take about a 1 ½ inch piece of fresh ginger root, slice the root into a mug, add some fresh mint leaves, pour boiling water over this, and steep at least ½ hour. Drink a cup before you retire for the night. This not only can help with joint pain but it may help you sleep more soundly. The mint is not necessary but it adds a different flavor. You can use the ginger root alone if you wish. Ginger helps to clean out the toxins in the liver and to aid in flushing them out of the body.

Lavender

The "Essential" Oil

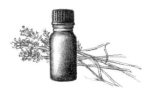

This is an oil I would not like to be without. The health benefits of lavender essential oil include its ability to remove nervous tension, relieve pain, disinfect scalp and skin, enhance blood circulation, and treat respiratory problems. Lavender comes from the Latin word "lavare," which means "to wash", due to its aroma. Lavender oil is extracted mostly from the flowers of the plant, primarily through steam distillation. Lavender oil has a soothing and calming effect on the nerves, relieving tension, depression, panic, hysteria, and nervous exhaustion in general, and is effective for headaches, migraines and insomnia.

It is also very beneficial for problems such as bronchitis, asthma, colds, laryngitis, halitosis (chronic bad breath), throat infections, and whooping cough, and helps the digestive system deal with colic, nausea, vomiting and flatulence.

Lavender oil relieves pain when used for rheumatism, arthritis, lumbago, and muscular aches and pains, especially those associated with sports.

Uses:

- burns

- bites & stings

- heart

  palpitations

- sleep aid

- calming

- respiratory

  problems

- revitalizes the

  skin

On the skin, lavender oil tones and revitalizes and it is useful for all types of skin problems such as abscesses, acne, oily skin, boils, burns, sunburn, wounds, psoriasis, lice, insect bites, stings, and also acts as an insect repellent.

Lavender is one of the few essential oils that can be applied to the skin without diluting it. They call this applying it "neat" and this is especially useful when treating a minor burn wound. It is a first aid kit in a bottle.

Insect Bites and Stings

Keep a small bottle of lavender oil in your purse or car for stings. When someone is stung, rub the area very well with a drop or two of lavender and the pain will disappear almost instantly!

This is a special blessing to your little ones who get stung running through the clover in your yard. If you apply it immediately and rub it in well, the area does not usually swell as much. This is because lavender neutralizes the poisons from the bite. I love this remedy. Works for mosquito bites, too!

We were at a campground for a weekend of church meetings and I was sitting outside the church because it was so warm inside. Suddenly a little fellow running down the drive way began to scream. I jumped up to go see if I could help him but his mother reached him first.

"He was stung," she said to me. Reaching into my purse I pulled out the bottle of lavender oil and offered it to her. She rubbed the swelling area with a few drops and the little one immediately stopped crying. It did not even take another application.

Half an hour later, during lunch break, the situation repeated itself with a different 6 year old. I offered the same help and the results were the same, instant relief.

Lavender for Burns

Treat minor burns and inflamed areas of the skin with a direct application of lavender oil. In addition to the soothing effect of the oil, the lavender acts as an antiseptic and antibacterial agent to guard against infection.

I often get burns in the kitchen from steam or touching a hot pan. Lavender works so well for this kind of burn that when I burn myself, I normally run it under cool water a couple of minutes and then grab the bottle of lavender essential oil and apply it neat even before I think of the aloe plant. It really does work! I've tried this more often then

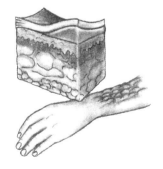

I'd like to admit. I like lavender on burns for it's antibiotic qualities, too. This helps to keep the burn from getting infected.

French chemist and perfumer Rene Maurice Gattefosse was not a believer of the natural health movement, but he was interested in the properties that essential oils exhibited. In 1910 he burnt his hand badly in his laboratory and being the first available compound handy, treated his badly burnt hand with pure, undiluted lavender oil, which not only immediately eased the pain, but also helped heal the hand without any sign of infection or scar. Lavender has long been known to work as an antiseptic and was utilized during World War I in hospitals as a disinfectant for surgical areas and wound dressings.

Lavender Oil for Headaches

Soothe headaches by rubbing lavender oil into your temples. Many find the oil to be effective in relieving sinus headaches as well as migraines. Try to apply the oil as soon as possible, as it works best when applied in the early stages before a headache has taken complete hold. Lie down in cool, dark room with good ventilation and massage the oil in circular motions on your temples. Take deep breaths and relax while the lavender begins to work.

Respiratory Illness

Use lavender oil mixed with water in a vaporizer to help heal respiratory illnesses and alleviate breathing difficulties. Add the lavender oil to your hot steam vaporizer (in the medication cup). Breathe in the vapors to treat coughs and congestion, as well as sore throat and sinus infections. Or moisten a handkerchief with a few drops of oil and lay it on your pillow when you go to bed to sleep.

Relieve Stress

Calm stressed nerves with oil of lavender. Lavender has relaxing properties useful in alleviating depression, moods swings, and restlessness, and helps one get a good night's sleep. Try placing a cloth soaked a with a FEW drops of lavender oil by your pillow at night. Or rub some on your head before you go to bed. Use a few drops since too much lavender is actually stimulating.

Aches and Pains

Rub lavender on your aching muscles and joints. This reduces muscular tension and relieves pain. You can use it to treat muscular aches, rheumatism, lumbago, and sprains. One of the family members who was suffering through the aches and pains that Lyme disease brings had an extremely tight muscle across the chest that was making it difficult for them to breathe comfortably, or even feel like eating. I suggested that rubbing that area with this oil might make a difference for them, but they resisted the idea because they do not like lavender's distinctive smell. After some time had passed and they were still extremely uncomfortable, I prevailed upon them to let me try my oil. It worked, the muscles relaxed, and the sufferer was relieved!

Tired Feet or Body

Put lavender in a foot soak with peppermint to relax those tired, aching feet. Fill a dishpan with hot water. Add two drops of peppermint and two drops of lavender and sit back and relax as you soak your feet. Or fill a tub and add three to ten drops of each for a pleasant, relaxing bath before you retire for the night. You will feel so refreshed and relaxed, and you will sleep well.

When I was going through a difficult time in my life and not sleeping well I decided to try this and see what it would do. I came away very relaxed and my feet felt cool and restful. This effect lasted well into the next day.

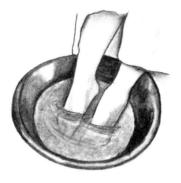

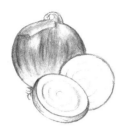
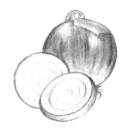

Onions

"Medicine in Your Kitchen"

The Value of Onions

Onions have a variety of medicinal effects. Early American settlers used onions to treat colds, coughs, and asthma, and to repel insects.

Uses:

- Antibiotic

- Relaxant

- Coughs

- High blood

pressure

- Coughs & colds

- Pneumonia

- High blood

 sugar

- Bacterial

infections

- Stops bruising

- Immune system

The World Health Organization (WHO) supports the use of onions for the treatment of poor appetite and to prevent atherosclerosis (the hardening of the arteries which contributes to heart disease). In addition, onion extracts are recognized by WHO for providing relief in the treatment of coughs and colds, asthma, and bronchitis.

*Onions are known to decrease bronchial spasms. An onion extract was found to decrease allergy-induced bronchial constriction in asthma patients.

Onions stimulate the growth of healthy bifido-bacteria and suppress the growth of potentially harmful bacteria in the colon. In addition, they can reduce the risk of tumors developing in the colon. Some of their beneficial properties are only seen after long-term usage.

Onion may be a useful herb for the prevention of cardiovascular disease, especially since they diminish the risk of blood clots. The more pungent varieties of onion appear to possess the greatest concentration of health-promoting phytochemicals. Since onions contain sulpher compounds they are super antiseptics. They also have an anti-inflammatory action, breaking up and drawing out fluid when correctly applied. *Excerpt from article "Natural Homemade Flu-Protection Preparation" - by Dr. Bruce Berkowsky, N.M.D., M.H., NCTMB

Onion for Bruising

The onion is an everyday item that will come in handy if you have little ones!

In the book, "Ten Essential Herbs" by Lalitha Thomas, I read that you can use onion slices for bruising. I really did not see how that would do anything for a bruise. But my chance to try it came when we had a toddler who lost his balance very easily. With a stair landing that is two steps up in our living room room, he often climbed up and fell face forward, getting a large bruise in the middle of his forehead.

One day when he had an especially hard fall, I remembered the onion. We quickly peeled one and sliced a thick slice. We pounded it a bit to make it slightly soft. Then we taped it over the bruise that had swelled and was rapidly turning purple. He was not too happy about the onion smell just over his nose, so 20 minutes later we took the onion off. To our surprise, there was a purple ring around a perfectly clear area where the onion had been. The onion had drawn the fluid out of the bruise and stopped the bleeding under the skin. The "goose egg" had disappeared! What an interesting experiment!

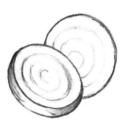

A bit later my husband was taking a bolt off an engine, and the wrench broke and hit him smack on the knuckles! He came in clutching his hand and asking for help. Unfortunately he had to leave in a few minutes for a meeting. I rubbed his hand with Deep Tissue Oil. Then I smashed up a piece of onion and laid it on the "egg" the wrench had made and bandaged it. These kind of "eggs" usually throb and ache, but this one did not, and when he came home we unwrapped his hand to find it tender, but the swelling and the bruising were all gone! Our estimation of the lowly onion went up quite a bit that day.

Stings and Bites

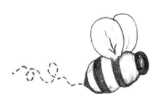

My books say that bruising onion slices and putting them on the sting or bite will take the sting and the swelling out of the area. I have not tried this personally since I usually go for lavender oil first. But if I were going to try onion for a sting, I would bruise it and apply it immediately. It probably works because it draws the poison out just like it did the fluid under the "egg."

Cardiovascular Help

Onions contain a number of sulfides, similar to those found in garlic, which lower blood lipids and blood pressure. In India, communities that never consumed onions or garlic had blood cholesterol and triglyceride levels substantially higher, and blood clotting times shorter, than the communities that ate liberal amounts of garlic and onions. Onions are a rich source of flavonoids, substances which are known to provide protection against cardiovascular disease. Onions are also natural anti-clotting agents since they possess substances with fibrinolytic activity and can suppress platelet-clumping. The anti-clotting effect of onions closely correlates with their sulfur content.

Onion/Salt Poultice for Inflammation

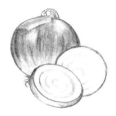

Onion breaks up congestion, fluid or inflammation under the skin that causes bruising or swelling. It helps to move the toxins out through the blood, lymph and the skin. If you use a poultice for water-on-the-knee, lung congestion, jammed limbs or other bruises and swellings you will often have dramatic, overnight results.

Grind or finely chop onions and mix it with salt using a 2:1 ratio, that is like 1 cup of onions to ½ cup of salt. Pile this mushy mixture around the joint, on the lungs or anywhere you need to use it. Wrap the area with a cloth and then an ace bandage to keep it in place. To keep in the moisture, finally wrap it all with a layer of plastic wrap and seal the edges with tape if you can. Allow the treatment to remain on the area at <u>least two hours or overnight.</u> In the morning throw the whole works into the trash and rub the area with lemon juice if the onion smell bothers you.

If you are treating lung or chest congestion you may have better results if you heat the poultice a bit before you apply it. DO NOT MAKE IT TOO HOT! Keep it warm with a heating pad or a warm rice sock.

Onion for Coughs

An onion poultice helps to quiet nasty coughs that keep you or your children from sleeping. It seems to break up the congestion and once again, clear out the fluid from the lungs.

Chop an onion finely. Mix it with salt in a 2/1 ratio. Put it on a saucer and heat in the microwave or place it in a frying pan, until the onion is somewhat soft. Put the mix on an old cloth and cool until you can rest your forearm on it. Oil the child's chest with olive oil, then flip the cloth onto his chest and bind it there. It can stay on all night if you wish.

This usually really helps an annoying nighttime cough. I always used this remedy until I found garlic salve, which is easier to work with. Be sure that you do NOT make the onion too hot or you will burn your child's chest like I once did. I had put on a poultice and the boy began to make an awful fuss. He was one that had a tendency to be fussy, so I told him that it would be fine. He would be OK even if it felt strange. But he kept on saying, "Mama, it burns." I checked him then and I was really sorry. He had a very red area from too much heat. So always test the temperature by applying your forearm to the warm poultice before you put it on the child.

Onion Syrup

A cough is the body's response to inflammation or irritation in the throat, larynx, bronchial tubes or lungs. For a congested cough try this recipe.

Materials - Onion - sugar (or honey) - glass jar (add a lemon for extra help if desired)

Preparation

1. *Cut a medium onion in half and then slice in 1/4" pieces.*

2. *Break into parts and layer one part onion and one part sugar in the glass jar.*

3. *Mash the onion up with the end of a spoon to begin juice extraction.*

4. *Let the preparation sit over-night or for 3 to 4 hours until a syrup is formed.*

5. *Strain out the pieces.*

Dosage: Give your child one teaspoon of syrup (half onion juice and half sugar) every few hours or as needed for relief of frequent coughing. This really works to loosen a cough and quiet it for rest at night. Adult dose: double or triple the amount. The sugar draws out the inter-cellular fluid, including a sulfur compound, that is both antibacterial and antiviral. The syrup tastes pretty good. You also can make a garlic syrup in the same fashion, which has similar properties to the onion and may even be more therapeutic.

Use the same recipe with fresh ginger root to produce syrup that likely will become a household staple for calming upset stomachs.

Stuffy Nose

If decongestants and anti-histamines are not something you prefer to use, then try Breathe Free Onion Syrup for your stopped-up, stuffy nose:

Chop one onion and place in a small bowl. Drizzle 2 tablespoons of honey over the chopped onion. Go to bed and place the bowl as close to your head as possible (on night stand or next to your pillow). You will breath freely all night. But wake up in time to shower because you will surely smell like onions!

Onion for Earaches

When a child begins to cry with earache, I immediately go for an onion.

Cut an onion in half and take out the center of each side. Then I heat it a bit until very warm but not soft and insert a piece in each ear. Finally I place moist heat, like a salt sock over the ears and have the child lie on the couch and rest. Almost always this procedure will stop the pain of the earache. To see more ideas for earache go to the chapter on respiratory illnesses.

Or you might want to try an onion compress for your earache.

Cut an onion in half, heat it slightly. Put the warm onion halves on the neck on either side just below the ears where the glands are. The soothing warmth of the onion and its drawing ability will often take the ear ache away quickly.

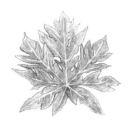

Papaya

"The Disease Chaser"

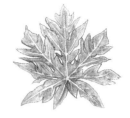

You can eat the tasty fruit, make tea out of the leaf, and take papaya enzymes. It is anti-bacterial, anti-viral, and anti-fungal. Perhaps it is the one of the medicines of tomorrow when antibiotics do not work. Some people are using it to cleanse the blood and aid in their battle to overcome cancer. There is an amazing amount of information about its effectiveness in that area. Papaya leaf contains a bitter that cleans out the blood.

Papaya fruit comes from the tropical tree, Carica papaya. It has been used orally and topically for many years to treat a variety of health ailments such as fungal infections, skin sores, cholesterol, and toothaches. Papaya is most widely recognized for the benefits it provides the gastrointestinal (GI) tract. Papain (the active compound in papaya) is also called vegetable pepsin on occasion, because papain is very similar to pepsin which is created by the stomach to digest food. Papaya encourages digestion, eases indigestion and constipation, can remove parasites from the intestines, and remedy heartburn.

Uses:

- Anti-fungal

- Blood Purifier

- Digestive Aid

- Antimalarial

- Anti-parasite

- Antibacterial

- Parasites

- Candida

Papaya for Indigestion

Troubled with heartburn and indigestion? Try using papaya fruit! Papaya contains papain, a remarkable, protein-dissolving enzyme that eases many stomach ailments and is an exceptional aid to digestion. A rich source of minerals and vitamins A, C, and E, papain also breaks down wheat gluten, which is a great help to those with Celiac disease. If you cannot get the fruit readily, take papaya enzymes found in most health food stores and at Walmart.

While there are many food remedies for heartburn, one fruit in particular that has been seen to be effective is papaya.

Heartburn Relief

Here are some ways you can use papaya to achieve heartburn relief: Eat ripe, raw fresh papaya fruit with your meal.

Drink papaya juice. You can get it at the health food store, or better yet, make it fresh daily to get the full value of the enzymes that heal your stomach and digest your food. Eat ripe, raw, fresh papaya fruit with honey to treat an attack of heartburn. You can also eat this sweet snack before meals and between meals as heartburn prevention.

Take papaya tablets or papaya seed extract to remedy heartburn symptoms. You can also take these products before you eat your meals to prevent heartburn from occurring.

Digestive Aid

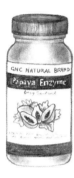

Our last child was born with autism from a mercury accident that we had at the dentist in early pregnancy, before I knew I was pregnant. He had lots of food issues, gluten intolerance, and digestive problems. We had a very difficult time helping him to gain weight as a toddler until we began papaya enzyme tablets. They were chewable, tasted nice, and were very inexpensive, but they did wonders for him. In just a few days his problems with diarrhea were over and his appetite became normal. He did fine as long as we gave him the enzymes, but when we ran out or stopped them, he began to have loose stools. He needed those pills until he was five or so and since then we have not had any problems with his digestion.

Interesting enough I have been working with a toddler who is seriously constipated and the remedy that has worked the best for her is papaya enzymes. Her mother noted that the ones from Wal-Mart do not work as well as the other brands she has tried. If the child is given two enzyme tablets with each meal she eliminates fairly well. There are definitely signs of gluten intolerance but that is a difficult issue and papaya seems to make a significant difference.

Papaya for Acid Reflux

Here is an account from a sufferer of acid reflux. "Recently I had developed a pretty bad case of acid reflux, to the point where I had to stop taking my supplements and ease up heavily on my exercise because I constantly felt like I was going to regurgitate my food.

Unfortunately acid reflux is a bodily malfunction, and I didn't think there was a whole lot that could be done without having to take medicines like Nexum. However, my manager suggested I first try aloe vera gel and a slice of fresh papaya with my meals, and let me tell you, I almost feel normal again already, and I just started doing this yesterday. My esophagus felt like there was a lot of damage from the acidity and excess belching that goes on with acid reflux, but the aloe vera gel provides a coating both of the throat and stomach, and the papaya seems to help my digestion."

You can mix the aloe vera with other beverages should you choose. And the enzymes in papaya are very powerful, so they do wonders to ease the digestion of foods. Therefore you don't necessarily need to take digestive enzymes as a supplement, you can eat the fruit. *See chapter on digestion for other ideas for acid reflux.

Papaya Leaf for Malaria

One missionary that I know volunteered to try papaya leaf tea for a malaria prophylactic (preventative measure), instead of Larium with its awful side effects. She took it as a prophylactic for 10 months and it worked very well for her. We have experimented with a number of folks now and it seems to work every time. The catch is that you must drink two cups of the tea every week at least 2 weeks before you are exposed, and keep on drinking the tea at least two weeks after danger of infection. They recommend that you drink a cup on Tuesday, and again on Thursday, weekly. I rather think that this is because the protective qualities build up in the blood stream thereby keeping you safe. My friend had no malaria while she was taking the tea, but she went on a small trip and forgot to take her tea along. She came down with malaria and took the tea. The malaria went away and she never had malaria again in the whole ten months, though others around her got it.

Papaya Leaf Tea

Bring 1 quart of water to a boil. Turn off heat. Add 2 heaping Tbls. papaya leaf and 2 heaping Tbls. peppermint leaf – (fresh in season). Steep for 20 minutes. Sweeten, ice, and drink.

Drink 1- 2 quarts daily for awhile if you are trying to purify the blood stream or help with Lyme.

Papaya Leaf for Dengue Fever

Here is are two interesting accounts from the web that agree with my thoughts on using papaya tea for malaria or parasitic infections.

"A friend of mine had dengue last year. It was a very serious situation for her as her platelet count had dropped to 28,000 after three days in hospital and water had started to fill up her lung. She had difficulty in breathing. She was only thirty-two years old. The Doctor told us that there is no cure for dengue. We just had to wait for her body's immune system to build up resistance against dengue and fight its own battle. She already had two blood transfusions and all of us were praying very hard as her platelets 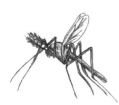 continued to drop since the first day she was admitted. Fortunately her mother-in-law heard that papaya leaf juice would help to reduce the fever and she got some papaya leaves, pounded them and squeezed the juice out for her. The next day, her platelet count started to increase and her fever subsided. We continued to feed her with papaya juice and she recovered after three days!"

"Two friends were admitted to the hospital last year and we helped out by making them fresh juice from papaya leaves. After taking the papaya leaf juice, their blood platelets count increased rapidly and they were out of the hospital within days. One of them reported their platelet count at a dangerous level of only 8 (normal count is 150 and above). One week after she was discharged, her platelets count shot up to 300."

This was interesting information to me since I was researching how to bring platelet counts up. I could not verify it but neither did I think that it would do any harm. I had been in contact with a young, pregnant mother who was desperate to bring up her platelet counts so that she would not need a transfusion. I knew about beets, some herbs, and red meats but I was not at all sure that they would work fast enough for her. I forwarded her the above account that I found on the web and she drank a quart a day of my papaya mint tea and her platelets came right up. We suspect that she had some blood disease from being in Africa on a mission's team before she was married. It seems that the bitters in the tea purify the blood, thus bringing up the platelet count. Will it always work? I do not know, but it worked for a number of people that I know personally. The tea does not taste bad and it does no harm.

Papaya Leaf for Lyme

We have had some success treating Lyme disease using papaya tea. The doctors may call it a home remedy, but they are not doing so well at eradicating this troublesome disease, either. If gotten quickly, the success of antibiotics is not too bad. But when a person has had Lyme for awhile, the cure is, at best, costly and lengthy.

Using papaya leaf seems to offer some hope to many Lyme sufferers without the side-effects of antibiotics. For some it may work alone, and for some it may need to be in conjunction with other herbs or antibiotics.

We have had a number of opportunities to try this treatment on our own family. Living in the heart of Lyme disease area, a number of us have contracted the disease and we 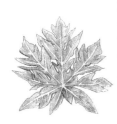 have all manifested the classic "bull's eye," so we did not need to do the testing. We contracted the disease at different times. Two of us began antibiotic treatments immediately. In the one case it worked, but the antibiotics gave her six-years worth of serious yeast problems. The other child did not respond to the antibiotic treatment at all, even after three rounds of it. In desperation we began to hunt for another method that would not assault the body's immune system.

In my research for our missionaries, I discovered that papaya leaf was used for many years as a prophylactic to keep malaria away. It seems that the bitters of the leaf, build up in the blood, and do not allow the bacterium and spirochetes to grow in the blood. The papaya also has components that digest any foreign protein in the body. How? I cannot tell you, but it does seem to work.

So when I came down with Lyme I opted to try the 2 qt. of the tea daily and see if it would help me. I added in high doses of vitamin C, (6 - 12 grams daily) 9 - Olive leaf capsules, lots of my Super Duper Tonic and hot echinacea tincture. Little by little the disease left me. I was doing it by trial and error and it took me about one year to get completely clear of symptoms. I also finished it by doing a few weeks of *Teasel Root tincture. In that time I learned a lot of valuable information. In the years that followed I have discovered that this treatment really helps some people and it does not do as much for others. Some of the keys are optimal nutrition, use of varied antibiotic herbs and liver cleaning herbs. *See *Healing Lyme* by Stephen Buhner and *Top Ten Lyme Disease Treatments* – Bryan Rosner. These books are full of helpful information. *Available at Natures Warehouse- see Suppliers

Papaya for Wounds

"Papaya fruit and juice have been reported to speed up the healing of wounds. Raw papaya also cures swellings and wounds infected by pus.

Healing speeds up when a piece of papaya is laid on wounds and surgical incisions. Papain is used in wound healing since it has the ability to break down proteins in the wounded area. Surgeons in the olden days spread papaya rinds on the skin after closing for quicker healing."

That was great information because I was dealing with a man who had a thumb with some gangrene and serious tissue damage. The doctor mentioned to him that he might need to amputate part of the thumb if he did not get healing to take place. The gentleman was NOT interested in that solution but he definitely needed help to resolve his problem.

He had a very thick eschar (scab) over the seriously infected area. The thumb had turned black and had the appearance and the feel of a roasted sausage. He took Complete Tissue caps in large amounts to help with the pain and we did hot and cold herbal soaks. The situation greatly improved but we needed to get that scab off. No amount of soaking served to loosen it. So following the previous suggestion, we put a piece of raw papaya over the wound and wrapped it well.

We repeated the process 2 times daily and it took us a number of days to get the whole thing to soften and come off. When it came off, there was a crater in to the bone. With more herbal soaks and applications of B&W Salve we were able to get the thumb to finally heal.

He needed to do therapy with his thumb to get it to limber up and be totally functional, but he is pleased that he has a thumb and that is becoming flexible again.

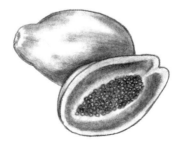

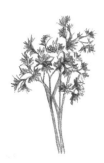
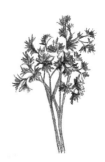

Parsley

"The Kidney and Bladder Herb"

Parsley has many uses as a medicinal herb but it is especially useful for assisting the kidneys and the bladder. It has great antibacterial action on the kidneys and bladder.

Parsley is a vitamin and mineral powerhouse, and as such should be part of every medicinal garden. It is incredibly high in Vitamin A and C. Indoors, it adds greenery and makes an attractive, edible garnish for the kitchen shelf during the winter. Outdoors, it can be planted with other herbs or flowers, and makes a pretty, green accent.

Parsley contains a large amount of chlorophyll, making it a natural breath sweetener. Eat the leaves right off the plant to combat breath odors. Throughout history, parsley been used mainly as a kidney stone, bladder infection, jaundice, and digestive aid.

Uses:

- kidneys

- bladder

- colds

- menstruation

- laxative

- blood pressure

- gall bladder

☒ *Drink parsley tea to help combat flatulence, relieve painful menstruation, and cystitis.*

☒ *Parsley is also a valuable addition to the diet of diabetics.*

☒ *As parsley has a strong iron content, it is ideal to be taken as an additional supplement if you suffer from anemia, rickets, jaundice, and arthritis.*

☒ *Parsley can be given as a supplement to anyone suffering from a lack of appetite since it acts as a stimulant.*

☒ *Some people are also finding parsley tea relieves some of their rheumatic pain.*

☒ *Nursing mothers may find relief of sore breasts by applying crushed parsley leaves.*

☒ *Crushed parsley leaves and seeds can be used to soothe and disinfect insect stings, bruises and wounds.*

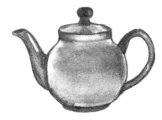

Parsley – A Diuretic

Its primary use is as an effective, mild, and gentle diuretic. Parsley is known to both detoxify and soothe the kidneys. When I see kidney problems in children, a parsley/raspberry tea is the first remedy I reach for, as it is quite easy to administer and very reliable. Parsley is helpful in the prevention and treatment of kidney stones.

Use one heaping teaspoon of parsley and one teaspoon of red raspberry leaf to each cup of tea. Steep ten minutes. Strain and sweeten.

Parsley helped us to keep a newborn out of the doctor's office. A day after the baby was born, the mother called us and reported that the baby had not urinated yet. His little abdomen was distended. The parents did not want to take him to the doctor and appealed to me for something to help him urinate. Kidney weakness is in their family so I suggested that they make parsley tea using dried parsley flakes that were in their cupboard. They were to give him two droppers of the tea and wait fifteen minutes and give him more. The parents called me back jubilantly an hour later to say that his plumbing was working very well indeed, now. Parsley to the rescue!

Parsley for the Common Cold

One of my all-time favorite uses of parsley is in a tea to clear up mucus during the first stage of colds and influenza.

To make the tea, steep one tablespoon of parsley leaves and one tablespoon of raspberry and one tablespoon peppermint leaves in four cups of boiled water for five to ten minutes. Strain and sweeten as desired.

Several cups of this tea have stopped many colds short in their tracks, making this one of the most simple, reliable cold remedies to use for children and adults alike. And the best thing about it is, you have parsley flakes in your cupboard for cooking,

Parsley for Menstruation

Menstrual complaints, including either a lack of flow, or an uncomfortable flow, can be treated with parsley. For uterine complaints, use the same parsley/raspberry/mint tea that I recommended for treating colds and flu. Drink at least three cups daily until the problem is resolved.

Parsley for Other Conditions

Parsley is mildly laxative, hypotensive (lowering blood pressure), and antimicrobial 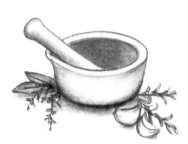 against a large array of organisms. The root can be used for gall bladder problems and is especially helpful in reducing gallstones. Parsley juice has been shown to mildly inhibit the secretion of histamine, making it useful in treating hives and relieving other allergy symptoms. Externally parsley poultices can help soothe tired, irritated eyes, and speed the healing of bruises. The juice or poultice will relieve the itch and sting of insect bites and serves well as a mosquito repellent.

How to Take Parsley

Aside from its uses in salads, as garnish, or as a tea, parsley can also be juiced and mixed with other juices such as carrot.

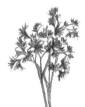

Use 1 oz. parsley juice to three carrots.

I take parsley almost daily to help with my blood pressure. I add it to my carrot, celery and cucumber juice.

This juice is a liver cleansing, blood purifying juice. Drink it daily when you are trying to clean up your system.

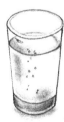

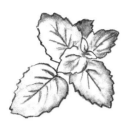

Peppermint

"The Cooling Herb"

Peppermint is easy to use and easy to grow. The herb is used to relieve the pain of rheumatism and neuralgia (nerve pain). The local anesthetic and antiseptic properties of its oil make it valuable in the relief of toothache and sore throat. In the treatment of cavities in the teeth, action of peppermint oil is exceptionally strong. It is a stimulant and disinfectant. Peppermint oil's pleasant cooling properties and muscle relaxing effects are helpful in external use. When used topically, it acts as a counterirritant and analgesic with the ability to reduce pain and tension. The bruised fresh leaves of the plant will, if applied, relieve local pains and headache.

It is inhaled for chest complaints, and nasal catarrh, laryngitis or bronchitis. It is also used internally as a stimulant or carminative. On account of its anesthetic effect on the nerve endings of the stomach, it is of use to prevent sea-sickness. Peppermint helps provide relief from muscular pains, varicose veins, sunburn and insect bites, lethargy and migraine headaches.

It works wonders for sluggish digestion or stopped up sinuses. Its potency comes from its oil. Peppermint is soothing to the nerves and stimulating to the circulation. The oil is stimulating and the tea is soothing.

Uses:

- digestion

- bad breath

- headache

- mastitis

- nausea

- laryngitis

- sinus

- sunburn

- sore muscles

- toothaches

- sore throat

- motion sickness

Peppermint for Digestion

When your stomach is not feeling comfortable after you have eaten, try a cup of peppermint tea, or a drop of peppermint oil in a glass of water. Peppermint calms the stomach, neutralizes the acid, eliminates gas, and helps to relieve heartburn.

Do not be surprised, if after you have taken a strong cup of peppermint tea or water, you begin to burp or pass gas. It increases the movement in your intestines and that will make you feel more comfortable. A **small drop** of peppermint **diluted** with some water can be helpful for a baby's colic or stomach distress.

Do not make the mistake that one grandmother did. She did not know that you must dilute the peppermint oil for a little one to take. She dropped the oil right into its mouth and then she received a terrible scare. The strong menthol of the oil made it very difficult for the little one to breathe. He gasped and gasped and turned blue. Finally he came around but it was a very difficult time for all of them.

Peppermint for Sunburn

Peppermint will greatly reduce the pain of sunburn.

Mix a few drops of peppermint oil into ¼ cup of olive or coconut oil and apply to your sensitive burned skin. Do not put to much peppermint into the oil or it will be too strong and irritate your skin.

We had a family sale after my grandfather died. It was a cold, windy day in early April and the day was overcast, so I never thought about the possibility of burning. We were out in the wind all day and when I came home in the evening I was painfully red on my face and my arms. I remembered that I had read somewhere that peppermint would help reduce the pain of the burn so I tried it. It was amazingly cooling and soothing. I have used this remedy many times since then.

Peppermint for Bad Breath

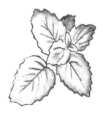

We all are familiar with this one. We take a breath mint or an Altoid to give us a nice, fresh breath. You can also chew on fresh peppermint leaves or put 3-4 drops of peppermint oil into a half glass of water to give you a nice fresh breath. Some people put 1 drop of peppermint right on their tongue, but for other folks this application is too strong.

Peppermint for Headaches

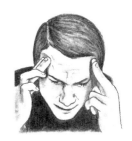

When you have a headache you might find it helpful to rub a drop of the oil mixed with a drop of olive oil directly onto your temples, behind your ears, and at the base of your skull on your neck. This often helps since it increases the circulation. In a tension headache it may help to cup your hand and tap over the skull. Do this by cupping your hand and resting your thumb on your head while you move around tapping gently with your fingers. This often works because it really increases the circulation to the brain, too.

Peppermint for Mastitis

Mastitis (breast infection) is characterized by a hard, tender area on the breast that quickly escalates into redness, pain, hardness, and fever. Whenever you feel an infection coming on, treat it immediately or you can become very sick. The key is to open up the duct that is clogged. Peppermint oil diluted with olive oil and rubbed firmly into the area, massaged toward the nipple vigorously, should help to open up the area. Yes, I know that it hurts, but it **must** be opened and you **must** do it. Cover the area with a very warm, almost hot washcloth. Heat helps to open up the clogged ducts, too. Drink lots of warm peppermint tea and go to bed and rest. Rest is imperative and so are massage and lots of liquid. I have always been able to resolve all my breast infections and most of my clients with natural remedies. **One of the keys is to catch it early and be aggressive in treating it.** Do not think that it is not serious. Left untreated these infections can make you quite sick. * See page 262 in the pregnancy chapters. They can also land you in the hospital for the doctor to lance an abscessed breast. This is quite painful, embarrassing and very expensive. So use simple measures aggressively and get well.

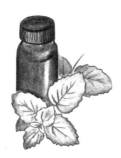

Red Raspberry Leaf

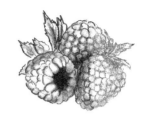

"The Mother's Herb"

The Red Raspberry (rubus idaeus) is native to many parts of Europe and North America. The leaves of this plant have been used as a medicinal herb for centuries. It is beneficial for pregnancy, childbirth and breastfeeding, and of general benefit to the family. I have seen raspberry leaf help tremendously, if taken regularly through pregnancy and labor.

It helps to:

- *Ease the morning sickness pregnant women experience.*
- *Relax the smooth muscles of the uterus when it is contracting.*
- *Assist with the birth of the baby and the placenta.*
- *Calm cramping of the uterus.*
- *Provide a rich source of iron, calcium, manganese, and magnesium. The magnesium content is helpful in strengthening the uterine muscle.*
- *Aid in fertility for both men and women.*
- *Promote a plentiful supply of breast milk.*
- *Stop excess bleeding after birth.*
- *Treat diarrhea.*
- *Regulate irregular menstrual cycle and decrease heavy periods.*
- *Relieve sore throats.*
- *Reduce fever and fight the flu.*

Uses:

- Morning sickness
- Eases labor
- Aids fertility
- Milk supply
- Diarrhea
- Menstrual difficulties
- Immune aid
- Hormonal problems
- Sore throats
- fevers

The tea is a valuable, inexpensive aid for families that has largely been overlooked in the twenty first century. Learn what it can do to simplify your life and help to keep you out of the doctor's office.

Red Raspberry in Pregnancy

Most of the benefits ascribed to regular use of raspberry tea through pregnancy are traced to the nourishing source of vitamins and minerals found in this plant and to the strengthening power of fragrine - an alkaloid which gives tone to the muscles of the pelvic region, including the uterus itself. Of special note are the rich concentration of vitamin C, the presence of vitamin E, and the easily assimilated calcium and iron. Raspberry leaves also contain vitamins A and B complex, and many minerals, including phosphorous and potassium. Raspberry leaf infusion contains calcium in its most assimilable form. Assimilation is further enhanced by the presence of phosphorous and vitamins A and C in the raspberry leaves.

Debbie Pearl from Bulk Herb Store says, "I was talking to a lady on the phone the other day concerning herbs, and she told me the most interesting story. She had ordered a large amount of red raspberry leaf. I thought she must be a midwife that delivered several babies a week. "No," she told me, "I raise goats." "Then," says Debbie, "I was really surprised."

"This lady adds two tablespoons of red raspberry to the feed of her female goats each morning for two weeks before the doe is bred. She says, "This aids in fertility." She also feeds pregnant goats two tablespoons per day for the last six weeks of pregnancy. This seemed a strange and expensive way to feed goats until she told me the amazing results she had achieved. She said they have many goats and have not had to call the vet in over four years. After commencing the red raspberry leaf, it has become normal for her goats to have three and even four kids at one birthing, with no complications. She said her goats yield record breaking volumes of milk that is creamy and delicious. Their little farm is known far and wide for the wonderful success they have had with goats. This lady believes the red raspberry is a very significant factor in their success." -used by permission of Bulk Herb Store

With all that I have read and seen in my midwifery experience, I am inclined to believe that ladies have much the same results when they use this simple herb regularly. Perhaps this information will help some couple to avoid the heartache of a childless marriage or repeated miscarriage.

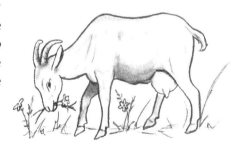

Pregnancy Tea Mix

Ingredients:

3 parts red raspberry leaf   1 part alfalfa leaf   1 part nettle leaf

Optional – 1 part peppermint for flavor (__do NOT add if you have trouble with premature labor. Mint can stimulate contractions.__)

Directions: Make a cup of hot tea by adding one tablespoon of the mixed herbs to one cup of boiling water. Let it steep for ten minutes, strain, and sweeten.

To make a pitcher of tea for storing in the refrigerator, use scant one-fourth cup to one quart, or scant one-half cup for two quarts. Follow the above directions. Or purchase empty tea bags and fill them. You can also purchase tea bags large enough to make two quarts of tea or use a drip coffee pot for ease. Check Mountain Rose Herbs and Bulk Herb Store for supplies.

Red Raspberry Supplies Calcium

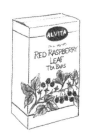

Red raspberry leaf is an absorbable source of many vitamins and minerals- especially calcium and magnesium. This relieves cramping and charley horses that pregnant women so often get. During the weeks after birth raspberry tea helps return the uterus to its normal size. Even post-menopausal women have found benefit from raspberry tea both as an aid in improving uterine tone and as a natural source of calcium. I think that this great source of available calcium is the reason why red raspberry made such a difference in my labors.

A Red Raspberry Story

For my first five babies I did not use red raspberry tea. I had tried the raspberry capsules and they did not do a thing for me. I still had long, poky labors of ten or more hours, with lots of false labor and cramping in the last six or so weeks. I also had lots of leg cramps, indicating low magnesium and calcium levels. I took lots of calcium but it did not really take all my problems away. I also had lots of leg cramps! Then I began helping other mothers at birth and I studied more and more about how to make labor the optimal experience.

A very experienced midwife told me that if I had my pregnant mothers drink a quart of red raspberry tea daily in the last half of the pregnancy, they would have shorter labors. "Usually," she said, "It cuts labor in half." I told her of my experience with the capsules. She looked at me and said, "Red raspberry is most soluble in water. Capsules are not very effective." At that time I was pregnant with baby number seven, so I began to faithfully drink the tea, a quart a day. She was right. My labors were never longer than five hours for my last three babies. My leg cramps completely disappeared. I began to tell others this good news and watch the tea benefit myself and other pregnant women in many ways. Even first-time mamas have good results with shorter, easier labors.

Fertility and Menstrual Difficulties

Red raspberry leaf can be used to increase progesterone levels. It's a phyto-progesterone, which means that it is a plant that acts like progesterone in the body. It acts as a precursor in the process of making the progesterone. If you take it with the herb chaste tree berry (vitex) it's effect is even more profound. However, you should go off the chaste tree berry as soon as you know you are pregnant. To regulate a menstrual cycle drink two to three cups of the red raspberry leaf tea a day. After two or three months the menstrual cycle should be right on schedule.

Red Raspberry for Cramps

Many people feel that PMS (pre-menstrual syndrome) is caused by hormonal imbalance. The rise and then sudden drop in estrogen levels through a woman's cycle can cause a variety of symptoms, including cramps. Red raspberry leaf is one of several herbs that has been used for many years to alleviate or eliminate this problem.

One of our friends makes a quart or more of red raspberry tea daily for herself and her girls. They tell me that drinking this tea helps a lot to eliminate PMS and cramping. When they forget to make it or get too busy, they can tell a real difference in how they feel emotionally. This agrees with all the studies that you can read.

Raspberry not only aids in bone development of the baby but also provides a needed source of calcium for young girls and boys. Do not forget that young boys have changing hormones, too and red raspberry can really help them. You will all benefit from it.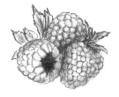

Tea for Acne and Puberty Problems

In "Herbal Home Health Care", Dr. Christopher says, "During puberty it would be wise to have the pre-teen boys and girls take at least one or more cups of red raspberry tea daily. This assists in helping the body make its own natural hormones. It helps in clearing up teen-age acne and in the irritability that often develops in the pre-teen youth.

Diarrhea

Red raspberry has health benefits beyond women's issues. The tannins in the leaf make it effective in soothing inflammation in the digestive tract and it can alleviate diarrhea, especially in children. When you use it for a child, give it by tablespoons or sips every ten minutes and after every loose bowel movement.

Make Red Raspberry Leaf Tea

Pour one cup of boiling water over one bag or one tablespoon of loose leaf. Let the tea steep for about twenty minutes. Strain and sweeten. Flavor it with lemon if you desire. If you use a tea ball or a tea hat, it is even easier. I think think that the tea is easier to drink if it is chilled and lemon is added. It tastes a bit like iced tea. We make a quart at a time to save the fuss.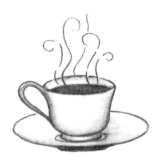

Flu and Digestive Upsets.

We use lots of red raspberry tea to keep the flu away and to help us over the flu when we get it. I first learned about this through Dr. John Christopher. He recommends fasting on red raspberry tea, fresh juices, and vitamin C, when one feels like he is coming down with the flu or cold. He suggests that you should use quarts of this tea and nothing else, and your headache, fever and runny nose will leave. Drink lots of this tea for the next two days. It does a wonderful job of cleansing the body and fighting the flu. Drink the tea as hot as you can.

He also tells the story of a family with a number of school children. One day one of the children came home with the "throwing up" disease. The mother groaned, thinking of all that was to come and called Doctor Christopher. He told her to give the sick child sips of red raspberry leaf tea to drink and nothing else. He then instructed her to make up gallons of the tea and give it to the rest of the family to drink. She followed his instructions and they all drank LOTS of tea for the next few days. The sick child was back in school the next day and no one else came down with the sickness, although the "bug" went through the whole school. When I read this I decided to try making a tea mix with raspberry leaf that would taste good and be helpful in flu. After researching a bit I came up with the following recipe.

Flu Tea

We drink this tea when flu season is here and our friends are coming down with it. We make it by the gallon, chill it, and drink it and it really helps. If someone does come down with the flu we drink it every hour. It has seen us through many a flu season with little or no flu. This tea is both inexpensive and tasty .

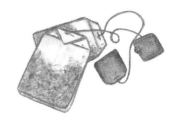

Mix together:

3 parts - Red Raspberry Leaf

2 parts - Peppermint leaf

1 part - Alfalfa leaf

1 part – Nettle leaf

¼ part –Yarrow flower or Boneset

Store in a glass jar to keep it fresh and flavorful. Use one-fourth cup to two quarts of boiling water. Steep twenty minutes and sweeten. You can drink the tea hot or cold. As you can see, the red raspberry leaves offer many healing abilities and everyone could benefit from drinking a cup or two of tea a day.

Sore Throat and Mouth Irritations

Red raspberry may also be used orally to soothe throat or mouth irritations and help with cold sores. You can gargle with red raspberry tea, or you can use herbal throat lozenges. These herbal lozenges are simple, easy to make, and effective in treating sore throats.

Mix together:

3 tablespoons each of powdered licorice, marshmallow or slippery elm and red raspberry leaves

1 teaspoon powdered cayenne pepper

1 teaspoon cornstarch

Mix together.

Add 10 drops rosemary essential oil.

Add enough honey to make the powders stick together. Form this moldable mixture into small lozenges of a comfortable size to suck on. Use these as often as needed when you have a sore throat. They are very soothing. <u>DO NOT use powdered licorice in the mix if you have high blood pressure since licorice tends to raise the pressure.</u>

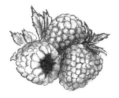

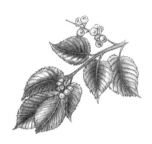

Slippery Elm

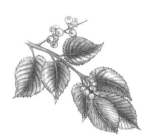

"The Soothing Herb"

Slippery elm is a member of the elm (Ulmus) family. Native to Canada and the US, it can be found growing in the Appalachian Mountains. The inner bark is collected from trees which are at least ten years old, and is mainly powdered for therapeutic use. It is a mucilaginous herb with properties similar to comfrey. It is gentle and soothing, yet it works extremely well. "Mucilaginous" means sticky and with an ability to coat. Slippery elm does this very well, coating the intestines and healing whatever it comes in contact with. It calms inflammation in the areas that it contacts, healing bladder infections, long-standing bowel problems, and sore appendixes.

It is especially helpful where there are inflammations like colitis, gastroenteritis, appendicitis or any other "itis." "Itis" means inflammation of.

Uses:

- constipation

- diarrhea

- abscesses

- wounds

- Irritable

Bowel Syndrome

- Croon's disease

- sore throat

Diarrhea

A teaspoon of slippery elm made into a thin gruel, sweetened a bit and given every time there is a loose stool, has an amazing effect on a baby or child's diarrhea. Use it a spoonful an hour, or after every loose stool, to stop potentially serious dehydration.

For an older child or adult who needs the same remedy just increase the dosage to a tablespoon or more an hour, or after every loose stool.

Slippery elm really absorbs liquid and helps to gel up the "runs". But there is another, almost unexplainable side to slippery elm. Read on.

Constipation

You can also give it to a child who is having problems moving his bowels because he is constipated. Slippery elm works very well for constipation because it lubricates the colon, adds bulk, and helps the child to move his bowels. When I first read this interesting fact, I had already used it to help quite a few mothers who had infants who were very sick with diarrhea and it always helped to clear up the problem. I was familiar with its success in that area, but I was quite skeptical about slippery elm's ability to aid in constipation. Then we had a child who developed a real difficulty with constipation so I decided to try the powder for her to see if it would work. Since she was old enough to swallow capsules, I gave her two or three capsules. They helped a little, but she still had some difficulty. A few more capsules remedied the problem. We discovered that a few capsules a day helped her keep her problem under control. She has nearly outgrown this and rarely ever needs her slippery elm capsules anymore. But when she does, she goes for slippery elm and her problems are over.

Wounds

Slippery elm is the binder that we use to hold our People's Paste together. We use People's Paste to hold together many a cut or wound. It is really great to stop the bleeding, fight infection and glue the wound together. When someone gets a nasty cut we let it bleed a little to flush out the wound and then we apply pressure beside the wound and fill it with People's Paste powder. This 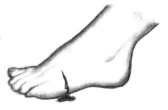 powder absorbs the blood and makes a really nice scab to aid in holding the wound shut.

People's Paste

Mix together equal parts of the following powdered herbs:

Slippery elm   Comfrey root   Myrrh root   ½ part Bayberry root   ¼ part Garlic

Store your ready-made mix in a jar to be prepared for any emergencies. Sprinkle the dry powder into the wound or mix it with a bit of oil or water to make a paste to apply to the wound. I use it most often in its dry form.

131

Slippery Elm and Wounds

The other day our youngest two children and their visitors were exploring in the woods and one of the boys had a machete. He was clearing the brush in the path to make it easier for the girls to follow. One of the girls tripped and fell just as he swung his machete and the blade caught her on the side of her knee and gave her a very deep, four inch gash. They carried her in bleeding and came for me. My first thought was People's Paste. (*page 137) The wound was bleeding liberally, so I applied pressure and poured a nice amount of the powder into it, cleaned the edges and taped it shut. When it was covered with a nice clean bandage, I called the parents and told them about the accident. They came to get their daughter and took her for stitches, and she got stitches down in the wound and then more to close the top layer. A week later when the stitches were taken out the child overused the knee and the wound began to split. Now she needs to heal without the stitches anyway. It would be very possible to use only the powder and have the wound heal nicely without stitches. We have done it for our family on various occasions. The healing begins down inside and works its way up through to the top layer of skin. To do this you would pack the wound and wrap it. Every day you would add more powder to the area, never removing the old paste or powder. The body absorbs it as it heals and the healing progresses from the inside out. You will be surprised at how quickly a wound will heal if treated this way. It heals especially fast if the powder contains a bit of cayenne. But test the cayenne in the area first to see if it will burn. In some places it is not a problem and in other places it will burn like fire. Be sensitive to this fact.

Irritable Bowel Syndrome

Slippery elm is such a specific remedy for helping this condition that it is almost a crime that doctors and hospitals don't make use of it. It will often soothe the pain of patients suffering these ailments within a couple of hours. This is not a case of the slippery elm hiding the pain, but by soothing the inflamed area, the pain, a signal from the body that something is wrong, simply goes away.

The cause of the condition must still be dealt with - maybe it's a congested colon; maybe it's a constitution which is easily stressed; but the slippery elm is a great herbal 'tool' to help deal with the symptoms, while the cause is being sorted out. Appropriate practitioners might be need to help sort out the causes.

One day my phone rang again. This time it was a man with Irritable Bowel Syndrome and quite a bit of pain. The pain was hindering his ability to work, what could he do? Of course there are a lot of things that one can do, like reducing the stress level and markedly increasing your fluid intake. But one of the next things on the list, simple, effective, and inexpensive, is slippery elm. Slippery elm covers the inside of the intestinal tract with a smooth slippery coating that both nourishes and heals the inflamed intestinal walls. He began adding slippery elm to his diet four times a day, and he started the road to recovery. It took him a few months to heal completely since he did not take comfrey tea, too. The last time I spoke with him, he was doing well, and only needed slippery elm occasionally. With the addition of two to three cups of comfrey tea daily, the time could have been cut at least in half.

Sore Throats

Lalitha Thomas, in Ten Essential Herbs, uses slippery elm in many, many of her herbal suggestions. We like to use it in a thin gruel to coat a sore throat. It has a slightly nutty, not unpleasant flavor, and it is very soothing to a raw throat.

Tooth Abscesses

If you have an abscess with a lot of swelling, you cannot get that tooth pulled until you get the abscess under control. This recipe works well to heal abscesses.

Mix together:

1 Tbsp. Slippery elm

4 drops clove oil

¼ teaspoon cayenne pepper

Add a little water, enough to make a paste. It will be gummy due to the slippery elm. Then pack this mixture around the gum. The slippery elm, like charcoal, draws out the inflammation, the cayenne stimulates the cells around the tooth to release toxins and the cloves are added as a pain remedy, especially in toothache. Take a clove of garlic every two hours, too. This should resolve your abscess and may actually save your tooth.

Notes

PART 2

WORKING WITH YOUR
FAMILY'S HEALTH

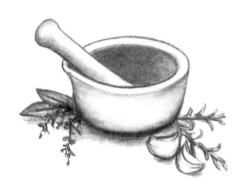

First Aid and Emergencies
In The Home

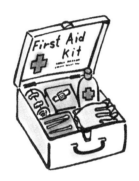

Learn how to deal with the small emergencies that come your way in normal home life and cut out a large portion of doctor and emergency room visits. This is not only cost-effective, but time saving and better for your health and emotional welfare.

Doctor Wootan, an older family doctor, was teaching a seminar of Family Health Care to a number of us who were in the middle of growing families. He was a father of nine or ten children and well versed in the common emergencies that a family faces. His first advice to us was, "Stop and drink a cup of tea." What he really meant is that when you stop and take the time to think rationally, many emergencies are not so hard to deal with as they first appeared. We have had many reasons to use this advice over the years. Of course there are times when you cannot stop and speed is imperative, but these are the exception rather than the norm.

Cuts and Wounds

People's Paste Powder

People's Paste is my back-up for cuts that might need stitches and cuts that need help to stop bleeding. Lalitha Thomas in <u>Ten Essential Herbs</u>, introduced me to it and I tweaked the recipe to suit me. You can always use cayenne, instead, but in places that are sensitive you might wish to use People's Paste. If you do this, in many, many cases you will not need stitches at all. Remember, facial wounds or scalp wounds really bleed for a short time. Stop the bleeding before you panic! If you stop the bleeding you will often see that the cut is small and you can pack it with People's Paste. We've used People's Paste for quite a few scalp wounds to eliminate the need for stitches. We have also glued some facial wounds that healed without scarring, while stitches tend to scar.

136

Recipe for People's Paste Powder

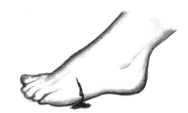

Mix together:

1 part - comfrey root powder

1 part - slippery elm powder

1 part -myrrh powder

½ part bayberry root powder

¼ part garlic powder

Store this mix in a tightly covered jar. Keep a tiny bag of this in your emergency kit, car, or purse.

When you have a wound that needs People's Paste, mix a small amount of powder with a bit of oil and pack it into the wound, or just pack the dry powder into the wound and apply pressure to stop the bleeding. When the bleeding is stopped, wrap it up and check it again the next day. Add more powder if you need to, but do NOT mess with the powder already there. Add more powder daily as needed. This mixture of herbs heals even big cuts very nicely, without stitches. We have tried it on facial wounds, too, with good results. Remember - facial wounds bleed profusely, immediately. They stop rather quickly if pressure is applied. But it usually looks a lot more serious than it is. Stop the bleeding and assess the damage. Never panic. People can lose a lot more blood than you might think, without it being serious.

Bleeding Wounds

Our daughter got a deep, triangular gash on her finger that did not want to stop bleeding. We applied pressure at the base of the finger, sprinkled in some cayenne powder and then liberally applied dry People's Paste between the loose flap and the finger. The bleeding stopped immediately and we bandaged it and sent her on to bed. The accident happened late in the evening. Unfortunately the bandage slid up during the night, pulling the flap of skin up slightly. I really wanted to move it down to its correct position so that it would heal without a scar but we decided to let it alone since so much healing had occurred overnight. There were lots of new skin cells forming and the area looked great. We added more powder to the outside of the wound and re-bandaged it in a way that it would not slide up. The wound healed quickly and left a scar that we treated with Complete Tissue Salve from Dr. Christopher. The finger looks really good now and we were saved a late-night expensive, emergency room visit for stitches.

Face Wounds – No Stitches!

One thing to remember about face wounds is that they bleed a lot and usually stop rather quickly. So, before you panic and run to the ER, take a bit of time to see what kind of wound you have. Stop the bleeding and clean up the area and you might find that you can handle the emergency yourself.

Another thing to remember is that stitches are hard on the skin, too. They make their own trauma that needs to heal. Two instances remind me of how the body heals. Two young men, both friends of ours, work for a shed building operation. On different occasions each of them gashed his forehead in approximately the same area and the same depth. One of them went to the local family doctor who does stitches in his office and had it repaired. The other one went home and had it cleaned and taped shut with steri-strips. Guess which healed without a scar? The one without the stitches looks the nicest by a long stretch. That was my first introduction to how well the skin can heal without stitches, if properly cared for.

Years ago, we were traveling a long distance and the little children were really tired of the car seats. We allowed the older children to take them out and sit on the floor bed that we had made behind the back seat of the van. A car stopped suddenly in front of us and my husband jammed on the brakes. The two year old hit her face against the back of the seat cutting her tiny nose across the bridge. The blood flowed freely and it looked terrible. I caught up a cloth diaper and applied pressure while my husband maneuvered us into a Walmart parking lot. By the time he got the van parked the bleeding had stopped and we could see that we had only a little cut. It was deep but small and we fastened it shut with a band aid as well as you can in the dip of the nose. This was long before I knew about People's Paste. It healed well anyway.

Let me tell you a story about bayberry root powder here. In the days before I met People's Paste, I encountered an emergency which showed me how effective the bayberry in the mixture is.

Bayberry Powder

I delivered my first grandchild only nine days before this incident, and he had had his circumcision the day before. I do not advocate circumcision. The personnel who did the circumcision neglected to tell my son not to immerse the baby in water until the site was healed. So, the helpful daddy put his strong little son into the sink for a bath. Somehow or other, his little hand caught the string on the end of the plastibell and pulled, and the whole works came off.

They called the doctor and wrapped it with gauze and Vaseline like he said. There was no bleeding, so they thought all was well. The little one was nursed and put to bed for his nap. When he woke two and one-half hours later, his daddy found a baby with blood dripping out of his soggy diaper and running down his legs. The area was not gushing, but it was dripping. Needless to say, he called me in a panic. I thought of cayenne, but the area is too sensitive to apply it there. Then I thought of bayberry which I had left on their dresser. "Open a capsule of bayberry and sprinkle it on the area and apply counter – pressure," I instructed. "Do it as often as you need and I will be there in ten minutes." I went in a hurry, not knowing how much blood the baby had lost or how much blood loss a newborn can sustain before going into shock.

When I arrived, a much relieved daddy met me. The first capsule of powder sprinkled onto the area had noticeably slowed the bleeding and the second one had stopped it. The little man looked stable to me but I did not want to take any risks, so we took him to the emergency room to be checked. When they looked him over, they declared him fine. When they saw his loaded diaper they wondered how in the world we had stopped the hemorrhage. They told us that hemorrhage after a circumcision often causes death to the infant. "What did you use to stop it?" they inquired. Bayberry! They shook their heads. "No," they had never heard of bayberry, but they were impressed with how well it worked. Since then, this great, blood-stopping herb is a valuable part of my People's Paste recipe and I usually keep some nearby for quick application if I cut myself in the kitchen and do not want to use cayenne. *See cayenne chapter.

Complete Tissue & Bone Formula

for Breaks and Sprains, Wounds and Damaged Nerves

Bad Sprains

When you have a bad sprain, you must be faithful with soaking and salve to heal the area. We soak the affected area in a strong tea of comfrey or Complete Tissue & Bone herbs (or we poultice it). It is preferable to use both hot and cold soaks. *See page 313. We give Complete Tissue capsules by mouth and rub the area (if possible) with Deep Tissue Oil. We do this every hour until the pain is gone, and then three to five times a day until the healing is complete. The afflicted person must NOT use the affected part! In a few days things begin to heal and you will be surprised how quickly your patient is up and running. Usually in a week your patient is up and going. A minor sprain can be healed a lot more quickly.

Breaks

Three years ago our eleven year-old daughter fell, while skating, and broke her arm just above the wrist. She was in great pain and her hand hung at a strange angle. My husband and our older children were gone. What should I do? I remembered one doctor's advice on how to deal with any skin or bone trauma. He instructs you to put crushed ice in a wet cloth on the area immediately. He promises that swelling and tissue damage will be greatly modified when you do this within five to seven minutes of the trauma. So, the first thing that I did was to go for the crushed ice. I applied that to her wrist and kept it there for about a half hour. While I was icing her she kept moaning in pain. Our thirteen year old reminded me of the pain relieving qualities of clove tea. Good idea!

We brewed up a quart of clove tea and put it in an insulated thermos for her to sip. We

---

Complete Tissue Ingredients

Marshmallow: high in "live" assimilable protein for muscle rebuilding.
Mullein: a special food for the glandular system. Unless the glands of the body are working properly, healing cannot be complete.

Lobelia: It is antispasmodic, a nervine, and an anti-infection herb as well.
Wormwood: relieves the body of pain.
Slippery Elm: a soothing herb.
Plantain: another herb that promotes healing.
Gravel root: for pain.
Aloe Vera: a cell proliferant.
Skullcap: known to help relax the body so that it can heal.
Black Walnut: high in potassium, calcium, iron, required for rebuilding the body.
White Oak Bark: tightens tissue.

gave her a handful (7-10) of Complete Tissue capsules for pain, too. The cloves and capsules made her amazingly comfortable and she was able to talk and laugh in about ten minutes. Then we made up a crude, homemade splint, and wrapped the whole thing with an ace bandage and set off for the clinic for the doctor to set it. In due time the bone was set and the splint applied. Doc said to come back on Wednesday for a cast, after the swelling went down. I was just about to tell him that this was three hours later and there was no swelling but I held my peace. He sent us home and we proceeded to use our own methods to speed up the whole healing process. We made our own half-cast with Sam splint wrapped onto the arm with an ace bandage.

For the first two days she sipped on clove tea for the pain and took Complete Tissue capsules every hour. She took a whole bottle of one hundred capsules that day. I instructed her to take a handful every time it hurt, and she did. This greatly reduced the pain and also took away her appetite (she was full of complete tissue capsules!).

We fed her comfrey–pineapple drink two or three times a day and kept a crushed comfrey root poultice on the area twenty-four seven. (We did not have a closed cast on, since I had made our own cast.) After the third day we began taking the arm carefully out of the splint and soaking it in a strong solution of comfrey root, two or three times a day.

By the fourth day the pain was gone unless we bumped her arm, so we reduced the number of capsules to half a bottle a day for the next three days and kept up the soaking. Movement returned to her fingers, and her wrist grew steadily stronger. Day number eight she began begging to use her arm and I refused, not wanting to damage the new growth of bone. We further reduced the amount of capsules to five, four times a day. Day number ten we put the splint away and put on a simple wrist brace that we got at Walmart. It was adult size so it came below her break and supported the area well. She kept taking her capsules, three times a day and was careful not to lift heavy things or twist her arm.

By the time two weeks rolled around she was able to use it well and we finished the next week, taking five capsule, three times a day. It was exciting to see the bone heal in ten to fourteen days rather than six weeks. It appears to correlate with the other experiences that I have read and heard about. Hence, the believable conclusion: "If properly nourished, the body speeds up the healing process remarkably!"

Another day we received a call from a young couple whose baby had fallen down the steps and broken his leg. They took him to their chiropractor for an x-ray and there was a green twig fracture. This means the bone was not broken off but there was a substantial crack in it. They brought the little fellow to us late Saturday afternoon when the doctor was not in his office to cast it. I fashioned a half-cast out of plaster casting tape and cotton lining. We laid his little leg in the cast and wrapped it well with an ace bandage. Every day she soaked his leg in a comfrey root tea and in two weeks he was crawling again. If I would have known about it then, I would have prescribed Complete Tissue Syrup to aid in the healing. This syrup is nice for little ones who cannot swallow the capsules. See Natures Warehouse on page 325, to order.

Pain in Your Mouth

A friend of ours heard about the benefits of Complete Tissue Formula. He had some teeth extracted and had a lot of pain. He began to take these capsules and his pain level greatly improved. We decided to try the same thing for a nerve in my husband's mouth that was quite painful. The dentist could not find the exact spot of the pain since nothing showed up on the x-ray. Myron began to take these capsules when he had pain and gradually the pain has subsided. Now he is taking them at mealtimes to try and finish healing the nerve so that it does not flare up and cause him problems again. * Note- the problem is nearly gone and he takes the capsules only occasionally if it flares up.

Damaged Nerves

Complete Tissue Formula capsules, herb or salve really help to heal damaged nerves. We have had a number of cases where nerves were damaged, such as an epidural gone wrong or a gash that severed a nerve and left some facial paralysis. In two cases direct application of Complete Tissue Salve healed the nerve after repeated applications to the area. In another case of root inflammation in the tooth, capsules taken repeatedly brought slow but sure relief without a root canal. In every case we have worked with it soothed inflamed nerves and rebuilt damaged ones. If I had any problem where nerves were damaged I would seriously consider using one or more forms of this product. It can be obtained from Natures Warehouse or you can make it yourself. If the area where the nerve is damaged can be soaked, the Complete Tissue Herb as a soak is very helpful. The powdered herb an be stirred into applesauce and given to children who cannot swallow capsules. See recipe for Complete Tissue Herb on the next page.

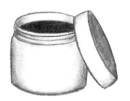

Torn Tissue

We have also seen a case where torn meniscus on both knees healed rapidly eliminating the need for surgery. The lady agreed to get off her feet for two weeks, except for bathroom privileges. We applied hot and cold compresses four times daily for a half hour each, (see p. 313)and she took a lot of Complete Tissue capsules. The hot soak was tea of complete tissue herb. After two weeks of intensive compresses her scan showed that she was healed and the doctor cancelled the surgery. Amazing!

Complete Tissue Herb

6 parts white oak bark
6 parts comfrey root
3 parts Marshmallow root
3 parts Mullein herb
3 parts Black Walnut hull
3 parts Gravel root
2 parts Wormwood
1 part Skullcap herb
1 part Lobelia herb and seed
1 part Slippery Elm bark

Get all the ingredients and mix them together. It will make a **large** amount so you may need to split it with friends. Use it as a soak for breaks, sprains, and wounds. Take ½ cup and simmer it for 20 minutes in 2 quarts of water. Strain and cool enough to soak affected part. If there is no infection in the area you can reuse this soak a number of times. Keep in the fridge. After two days make a new soak. (A "part" can be ¼ cup if you can obtain that small an amount.) This tea can be taken internally but it tastes awful.

Complete Tissue Salve

Fill a pint jar with the above mixed herbs. Fill the jar the second time with olive oil. Get out all the bubbles and cover all the plant material. Set the jar in a crock pot and add water to the neck of the jar. Set on lowest heat setting. DO NOT BOIL. Heat for 1 ½ days stirring at least one time daily. Strain out herbal material and thicken with beeswax.

*To **every** ounce of oil add 1 tablespoon of grated beeswax and a capsule of vitamin E to prevent spoilage. Heat the oil stirring until the wax melts. This happens very quickly. Test by putting one spoonful of oil into the freezer. If it is too soft, add more wax. If it is too hard add more oil. Pour into jars and cool. A cup of oil makes a cup of salve.*

Concussions

A hard blow to the head that knocks your child out can be quite frightening to any parent. But do as one doctor told us. Stop and take a deep breath. Panic never helps in any situation. Observe your child carefully.

- ☒ *Is he awake and alert now?*
- ☒ *Are the pupils of his eyes the same size? If they are different it may mean that there is pressure on the optic nerve. Do they respond to light normally?*
- ☒ *Is the person nauseous?*
- ☒ *Is there still loss of consciousness?*
- ☒ *Is there blurred vision?*
- ☒ *Does he have loss of short-term memory, such as difficulty remembering the events that lead right up to and through the traumatic event?*
- ☒ *Is his speech slurred?*
- ☒ *Does he have difficulty walking?*
- ☒ *Is his skin abnormally pale?*
- ☒ *Does he have seizures?*

Watch for bleeding into eyes, ears, and noses. Obviously if they have seizures you'll take them to the hospital. If you go to the hospital they will take an x-ray to check for a fracture and they will check all the above symptoms. Then they will keep you overnight so that they can monitor the symptoms. That's all they'll do. Finally they will send you home with a list like the above one and say come back if any of these symptoms happen. Of course your child will have a headache and probably a severe one because of the blow to the head.

Lay him down and let him rest a few minutes and reassess him. Give him plenty of water and very gently apply arnica oil to the area where the blow was. This will help with the hemorrhaging under the skin. That is part of what causes the pressure. DO NOT take arnica oil internally. You can reapply the oil every half hour if you wish. Do not use it where the skin is broken. If you are faithful with this you will really help the swelling.

Give Tylenol for the pain, but nothing stronger and absolutely NO ASPIRIN since it causes bleeding. Rest and quietness is imperative because the brain is traumatized. People tend to freak out and do not want the child to sleep. But sleep is what happens when a child has been hurt badly and cried a lot. People worry that you cannot let a person sleep after a concussion. But the medical community is saying the opposite. This is what they say. *"You do not need to keep a person with a recent concussion awake. This was recommended for years, to observe a person for any changes after a concussion. People worried that the person may go into a coma and never wake up. This is no longer believed to be true. You can allow someone to sleep after a concussion. This should cut down on sleep deprivation for all involved. People with concussion should be seen by a doctor if they were unconscious for more than five minutes, or amnesia persists, or if they do not appear to behave normally."*

After a day or two you may find that giving Dr. Schultz' brain formula (p 324) will really make a difference in the headaches, the dizziness, the brain fog and the vision problems. Repeat a couple of times a day if needed. It takes months to fully heal up from a real concussion. If it is a child playing a competitive sport, a concussion probably means the end of the season for them, or it should. A good knock on the head is different from a concussion.. A day or two later it might be sore where you got hit but everything else is fine. With a concussion things will seem strange. Sensory inputs may feel blurred or like they are coming from far far away. Reactions and thought processes are much slower. There may be loss of short-term memory. For a few days the person may seem lethargic. Strong headaches will come periodically. Vision may be not quite right. It may be really blurred for a bit. The worst is over in a few weeks but some mild symptoms will usually persist for a few months. You will usually find that a storm front moving in will produce a rather severe headache. This is probably due to different atmospheric pressure. This occurrence may last for a few months or years, depending on the severity of the concussion.

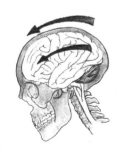

Concussions and Brain Formula

We worked with a friend who had been in a car accident and hit the side post of the car at the windshield. She was taken by ambulance to the hospital and we followed. They took her for an x-ray and said that she had definitely had a concussion but they released her and told the family to watch for any of the above symptoms that I listed.

She had no short term memory and the family was terrified as she kept asking the same questions over and over. She was so dizzy that she could hardly walk and she was experiencing blinding headaches. This continued and they took her back to the hospital two days later but received the same diagnosis. I took some arnica oil to them and they began to use it throughout the day to reduce the swelling (which also reduces the pressure). She took Brain Formula and found real relief in using this. I was amazed to see the way it increased the healing. This was because that particular formula really increases circulation to the brain. Even with these measures, my friend could not shop or attend church for nearly a month. Healing a brain injury takes time.

A few months later our daughter was hit in the temple with a hoe. It knocked her out and she exhibited blurred vision, slurred speech, dizziness, and severe headaches. She spent the greater part of four days on the couch until she felt well enough to be up and around a little. At the end of a week she looked terrible because of extensive green and yellow bruising, but she was feeling much better. We used arnica to dissipate the bruising. Unfortunately, when she went outside to watch a group of children playing, she accidentally received another blow right on the same temple. This one, coming on the heels of the other, slurred her speech and gave her all her other problems again, at which time I remembered the arnica oil and the Brain Formula. We used both of them frequently, with very good success. She felt immediate clearing in her eyesight. Her headaches became less severe and her dizziness was much improved. This is a formula that I do not want to be without.

Black Salve

"Drawing Ointment"

I often recommend black salve when someone has something under their skin that does not want to some out. Here is a story that a mother told me after she followed my recommendation to use black salve on her daughter's foot.

She had an angry festering sore there that looked like a splinter, but they did not know what had made it. This is what she wrote:

"You said that the wood sliver would come out in two to three days. Well, it did. It turned out to be a one-half inch long thorn---much larger than I would have guessed by just looking at her foot. Today, it had risen to the surface and with just a nudge with the tweezers, it came all the way out. We were surprised how long it was and how easily it came out. Before we started the salve and soaks, she had a red raised welt that looked infected and angry. After soaking with epsom salts and applying band-aids with salve, it went back to looking soft and white and just a bit raised. Needless to say,

I was pretty impressed with how well that worked. I just thought you would like to know." I did want to know and I was so glad to hear that the inexpensive, black salve had won the day again.

You can get a large amount (10 oz.) of it for a few dollars by going to your local farm store. The farmers use this on their animals when they have sores or something that is stuck in their hoofs, and it works just as well on people. It will save you many a doctor visit.

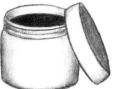

You can also order it from Natures Warehouse. This jar will contain only two to four ounces.

Flu Tea

I keep a jar of this tea mix, on my pantry shelf all winter. The children love the taste of it if I add enough of peppermint to it for good flavor. Red raspberry alone can do a wonderful job of eliminating flu, but when you add the others it makes a great flu buster. Mix together:

3 parts - Red raspberry - anti flu,

1 part - Nettles - strengthens the immune system,

¼ part - Elder flower - immune system,

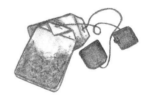

1 part - Peppermint - circulatory enhancer, flavor aid,

¼ part - Boneset or yarrow flower - fever breaker

At the first sign of illness, or if we have been exposed to some particularly nasty flu, we brew six to eight quarts of flu tea. We sweeten and ice it and then everyone can have all they want for the next two or three days. Since we have begun to do this we have not had any extended illnesses. It is good and it helps! No longer do we spend a week or two sick! This tea is also very helpful for young ladies with cramps and other monthly type difficulties.

Honey Heals Wounds

Honey is proven to have a natural anti-microbial effect against many bacteria and fungi. The current research has its origins in the experience of a University of Wisconsin School of Medicine and Public Health professor and doctor, who successfully used honey to treat a borderline diabetic's open wounds.

The doctor prescribed topical honey after a strong staph infection that the patient had been fighting for eight months continued to fester, despite the use of oral antibiotics. Once the honey treatment started, the wound healed completely within months, without the use of drugs, including antibiotics.

Honey can also help with diarrhea, insomnia, sunburn, and sore throats. Raw honey seems to be more effective than processed honey since it has not been pasteurized, thus killing the bacteria fighting enzymes.

Large burn centers in the United States are researching the usefulness of honey to help fight infections and heal serious burns. Old timers are way of ahead of them in that area. They have been using honey to heal burns for many, many years. Raw honey even seems to help to fight off serious bacterial and viral infections.

Here is a story from the time of the 1918 Spanish Flu epidemic:

"During the 1918 Spanish Flu epidemic, my dad was a little boy, 8 years old, in Stockton, California. His dad was a beekeeper, and kept some filled honeycombs in a closet in the house. During the epidemic, the family members would go into that closet and eat some of the fresh honey every day, whenever they wanted.

The flu decimated the population of Stockton, including the families of our neighbors. Next door, only one little boy survived, and when he came out of the house, they couldn't recognize him, he was so emaciated. Other whole families were entirely wiped out. They piled corpses in the streets, as there weren't enough healthy men to bury them. Dad's (large) family escaped the flu intact. It skipped their house

> Honey is more effective in treating difficult-to-heal wounds than antibiotics, says Jennifer Eddy, a professor at the University of Wisconsin School of Medicine and Public Health. Even methicillin-resistant Staphylococcus aureus, the so-called flesh eating bacterium is no match for the antibiotic compounds the bees manufacture for us - for free.

completely. Dad always said he thought it was something in the honey they ate that helped them."

Honey is very acidic (antibacterial), and it produces its own hydrogen peroxide when combined with the fluid which drains from a wound! The extremely high sugar content of honey means it contains very little water. So, it draws the pus and fluid from the wound, thereby speeding the healing process. Furthermore, the honey contains powerful germ-fighting phyto-chemicals from the plants that produced the pollen harvested by the honeybees. This has already been accepted by the overseas mainstream medical community for some time. North America finally caught on.

Deep Tissue Oil

This oil could be called "first aid in a bottle." I use it for so many things. This oil increases circulation, breaks up congestion and speeds healing. It is an incredible aid to aches and pains and sprains and what ever ails your muscles and tendons. Since the oil is so strong, rub it on a small area first to be sure that it does not cause lasting skin irritation. A few people simply cannot use this without diluting it with olive oil, because of sensitive skin. *Natures Warehouse

Ingredients:

Wintergreen oil, Peppermint oil, menthol, Cayenne pepper, Ginger root, Arnica, Saint Johns' wort, Calendula and Organic Virgin Olive oil.

Therapeutic Action: This is a deep penetrating, heating oil that relieves pain, inflammation and stiffness in joints, tendons, ligaments and muscles. For arthritis, bursitis, or any muscle or bone pain. For sprains. It helps move the lymph and increases circulation.

Chest Congestion

Deep Tissue Oil rubbed onto the chest relieves congestion and helps clear up nagging coughs. Whenever you use it on a baby or small child dilute it by **more than half** with olive oil. Use at least two droppers of olive oil to one dropper of Deep Tissue Oil. Be careful not to get it in the eyes or any sensitive area. It will not damage these areas but they will smart for awhile.

Swollen Lymph Nodes

Massage it into sore and swollen lymph glands to get them flowing again. It really helps to heal a stiff neck and any sore muscles. The children come for it with every bruise and swollen gland. They know from experience that it makes a difference! I rub it on liberally around my ears when I get earache or swollen glands and it really helps ease the pain and reduce the swelling.

Coughs and Sore Throats

Rub well into the throat, neck and ear area for relief from congestion. The oil penetrates the tissues and increases circulation to the area.

Sprained Ankle, Back or Muscle Pain

Try rubbing it on a sprained ankle a few times a day after soaking it in BF&C and you will find the ankle healing up very quickly. It is a great help for any bruised, sprained, or damaged muscle or cartilage.

Rub the afflicted muscle area well for about five minutes and you will find a great amount of relief. For extra help, cover the area with a warm rice sock. When I overuse my muscles and have those very achy feelings in bed at night, I get out the Deep Tissue Oil and massage my sore muscles. It helps a lot!

Headaches

I like to rub it on my temples and forehead when I get a headache. It improves the circulation, relaxes my head and eases the headache. The smell of it is relaxing and refreshing to me.

Leg and Muscle Cramps

We used large amounts of Deep Tissue Oil on our six year old's legs when she had Lyme. She would come down at night crying with severely cramped muscles under her knees and in her calves. I would heat a rice sock and get the Deep Tissue Oil and deeply massage her cramping muscles until they relaxed. We would use the warm rice sock for the leg I was not rubbing. Today she is fourteen and we laugh together at the memory of how she would hold the bottle of oil for me and get some on her fingers. Then, because she was crying, she would rub her eyes with those fingers and get the oil in her eyes. This would make her eyes burn and she would cry even louder. Deep Tissue Oil in the eyes really does make them smart but it does not damage them in any lasting way.

Note: Some folks have sensitive skin and this oil irritates the area causing redness and burning. Try only a small bit of oil on a little area first. For children dilute it by half with olive oil to prevent irritation. Order from Natures Warehouse. 1-800-215-4372

Or you can make your own. In this third printing we have included the recipe- p. 161.

Pantothenic Acid and Maximizer

"Antihistamine Duo" for Bites & Stings

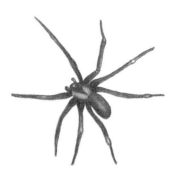

I keep these two supplements on hand to deal with allergic reactions to bites and stings. Large doses of these two have helped us clear up two serious spider bites and a number of other cases where the child was reacting and swelling and beginning to feel dizzy. One example was a spider bite that had started as what we thought was a mosquito bite acquired in the night. We thought nothing of it, but each day it enlarged until it was very painful and the size of a man's hand. At that time I did not have extensive herbal knowledge but I did try quite a few things. None of these helped.

Then the center of the bite began to turn darker and somewhat purplish, as though the circulation was being impeded. She also began to run a fever. This was, of course, on a weekend and late at night. I knew that we were fighting infection now, and I began to worry. We finally decided that we should head for the emergency room. Late Saturday night they examined her and drew an ink line around the huge bite to be able to check improvement. Then they set up an IV antibiotic drip saying, "It is probably Lyme."

Now we had had two daughters who had had a bout with Lyme and this did not look or act at all like the same thing. At the end of the drip they released us and we went home and nothing had changed. The swelling continued to increase. This was discouraging. Finally I made a call to an herbalist that I knew and she told me to use pantothenic acid and Maximizer (an enzyme supplement). She was ready to leave for church, so she put them in her mailbox for me to come and pick up. We started the child on intensive doses immediately, every ten minutes, and we began to see improvement. We switched to a capsule of each, every half hour for the next six hours. Hour by hour the redness receded, visible because of the pen line that the doctor had drawn at the emergency room. By night fall much of the redness was gone and the wound was the right

> The reason **Maximizer** works is this – it helps your body to get rid of and digest the foreign protein injected by the bite, more efficiently.
>
> **Pantothenic Acid** is a natural form of antihistamine, and it helps to counteract allergic reactions. We have not tried it on allergic reactions to bee stings yet, but the company who produces them says that it is effective for this, too.

color. I was not sure, then, whether it was just the herbal remedies, or whether it was the IV antibiotic.

As it often happens to me, two weeks later, an older woman came to my door. She had been out picking beans in her garden when a spider bit her and her bite looked much like our daughter's. She put the same things to practice (without the IV), with the same good results. Now I was sure that my treatment really worked like my herbalist friend had said it would.

A few years later the girls went to a church camp meeting for the weekend. They were going to sleep in a tent for a few days. Knowing her severe reaction to bites, the younger one took her Maximizer duo along in case of bites or stings. The first night in the tent she got fifteen spider bites in a row up her leg. When she woke up they were beginning to itch and swell and she got out her pills. She took them like recommended and in a short time they were gone, and she suffered no ill effects.

Hives

Recently one of the children woke up with a case of giant hives. We have no idea what triggered this reaction unless it was a response to the varnishing she was doing the day before. She swelled and itched and was very uncomfortable so I gave her a dose of Benadryl since I did not have what I needed on hand. It helped but made her extremely drowsy. When the dose wore off, she was worse again. I knew that I needed to go get something to get to the root of the problem so I went for my helpful duo. We gave her a different, good quality digestive enzyme that I had on hand and pantothenic acid. We gave her a dose every fifteen minutes, and in an hour she was much improved so we switched to a dose every hour for a few hours. That was the end of it for that day. The next morning she woke with some itching and took a few doses and everything cleared up. She said she liked the pantothenic acid treatment much better than the groggy feeling that accompanied the Benadryl.

Dosage: Adult – 2 capsules of maximizer and 2 of pantothenic acid every ten to fifteen minutes for an hour. Then use 2 capsules every half hour for a few hours. After that take it four times a day until your problem is completely resolved.

Child dose: Put their weight over 150 pounds and compute. Ex. 75/150 = ½ dose.

Drink lots of water with this to help flush out the poisons that you are dealing with. Extra vitamin C would be very helpful too. Use 1000 mg per hour until the problem is cleared up.

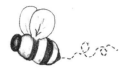

Other good, protein digestive enzymes will also work. But Maximizer seems to work well and be cheaper.

Pantothenic acid and Maximizer both store well on your medicine shelf and I never want to be without them if possible. You may save yourself an emergency room bill. Pantothenic Acid can be purchased at health food stores. Maximizer can be ordered from: *R Garden - 14 Enzyme Lane, Kettle Falls, WA 99141. Phone (800)800-1927*

Poison Ivy and Oak

If you take pantothenic acid and vitamin C for poison ivy you will usually find some relief. For some people the relief is marked and they would not be without it. For others it simply relieves some of the symptoms. You will probably need to get it from your health food store since it is not readily available. Take a capsule of pantothenic acid every fifteen minutes for two hours, along with one-thousand milligrams of vitamin C. The brand of vitamin C that I like best for this is Alacer brand's Emergen-C in the powdered form that you stir into water and drink.

This goes into your system more quickly. If you take this faithfully every fifteen minutes for two hours, and then switch to every two hours for the rest of the day, you should be able to tell a great difference. The next day repeat the dose at least four times unless you need to do it the same as the day before.

Some folks also take strong doses of echinacea to boost their immune system and help them fight this off.

The juice of the jewel weed plant smeared over the poison spots is an herbal remedy. Reapply as often as you need it.

The young daughter of our friend is extremely sensitive to poison ivy. They called for some suggestions and I recommended the above duo. Her face and eyes were swollen and so were her hands and legs. They took my recommendations faithfully and found a great measure of relief. This seems to work better for her than most things that she has tried.

Vinegar for Poison Ivy

One family declares that it has cured poison ivy every time. They just apply liberal amounts of 100% pure apple cider vinegar to the affected area whenever it began to itch. It stops the itching and clears it up in no time. This makes sense to me since the acid probably deals with the oils, and I would like to try this remedy.

Poison Ivy On the Run

Revised and used by permission of Bulk Herb Store ". . . My seven year old got into poison ivy almost a week ago. I'm ashamed to say it, but we have been so busy that it was two days before I even realized it! As soon as I realized what we were dealing with, I got out my burdock, comfrey leaf, and plantain and made some healing oil. Each time I treat my son (about 4 times a day) the rash looks a bit better than the previous time; some spots are completely healed already! Considering that my husband got progressively worse for several days before showing improvement (using Caladryl) we've been very impressed with these results. I'm fairly certain that if I'd have caught it sooner, the rashes would be gone by now. Below is our oil extract, which I expect to be good for all sorts of rashes and skin irritations. (I used it on my baby's irritated bottom with equally impressive results!) I also made a wash by simmering the same herbal blend in water for several minutes. I wiped down his skin with the wash before applying the oil."

Rescue Oil for Poison Ivy or Oak

Mix 1/3 cup each of:
burdock, comfrey and plantain herb mixture in a small saucepan and cover with extra virgin olive oil. Simmer until herbs are crispy (about 1 - 2 hours). Strain. Add 5 drops lavender oil (acts as a preservative) for each ounce of oil extract. Use as needed and watch healing take place.

Chickweed Salve

Chickweed salve will also take the redness and swelling out of the poison and make it bearable. You can make a nice salve from the chickweed in your flower bed. Use the Plantain Salve recipe in the Making Medicine section and substitute chickweed and you will have a lovely green salve that will take the fire out of the poison.

Epson Salts or Table Salt

Infection

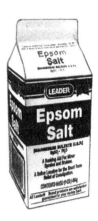

Epsom salt is a very healing, inexpensive soak to get rid of most infections. My mother never took us for tetanus shots. When we stepped on rusty nail, or cut our foot in the barnyard, the first thing she did was dissolve salt or epson salt in very hot water and make us soak it for thirty minutes. We had to soak it whether we felt like it or not. She made us soak it at least two times a day for the next two days. If we showed any signs of infection we soaked oftener. The water was HOT, hotter than we thought we could stand it and she kept it HOT! None of us ever developed a bad infection.

This old fashioned treatment still works today as a disinfectant for any cut or wound.

I would add heavy doses of echinacea and garlic to the treatment just to boost the immune system, but she never did, and we lived on a farm and stepped on nails and pitch forks. Here is a word of advice for you. **Never, never, mess around with a red streak coming from an infected area**. **Get aggressive with your treatment** or go to the doctor for antibiotics.

Salt for Infection

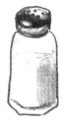

When we were in Haiti, I scratched myself on the truck cage as we were driving out to the city. In the course of the six hours that it took to get out to the city, the scratch became red and painful. Must have gotten some foreign bug in it! By the time we sat down to eat, seven hours later, there was a red streak going from my scratched wrist halfway up my arm. I had none of my stuff there, so I soaked it in plain, HOT, salt water. There was no epsom salt to be gotten either. I soaked it at the house where we stayed overnight. I soaked it in the middle of the night when I woke up feeling very ill and the streak had appeared again and run up to my elbow. I soaked it in the airport restaurant because the streak began to run upward again and I felt really ill.

There was no place to go and we were due to board our plane in an hour. So I asked for a cup of hot water for tea, dumped the whole salt shaker into the cup and soaked my finger till it was time to get on the plane.

On the plane I asked the stewardess for hot water and salt and repeated the procedure on both flights. By the time I arrived home, the infection was gone and I had no more problems with that finger. I was "salt cured." The infection was bad enough that I had been feeling really ill but salt water did the trick! Let me remind you again, that a red streak means serious infection and you dare not let it go or it will make you very ill.

Sore Muscles

Soak in a warm tub of epsom salts to relieve the pain of sore muscles. Use one to two cups of epsom salt and soak for at least twenty to thirty minutes.

High Blood Pressure

If you are dealing with blood pressure that just will not go down, soak in a tub with one-half cup of Epsom salts for fifteen to twenty minutes. This is especially helpful for a mama who is pregnant and needs to bring her blood pressure down.

Hyperactive Child

To calm a hyper child and relax him for bed, give him a soak in a tub of epson salts for about twenty minutes before his bedtime. This will calm him and help him to rest better for the night.

Aloe Vera Gel

Aloe vera promotes the rates of healing in many wounds and in stomach ulcers. The cumulative evidence supports the use of aloe vera for the healing of first to second degree burns. In addition to topical use in wound or burn healing, internal intake of aloe vera has been linked with improved blood glucose levels in diabetics. Studies have suggested oral aloe vera gel may reduce symptoms and inflammation in patients with colitis.

Aloe vera extracts have antibacterial and anti-fungal activities. For its anti-fungal properties, aloe vera is used as a fish tank water conditioner. For bacteria, inner-leaf gel from aloe vera was also shown to inhibit growth of streptococcus and shigella.

Aloe vera gel is a must to have on hand for every home. A pint of the gel at the health food store costs less than five dollars. Get the kind that says ninety-nine percent pure. I like the gel best, but the juice will also work. I keep at least two quarts in my fridge since I get emergency calls from other people.

Burns

Keep the aloe vera in the fridge and you will always be prepared for any sunburn or kitchen burn. As soon as you get a burn, run it under cool water or hold it in cool water. Do this for a few minutes while someone is getting the aloe gel. Then put cool gel on the burned area or immerse it in gel. Do this until the heat and pain is out of the burn. This may take an hour or even three if the burn is deep or large. Do it anyway. You may need to keep changing the gel to keep it cool. I use two containers and switch them in the freezing compartment so that the burn stays cool. When you take the burn out of the gel, cover it with a comfrey paste.

Use equal parts of wheat germ oil - raw honey - comfrey root powder to make a salve, or use B & W salve. (see burn chapter)

I keep a small bottle of wheat germ oil in the fridge so it is always there to mix with the honey and comfrey root powder. Put a good quantity of the comfrey paste on gauze and lay it on the burn. Wrap it lightly in more gauze and treat at least two times a day if you have second or third-degree burns. This paste has a great, healing effect. You can cover the burn with lavender oil before adding the paste if you wish. Studies show that lavender really inhibits the infection and speeds healing. *See burn chapter for more information.

Intestinal Distress, & Ulcers

Aloe is a great healer for intestinal problems because it soothes and heals. A friend of mine had taken an antibiotic because of some virus that left her ill in the hospital. The antibiotics left her with terrible diarrhea and a seriously messed up digestive system. She tried all sorts of things but nothing was working. Her weight dropped steadily and she got very thin. Then someone suggested aloe vera to her. They tried it in desperation and it worked! In a few days there was definite healing taking place. It took a bit of time, but she continued to take the aloe vera and gradually her digestive system was healed and she gained the needed weight back. She still uses it occasionally today.

People also use it to heal stomach ulcers with good results. The soothing properties of the aloe helps with healing in colitis, too.

Boils and MRSA

Red Beets

Did you know that the common red beet or potato can safely, swiftly help to get rid of the pain of a boil or carbuncle? Grate a fresh red beet or a potato and place it over that painful boil. Leave it on overnight and usually in the morning the boil will have come to a head. If it has, take off the poultice and empty the boil. The core should come right out and it will drain. Now disinfect the area with salt water or any disinfectant that you like. If it has not come to a head overnight, repeat the process until it does. Amazingly enough it does not usually take very long to clear up. If you have a systemic case of boils this will not be enough. Remember to wash your hands well so that you do not spread this highly contagious staph infection.

Turmeric

Without a doubt, the spice turmeric is the very best remedy to take when you have boils, staph infections, or MRSA.

Instructions: Take internally, one teaspoon of turmeric powder in half a glass of warm water three times a day, or take five capsules of turmeric.

Continue for several days or more if you have recurring MRSA boils. Turmeric, a traditional spice of India, is anti-inflammatory and a blood purifier. You will see healing begin within a matter of hours. You do NOT have to touch the boil whatsoever or apply anything topically.

NOTE: Regular high doses of turmeric can lead to dehydration and constipation, so be sure to take the above remedy only when necessary, such as when you begin to see signs of a boil. A single weekly dosage of the remedy is also acceptable at other times as a preventative measure.

Note #1: It is best to take turmeric internally at the earliest sign of a boil (i.e., before it breaks the skin). If you do, the boil will literally disappear overnight.

A friend of mine was diagnosed with MRSA after having a MRSA infected child stay in her home. She broke out on her face with painful boils that hurt the whole side of her face. After the diagnosis she came to me for help and I recommended turmeric to clear up the boils. The directions said, *one teaspoon of turmeric in ½ cup of warm water, 3 times a day.* I suggested that it might taste nicer and work just as well to put the turmeric in *5 capsules and take 3 times daily.* She did this faithfully and in three days the boils were dried up and the pain was gone. It is almost astounding to see how fast this treatment worked. The doctor who had cultured her boils then called to say that she should come in for a round of antibiotics. He gave her Bactrim to take for fifteen days. As a safeguard she decided to take the antibiotics, since MSRA is so contagious. Soon after beginning the Bactrim, she developed an annoying rash and then began to run a low grade fever. I suggested that it was a reaction to the antibiotic. She returned to the doctor who told her to keep on with it anyway. That night when I saw her she was not comfortable and she was beginning to feel rather sick. I suggested again, that she stop the course of Bactrim for forty-eight hours to see whether Bactrim was the cause. Indeed – she began to feel better and in a day the symptoms were nearly gone. To replace that medicine she purchased garlic capsules and some grapefruit seed extract (GSE) tablets, which she took every four hours for the next week. This treatment got rid of anything that was still lurking in her system without harming her.

Remedy for MRSA Boils

Used by permission from Enlydia/BulkHerbStore.com

Mix in a little dish some activated charcoal powder, turmeric powder, few drops of tea tree oil and a white willow bark capsule. This kills the bacteria and takes away the pain while the charcoal draws it out of the system. Rub on sore until healed. This has worked successfully for us on numerous boils. It also helps to take turmeric, activated charcoal, and white willow bark capsules internally as that will fight the toxins released inside the body. Please note that if the person has a high fever (over 102) or if there are red streaks going from the site with their boils they should see a doctor. There may be serious infection going on.

NOTE: When you take tumeric internally, you should also take acidophilus or another probiotic to keep your bowel flora healthy.

Kerosene Opens Bronchial Tubes

Croup

Our first baby came down with a distressing case of croup when he was six weeks old. Nothing I did helped, so I took him to our family doctor who had delivered the babies for my husband's mother. That old gentleman gave him some tiny black croup tablets and they were very effective. I never went away without them since the baby often struggled with this distressing malady. When we used the last of the tablets, we called him to ask for more.

"I'll tell you what," he said. "My grandmother used a drop of kerosene on a lump of brown sugar and that opened the bronchial tubes."

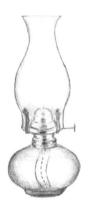

When I protested, he told me that most bronchial dilating medicines, like the tablets he had given me, were made largely from petroleum products. I was not sure about this, but we were poor, and simple kerosene and brown sugar lumps were things that I had on hand. The next bout of croup came and I took a pea-sized lump of hardened brown sugar and dropped **2 drops** of kerosene onto it and tasted it. I did not like the taste but it was do-able. So, in went a lump of sugar with it's kerosene. And it did the trick! The sugar is only a vehicle for the medicine. I never went away for the next two or so years without a tiny bottle of sugar lumps and one of kerosene. Many a person got a laugh out of how we "oiled" our baby, but it worked. **Be sure you do not use colored or scented kerosene.**

After two more babies I learned that milk sensitivities can bring on croup and that if I did not use milk, etc., my babies usually did not get that nasty disease. Diet is a much better way to work with croup and asthma but 2 drops of kerosene may save you an emergency room visit.

Asthma

Recently I was with a family when a little boy had an asthma attack. I remembered the bronchial dilating characteristics of kerosene and suggested that she try it on her wheezing child. The effect was almost instant. The wheezing left and he began to breathe freely. Once again, I must say, that I believe diet changes will make a tremendous difference in helping with asthma and that should be implemented, but kerosene can be used to clear up a problem in an emergency for many children. *See respiratory chapter for other ways to work with asthma.

Cayenne for Stroke or Heart Attack

If someone begins to have heart attack symptoms, mix 1 teaspoon of cayenne powder into a glass of warm water. Drink it and go to the emergency room. Take another glass of it along to drink while you wait. Repeat this as often as necessary with out problems. Here is story to illustrate this.

A friend was in Belize, visiting and saw an elderly women in the yard, moaning, groaning, and complaining that she's going to have another heart attack. She didn't want to go to the hospital. Nathan told her, "My sister says cayenne pepper can stop a heart attack". They immediately sent to the house for cayenne. The woman began to scoop the cayenne into her mouth using her fingers like a little shovel. She was immensely grateful to him, saying the pain was gone and she felt much better.

I really like American Botanical Pharmacy's (p. 324) heart tonic to help people with heart problems. We have used it quite a bit to deal with persons who were scheduled for quadruple by-pass surgery with really good success. The surgeries were cancelled. The pain was gone and they were back to work again. I will discuss this in an upcoming book but perhaps someone needs the information now. To cancel the surgeries we used 2-4 droppers at least 5 times daily, or as often as needed. This medicine relaxes the arteries, helps to unclog them and steadies the heart beat, all the while nourishing the heart. It even helps to lower blood pressure and stop arythmias.

Deep Tissue Oil from p 149

Fill a jar with:
   ¼ cup each habenero peppers (dried) and ginger root grated
   ½ cup each calendula flowers, St. Johns Wort flowers and Arnica flowers
Cover with olive oil – at least 6 oz. Set for 6 weeks, shaking occasionally. Strain out herbs. Heat the oil till warm and add - 1oz. - Botanical Menthol Crystals. (cover container)
Now add and stir well: 4 oz. - Wintergreen Oil and 2 oz - Peppermint oil.
Bottle tightly in glass bottles only. Keeps for years. This oil will burn any sensitive mucous membranes. It will not damage them though the eyes will really burn!

Respiratory Difficulties

Pneumonia – Croup – Whooping Cough - Asthma

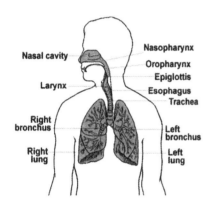

What About Antibiotics?

Giving antibiotics for a non-respiratory tract infection to an infant younger than one greatly increases the odds that the child will develop asthma, according to new research reported by "Health Day News" June 11.

The study found that the risk was highest for those infants who received multiple courses of antibiotics and those who received prescriptions for broad-spectrum antibiotics.

"Asthma is a multi-factorial disease, and we've found evidence of an association with first-year-of-life antibiotic use and asthma," said the study's lead author.

Antibiotics are not necessarily a good choice for respiratory problems. If the problems are viral in nature, the antibiotic will do no good. If they are bacterial in nature, common garlic may do you as much good as the antibiotic with none of the harmful effects.

Pneumonia

Pneumonia usually begins with the flu or another illness and progresses into pneumonia. Your job is to keep this from happening. Give your sick child **lots of liquids** to keep him hydrated and thin the mucus secretions that are in his chest and nasal cavity, thus allowing the body to get rid of it properly. Keep the child on mostly herbal teas and non-sweetened juices. **Do not give any MILK PRODUCTS.** Dairy makes mucous, and you are trying to clear up their respiratory system. Give herbs designed to help stimulate the immune system to work. Make sure the child gets plenty of rest.

If the simple measures do not work and the child becomes sicker, then you must immediately become more aggressive with the treatment. **I usually like to get aggressive with the herbal treatment immediately so that we so not have a really sick child.**

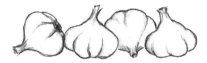

Herbal Treatment

For a 75- 100 lb. child. Treat every hour when awake. 7Am – 7PM
> *1000 mg. vitamin C*
> *2 droppers of echinacea tincture*
> **"Garlic salve" rubbed on chest and fresh garlic - (½ clove, with bread)*
> *1 cup of respiratory tea*

40 – 70 lbs.
> *500 mg. vitamin C*
> *2 droppers of echinacea tincture*
> **"Garlic salve" rubbed on chest and fresh chopped garlic (½ clove)*
> *½ cup of respiratory tea*

25- 30 lbs.
> *100 mg. vitamin C*
> *½ dropper echinacea tincture*
> **"Garlic salve" rubbed on chests, back and feet 3 times a day.*
> *1/4 cup of respiratory tea – 4 Tablespoons*

Do this for a day intensively, or longer if the child is still really sick. Then switch to every three hours for the next two days.

After that give every four hours for a day if the child has made good improvement. I would treat at least a week if the child is not completely well. If you suspect pneumonia you must get help from the doctor or another person who is able to recognize the symptoms and tell you how to deal with them.

Do not try to do it yourself if the child is blue around the lips or the fingernails and his chest is retracting with grunts when he breathes and he has a rising fever. With this group of symptoms you need to get *immediate* medical attention. This is probably bacterial pneumonia.

*See directions on how to make "Garlic Salve" in the garlic chapter.

Respiratory Tea

Make a tea to clear out the respiratory system and help the immune system to work efficiently. Use:

2 parts – peppermint

1 part - oregano

1/2 part – echinacea

1/2 part - mullein

1/2 part - comfrey leaf

Bring a half gallon of water to a boil. Turn off the heat. Do not continue to boil! Boiling makes the tea bitter and lessens the medicinal value, as the essential oils are evaporated into the atmosphere. Add one half cup of tea mixture to the water. Let it steep with the lid on, for twenty minutes. Strain and sweeten. Chill with ice and drink. This tastes nice enough to enjoy. Give them a cup every hour or oftener.

Viral or Bacterial Pneumonia – How To Decide

Viral pneumonia is usually mild and you can treat it successfully yourself. This is not true with bacterial pneumonia. Bacterial pneumonia can usually be detected by a fever over 102, accompanied by pain and difficulty breathing, often followed by blueness of skin. **There is no doubt that this is an emergency and needs immediate treatment.** Take the child to the emergency room immediately.

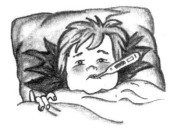

Viral pneumonia can turn into the more serious bacterial pneumonia if not tended, so be aggressive with your treatments of viral pneumonia.

Hot Ginger Baths

Give your sick one a hot ginger bath, (not under age 6) keeping him completely covered. (Ginger is a circulatory herb. It gets that lymph flowing in the body!) Stay close to him (stay right with a child) during the bath and give him hot peppermint or ginger tea to drink while he is in the bath. Do not leave him, and if he feels faint or dizzy give him a cool drink. Put a cool washcloth on his head and get him out of the bath. Make sure the room is warm, dry him well and put him to bed, covered very warmly. Rub his chest with menthol salve or Deep Tissue Oil and garlic salve. There are all kinds of these salves out there. I like Deep Tissue Oil the best. (Dilute it by ½ with olive oil for a child.) Top the rub off with a nice, warm rice sock. Repeat this performance a few times daily if needed. (Three to four times a day if needed.)

Onion Poultice

You can treat chest congestion by applying a warm onion poultice to the chest in the front and the same in the back. Give the child immune support every hour with lots of fluids. (Mullein, comfrey & peppermint tea is very helpful for chest congestion.) Use moist air to make it easier for him to breathe. I like the cold mist vaporizer the best for nighttime, but warm steam with eucalyptus and mint in it really helps to break up congestion and make breathing easier. NOTE: Many of our houses are too DRY! If the weather outside is cold, and the windows have no condensation on them, your house is probably too dry. This adversely affects your mucous membranes, making you much more susceptible to respiratory illnesses.

Short of obviously severe respiratory difficulties, do not go to the the doctor or give over the counter medications to treat the symptoms. These drugs include: decongestants, expectorants, antihistamines, cough suppressors, pain relievers, and antibiotics. They are unnecessary, they interfere with the body's own working mechanisms, and they may have side affects that can be serious. Study Mendelson's book, (he's a pediatrician) to see what he says about these over-the-counter drugs for your child! He believes that they are not helpful for your child, and recommends that you do not use them.

When I was sixteen I developed pneumonia, and since my parents seldom used the doctor, they put me to bed, gave me lots of tea and chicken broth to drink, and lots of vitamin C. I was unable to work for two weeks and had a terrible cough, but I pulled through just fine without antibiotics. However, my mother was a strict nurse and I was on bed rest and liquids to thin the mucus and get it out of my lungs. She did not let me go away until my fever was gone for a few days.

One of the things that Americans do these days is to take Tylenol or its counterpart so that the fever goes down, and then they keep on working or playing, etc. This really works against the body and hinders its ability to heal and aids illness in really setting in.

When the body is rested and given the proper liquids and healing aids it will usually rally and heal without drugs. Occasionally you will need assistance, but this should be the exception rather than the norm.

As I said before, it is of utmost importance to hydrate that sick child. How do you do it? Be persistent and creative. Get a tablespoon in every 10 minutes. That will do it. There are four tablespoons in one fourth a cup. Sick children need that much every hour if they are ages two to four. If they are older they need half a cup. Sick adults need about one cup hourly. Use ice, juice pops, warm chicken broth, and love. Just do it. And remember, almost no child is too sick to drink, or they should be in the hospital. A baby, maybe, but a child needs to obey even when he does not feel good. So work on that obedience and expect it in sickness. Just do it in gentleness and love.

Cold and Flu Tea

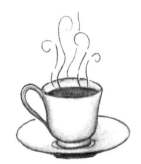

"Kill-or-Cure Cold Remedy"
2 cinnamon sticks
a few peppercorns
2 Tablespoons fresh ginger, grated
Add to 2 quarts cold water. Bring to boil and simmer for 5 minutes.
Add:

1 tsp dried or 1 sprig fresh (each) thyme, sage and marjoram and 1 tsp
fenugreek seeds

Let steep for 5 more minutes, strain and sweeten.
Take a half cup of the mixture and dilute half and half with hot water.

Drink as hot as you can bear with honey, orange zest, and/or lemon juice to taste. Take quarts of water to bed, dress warmly, and get under the blankets. Drink a few cups of remedy throughout the day, reheating only as much as you'll drink at a time.

Whooping Cough

Whooping cough has made its comeback in the USA. Despite the immunizations, there is widespread pertussis and the doctors are distressed. They have to re-educate themselves on this disease. Remember, it starts very simply and grows in intensity. What are the stages, symptoms, and signs of whooping cough?

Stages of Whooping Cough

The **first stage of whooping cough** is known as the catarrhal stage. In this stage, which typically lasts two weeks, an infected person has symptoms characteristic of an upper respiratory infection, including:

- ☒ runny nose

- ☒ sneezing

- ☒ low-grade fever

- ☒ mild, occasional cough, similar to the common cold

The cough gradually becomes more severe, and after one to two weeks, the second stage begins. The disease is very contagious in this stage but people often do not know that they have it. That is why whooping cough tends to spread so rapidly.

It is during the **second stage (the paroxysmal stage)** (bursts of coughing) that the diagnosis of whooping cough usually is suspected.

The most serious symptoms develop during this phase and last about two to four weeks or longer. As cold-like symptoms fade, the cough gets worse. A dry, hacking cough turns into bursts of uncontrollable, often violent coughing that may make it temporarily impossible to breathe. This may happen up to thirty times a day and tends to be more noticeable at night. The person may quickly inhale when trying to take a breath through airways narrowed by inflammation, which sometimes creates a whooping noise. The second stage is characterized by:

- ☒ bursts of coughing.

- ☒ at the end of the bursts of rapid coughs, a long inspiratory effort (breathing in) is often (**but not always**) accompanied by a characteristic high-pitched "whoop"

167

- [x] during an attack, the individual may turn blue from lack of oxygen

- [x] vomiting (referred to by doctors as post-tussive vomiting) and exhaustion often follow the episodes of coughing. This vomiting happens, not because the stomach is upset, but because the violent cough expels the contents of the stomach

- [x] the person usually appears normal (and well) between episodes

- [x] paroxysmal attacks occur more frequently at night, with an average of fifteen to twenty attacks per twenty-four hours

- [x] the paroxysmal stage usually lasts from one to six weeks but may persist for up to ten weeks. This stage is referred to as the wet stage because of the droplets that leave the mouth while coughing. It is a contagious stage!

Infants under six months of age may not have the strength to have a whoop, but they do have paroxysms of coughing.

In babies, coughing spells:

- [x] May be triggered by very slight stimulation, such as taking in food or milk, sucking, exposure to a sudden sound or light, or stretching.

- [x] May cause symptoms of flushed cheeks, pale or bluish complexion from lack of oxygen, and bulging or watery eyes. A baby may also stick out his or her tongue, push the chest forward, or flail arms and legs in distress.

- [x] May be frightening to watch, although most babies recover and regain control of their breathing on their own. Babies generally feel well between coughing spells but may become exhausted from the physical effort of coughing. It's also possible that your baby's breathing could stop for a short time during the coughing spells. This is called apnea.

The third stage of whooping cough is the recovery or convalescent stage. In the convalescent stage, recovery is gradual. The cough becomes less paroxysmal and usually disappears over two to three weeks; however, paroxysms often recur with subsequent respiratory infections for many months, especially in the winter. Although the person gains strength and begins to feel better, the cough may become louder and sound worse.

How is Whooping Cough Transmitted?

Whooping cough is highly contagious and is spread among people by direct contact with fluids from the nose or mouth of infected people. People contaminate their hands with respiratory secretions from an infected person and then touch their own mouth or nose, or that of their children or friends. In addition, small bacteria-containing droplets enter the air during coughing or sneezing. People can become infected by breathing in these drops.

How is Whooping Cough Treated?

Antibiotics directed against Bordetella pertussis can be effective in reducing the severity of pertussis when administered early (the first five days) in the course of the disease. **Antibiotic therapy can also help reduce the risk of transmission of the bacterium to other household members as well as to others who may come into contact with an infected person.** Unfortunately, most people with pertussis are diagnosed only later when the condition is in the second (paroxysmal) stage of the disease. **Erythromycin** is an antibiotic which has been shown to be effective in treating whooping cough in the first five days. It does not appear that antibiotics have any benefit for people who have been ill with pertussis for longer than five days. There is no medically proven, effective treatment for the paroxysms of coughing that accompany pertussis, although there are some herbal remedies that do make a great difference.

Antibiotics are also routinely administered to people who have had close contact with an infected person, regardless of their vaccination status.

The most common, serious complication is secondary bacterial pneumonia. (Secondary bacterial pneumonia is bacterial pneumonia that follows another infection of the lung, be it viral or bacterial. Secondary pneumonia is caused by a different virus or bacterium than the original infection.)

Symptoms of bacterial pneumonia are blueness of lips and fingernails, difficulty breathing (chest retracts) and weakness and listlessness (because of lack of oxygen). This needs **immediate, emergency, medical attention**! Thankfully, most cases do not lead to this kind of problem.

- ☒ Pertussis resolves on its own in the majority of cases.

- ☒ The antibiotic, erythromycin, has been shown to lessen the transmission from the host to others but doesn't do a great job in shortening the course of illness.

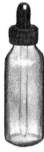 Pertussis is increasingly recognized as a disease that affects older children and adults, including fully vaccinated persons. Possibly the disease may have mutated making the vaccines ineffective.

How Long is a Person with Pertussis Contagious?

Persons with pertussis are most infectious during the second stage (two to four weeks) and during the first two weeks after onset of the cough (approximately twenty-one days).

Herbal Remedies for Pertussis

Resp-aid Syrup

Mix together equal parts:

mullein leaf (fresh if possible) - horseradish root - fennel seed

colts foot leaf (optional, but so helpful) - fenugreek seed

Add: ¼ part boneset leaf and ½ part comfrey leaf (optional)

Fill a quart jar a little more than half full of the mixture. Cover it with a mix of glycerin and water. (See Making Medicine chapter.) Let it set for two to four weeks. Strain and bottle. If you need it in a hurry, fill two pint jars with the mixture and put them in your crock pot. Fill the pot with water up to the neck of the jars. Put the lid on and turn the heat to the lowest setting. Heat on low for two to three days. Strain and use.

Dosages:

Baby - a few drops at each nursing,

2-4 year old - 1 dropper every 2 hours, or as often as needed.

Children- 2 droppers every 2 hours or as needed

Adults – 4 droppers (4 droppers are in a teaspoon) or more as needed (hourly if needed)

This works for any bronchial type, irritating cough, as well as for pertussis. It helps to give the syrup to children with respiratory weaknesses at least three times daily, for awhile to build up their systems, especially in the fall before flu season comes. Then if they get croup, whooping cough, asthma, or just a nasty respiratory infection you can increase the dose to every two hours or more often if needed.

Here is another syrup that helps and is easy to make. This one is especially helpful with mucous and phlegm.

Thyme Syrup

Mix together:

2 oz. thyme leaf   2 oz. marshmallow root

2 oz. red raspberry leaf   1 oz. bayberry

1 oz. fenugreek seed

Cover well with boiling water (5 cups or more). Let set for twelve hours. Bring to a low boil, turn heat on low and simmer for five minutes. Strain and add and an equal amount of honey to the liquid. Simmer on low for ten minutes. Bottle and use as needed to thin phlegm and act as an expectorant. Use the doses suggested for Resp-Aid.

Our Experience with Pertussis

One of the things that helped us the most when we had the whooping cough, was ALJ syrup from Nature's Sunshine. This syrup really helped to loosen the mucus so that the child did not cough as hard. We used the cold mist vaporizer and when they had a paroxysm of coughing they ran and put their head into the cold mist. This helped to loosen that phlegm so that they did not choke on it. We gave them the syrup and used percussion (patting their back like a drum) so the stuff would break up and come out. It was a hard three months because five of the children and I had it at the same time, and one on them was a three month old baby! I was so impressed with the ALJ that I researched the ingredients and came up with a similar syrup that I call Resp-Aid. See the recipe for this. We coughed until warm weather came! Those were four long months! I was really ready for summer that year. One interesting side note is this- our nineteen year old daughter was the first one to get this cough. She went to Africa on a mission's team with her cough. (We did not know it was whooping cough for a few more weeks.) She told me that her annoying cough simply disappeared when she reached the hot, dry climate of Ghana. I found that very interesting since pertussis usually goes underground in the summer in the USA. Apparently warmth and sun do something to alleviate the disease.

Winter whooping cough has far more problems than summer and fall whooping cough. I cannot tell you why, but it is true. Spring and summer whooping cough tends to be annoying coughing but not the serious "think you are going to suffocate" kind. Winter time whooping cough can be really nasty for some children, especially those with respiratory weakness. They often panic and cry, which makes the episodes even more difficult.

Even as an adult, I thought, quite a few times, that I was going to die from lack of air. It was an absolutely scary feeling. By all means, be courteous and stay away from everyone. Pertussis is very contagious. Did you ever watch a person cough in the bright sunlight, and see how far the spray of droplets go? They really spread! That is how pertussis spreads. When you cover your mouth with your hands, you transfer the germs to everything that you touch! So be considerate and stay away from others. And in case you wondered, you can get pertussis even if you have been immunized.

Asthma

Asthma is a chronic lung condition in which inflammation of the airways or bronchi, affects the way air enters and leaves the lungs, disrupting breathing. Asthma is an ancient Greek word meaning "panting or short drawn breath." It is the most troublesome of the respiratory diseases, affecting twice as many boys as girls in childhood, more girls than boys in teenage, and in adulthood, the ratio becomes 1:1 males to females. People with asthma have extra sensitive or hyper-responsive airways. The airways react by narrowing or obstructing when they become irritated. This makes it difficult for the air to move in and out.

Asthma is a very frightening experience for both the child and the parent. When you cannot breathe well, you tend to panic, and when you panic the situation worsens.

For children with asthma, 200 milligrams of vitamin C, three times daily (for a 50-pound child) is recommended as an antihistamine. Increase the dose for older children. To support their adrenal glands, children with asthma can also take pantothenic acid one and one-half hours before exercising.

Other vitamins recommended for children with asthma, include magnesium and the B complex vitamins, particularly B6, which has been shown in various studies to reduce the severity of asthma attacks.

This tea brings some relief to many asthma sufferers:

BreatheEasy Tea

1 quart boiling water

1 teaspoon each:

chamomile flowers, echinacea root, mullein leaves, passionflower leaves (not optional)

½ teaspoon each:

elecampane root and lemon verbena leaves (if available)

Pour boiling water over the herbs in a saucepan and steep for 10 to 15 minutes. Strain out herbs.

For a 50-pound child, give a half cup of tea twice a day as a preventive, a few times a day when breathing becomes strained or when emotional conditions may lead to an attack. If you use a tincture of these herbs, give ½ dropper (30 drops) to replace each half-cup of tea. Store extra tea in the refrigerator.

To tincture the herbs:

2 oz. Each:

chamomile flowers, echinacea root, mullein leaves, and passionflower leaves (not optional)

1 oz. teaspoon each elecampane root and lemon verbena leaves (if available)

Fill a quart jar a little more than ½ full of the mixture. Cover it with a mix of glycerin and water. (See Making Medicine chapter) Let set for 2-4 weeks. Strain and bottle. If you need it in a hurry, fill 2 pint jars with the mixture and put them in your crock pot. Fill the pot with water up to the neck of the jars. Put the lid on and turn the heat to the lowest setting. Heat on low for 2 - 3 days. Strain and use.

Janet, a registered nurse, used both medical and herbal approaches to treat her son Ryan's asthma. Janet and her husband, Dan, say that the best prevention for seven-year-old Ryan's asthma attacks is a lavender chest rub just before he goes to sleep. The lavender does double duty: as a muscle relaxant, it keeps chest muscles and bronchial passages from constricting; as a mind relaxer, it reduces the stress that might trigger an attack. If the child tends to become congested while sleeping, Breath-Easy tincture can be used in conjunction with the lavender.

Lavender Chest Rub

8 drops lavender essential oil

2 drops chamomile essential oil (optional)

¼ cup olive (or almond) oil

Combine ingredients. Rub on chest as needed, especially before bedtime. If you wish to add chamomile as an antihistamine, replace 2 drops of the lavender essential oil with 2 drops of chamomile essential oil.

An alternative to the chest rub is an herbal steam that uses these same essential oils. Add two drops of lavender essential oil to a humidifier (check the instructions to make sure yours will not clog or otherwise be damaged by essential oils) in your child's room or have your child inhale the steam from a pan of water containing four drops of lavender essential oil.

Janet and Dan tried a lavender steam with Ryan but he did not like putting his head over the hot steam. In exploring other ways to administer this herb, they eventually discovered that if they put him in a hot bath containing a few drops of lavender essential oil at the first signs of a serious attack, Ryan breathed easily for at least an hour. Dan says that it is amazing how dramatically the herbal bath works in halting even the worst attacks—a great relief, since Ryan's asthma is so bad that he has ended

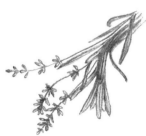

up in the hospital a few times, once in intensive care. Since the herbal treatments began, there have been no hospital visits, and Janet and Dan have been able to reduce Ryan's medication.

To play it safe, have your child sniff the oils before you use the chest rub, steam or bath for the first time—some asthma sufferers are sensitive to any fragrance.

Quercetin for Asthma

Quercetin has been proven helpful in reducing allergy symptoms and asthma attacks. Quercetin is a bio-flavonoid found mainly in apples, onions, berries, cauliflower, and nuts. It has significant anti-inflammatory, antihistamine, and antioxidant properties.

In one study in 2002, in the American Journal of Clinical Nutrition, higher Quercetin intakes were associated with lower incidences of asthma.

"Flavonoids, particularly Quercetin, appear to be key antioxidants in the treatment of asthma. Quercetin is known to inhibit mast cells from releasing pro-inflammatory compounds that cause allergy symptoms. . . . it relaxes the mast cells, calming them down. Quercetin also spares vitamin C and stabilizes cell membranes, including those of mast cells.

"Quercetin is available in powder and capsule form. When Quercetin is being used for its anti-inflammatory properties (which may even extend to cancer therapeutics), it should be combined with the pineapple enzyme bromelain for its own anti-inflammatory activity and possibly enhanced absorption of Quercetin. If used in combination, then the amount of bromelain should equal the amount of Quercetin. Most recently, a new water-soluble form of the Quercetin molecule has been developed which may enhance absorption." Excerpts from "Quercetin: A Review of Clinical Applications" - compiled by Frank M. Painter, D.C.

Dosages
Asthma and hay fever: Adults - take 400 mg 20 minutes before each meal.
Children – weight/150 i.e. 50/150 = 1/3 dose = 100- 130 mg.
Also take Bromelain with it for enhanced digestion and absorption.

One Mother's Experience

I first heard of Quercetin when a mother shared about asthma attacks in one of my herb classes. She said, " I want to share my experience so that other mothers can benefit from it." Her daughter, a premie at birth, developed serious asthma. They ran her into the Emergency Room more times than they wanted to count for serious difficulties in breathing, despite the fact that she was on medication and inhalers. Nothing was working and the attacks were becoming more and more frequent. This mother was desperate for help. She began to research natural means for alleviating asthma and came across Quercetin Having never been a health minded person she went to the drug store to buy this bioflavonoid. Fortunately her druggist was well versed in the use of Quercetin.
"For asthma?" he inquired as he handed her the small white tablets.
"Yes," she responded.
"You will be surprised how well this works," he returned, leaving her to wonder why her doctor had not recommended it long before. It worked wonders, in fact it worked so well that when she told us about it, she had never had another emergency room visit. I was duly impressed and began to look at this helpful bio-flavonoid.

As I studied it I noticed that it was very helpful in reducing any swelling. I experimented, trying it on hives with good success.

Then a few years later I had the opportunity to use it on a mother with DIE (drug-induced encephalitis). This young lady had gone to the dentist for a normal procedure and ended up in bed for more than a week with encephalitis resulting from the Novocaine that the dentist had injected. It seems that the numbing shot containing chlorine (to which she is extremely sensitive) as a stabilizer, had gone through a blood vessel up into her brain, swelling her brain in response.

What to do now? She manifested an extreme headache. She could not tolerate any light or movement and she was a very sick girl. We did a number of things to relieve her, but the thing that helped the most were high doses of Quercetin and vitamin C. I was really impressed with the way they reduced the headache and the light sensitivity. Two days later we added hot ginger foot baths to pull the blood away from her head and ice packs on the back of her neck. These helped to make her more comfortable, too. But the Quercetin came to the rescue first to reduce the initial symptoms. I have since learned about the incredible effects of 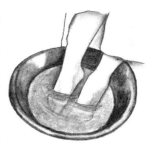 charcoal and would use charcoal by mouth and as a poultice on the forehead and the temples if I had it to do over.

We learn as we go and every little bit makes a difference. That is the main object of all the stories in my book. They will help you to better remember the treatments.

Croup

Croup is a viral infection or an allergic response to food taken in. There is a distinct barking cough, trouble with breathing, tightness in the lungs, and a mucous build up. Croup is a group of conditions involving inflammation of the upper airway and leading to a harsh cough that sounds like the barking of a dog particularly when the child is crying. Most croup is caused by a viral infection, but some is triggered by an allergic response. Children 3 months to 5 years are most susceptible to this difficulty, and the smaller they are the harder it is to deal with it. Most croup is mild and can be treated at home, but occasionally it is life-threatening. It frequently begins at night with sudden onset, frightening both the child and the parents. The child may have cold-like symptoms with runny nose and even a low grade fever. As the upper airway becomes swollen, a harsh, bark-like cough begins. At night the symptoms worsen and any crying also makes it worse.

Humidify the environment with a cool mist humidifier or sit in the bathroom with the steam of a hot shower surrounding you for about 10 minutes to break up the onset of the cough. Viral croup will usually disappear in 3 or so days. Give the child some Tasty Echinacea every hour and rub his throat and chest with garlic salve a few times daily.

You can give a small bit of lobelia by mouth to soothe the bronchial muscles and loosen the mucous, or rub it on their throat and feet. This does not taste so nice but it is helpful. Taste it before you make your child take it. Resp-Aid Syrup given every fifteen minutes for an hour may help you. Some folks find that a few drops of eucalyptus oil in a steaming kettle on the stove brings relief, and other children cannot tolerate it. We use 2 drops of kerosene for immediate relief. (See page 151 for instructions)

Eyes, Noses, Sinus and Ears

Pink Eye

Pink eye, or conjunctivitis, is a common childhood ailment. Here are some pink eye remedies. Conjunctivitis is a very contagious ailment, so keep you child away from other children. It is important to treat this right away so that the condition does not worsen.
This is a very contagious children's disease which you can get yourself if you are not very careful about hygiene when working with and caring for children who have it. It spreads quickly in a family with little ones. Always wash the infected eye carefully, one at a time, using a clean cloth for each eye so that you do not move the infection around.

My favorite, simple pink eye remedy is chamomile! Place cool, moist chamomile tea bag on each closed eye for about ten minutes. Repeat this every couple hours. You can buy these tea bags at any supermarket. Make sure chamomile is the only ingredient. If you have bulk chamomile flowers, use a muslin tea bag to make the tea.

You can also use three to five drops of lavender diluted with one teaspoon of oil to wash around the eye and disinfect it. Do not get it in the eye. If you do, rinse it with milk and wipe the eye out.

I have used salt water and a bit of strained goldenseal-water to wash the eyes. *Empty a capsule of goldenseal powder into 1/4 cup of boiling water (or you could use eyebright). Stir. Let set and then strain through a cloth. Dab it on the eyes with a cotton ball or a bit of clean cloth.* You could also use a weak eyebright tea for a wash, too.

If you are a nursing mother, you may be surprised to know that breast milk will do wonders for clearing up pink eye.

The older grandmothers washed the eyes out with a diluted solution of Boric acid. Today some folks say that is not good. I know that it worked since I have used it for our older children when they were small, but I do not have scientific research on this. I am sure it is no harder on the eyes than the current drugs prescribed for pink eye, which burn a lot, when applied to the eye. All of these things are healing so any of 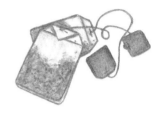 them could be helpful. Remember that it takes a bit of time for this disease to clear up. Be patient and consistent with cleanliness.

Sinus Infections

Sinus problems can be viral or bacterial in nature, or they can be triggered by allergic responses. Sinus problems are usually easy to deal with if you address the problem properly. Do not take decongestants, etc. Mix up a saline solution: ¼ cup of warm water with ¼ teaspoon of salt. Put a puddle of that solution in your one hand, and hold one nostril shut with the opposite hand. Now inhale deeply with the open nostril. Pull the salt water up into your sinus as far as you can. It will burn a bit, but never fear, it will not damage you. Now switch hands and hold the opposite nostril shut and sniff again. You will be able to blow quite a bit of stuff out immediately. If you are still clogged, repeat the procedure as often as needed. When I am struggling with clogged sinuses, I wait about a half hour and do it again. This will open up your sinuses immediately and usually help relieve a sinus headache. I usually also massage all the aching sinuses and the temples and forehead with Sen-sei salve, or my Deep Tissue Oil. These menthol products open up the sinuses, are relaxing, and smell so nice. **Remember to cut out the dairy products until your sinuses clear up since these things make a lot of mucus.**

Irrigation with a Neti Pot

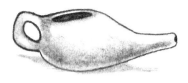

Sue uses a neti pot (aka 'nasal irrigation') for general sinus health. She battled with chronic sinusitis for quite a few years, darkening the doctor's door many times without success. She told me that she had tried every remedy out there and spent a good bit of money at the doctor's office. When she started irrigating with saline solution about 5 years ago, her chronic sinus issues improved by 90%. She mixed ¼ teaspoon salt (with a pinch of baking soda) per cup of warm water, put it in a neti pot and poured it through one nostril, out the other. This helped moisturize her sinuses, flush out the allergens, and improve the health of the cilia and mucous membranes. Sue was so excited that such a simple thing would do what no medicine had done for her. As long as she continues to irrigate she does not have anymore problems with her sinuses.

Some neti suggestions include adding a drop or two of sesame or sunflower oil to moisturize the membranes when humidity is low, or diluted herbal teas with salt to directly treat the sinuses.

Neti pots are available in most drug and grocery stores today.

Instructions for Neti Pot Users:

1. *Mix a 1/4 teaspoon of finely ground non-iodized salt. Use the purest salt available because impurities in the salt can be irritating.*

2. *Lean forward and turn your head to one side over the sink, keeping the forehead at the same height as the chin, or slightly higher.*

3. *Gently insert the spout in the nostril so it forms a comfortable seal.*

4. *Raise the Neti Pot™ gradually so the saline solution flows in through your upper nostril and out of the lower nostril. Breathe through your mouth.*

5. *When the Neti Pot™ is empty, face the sink and exhale vigorously without pinching the nostrils.*

6. *Refill the Neti Pot™ and repeat on the other side. Again, exhale vigorously to clear the nasal passages.*

Ear Infections

So many children have ear infections. Ear infections can come from viral or bacterial infections. They are likely, more often caused by diet.

If your child has re-occurring ear infections, change his diet. Cut out all dairy and most wheat for at least a week, two is much better. Sensitivities to foods can cause extra fluids that build up behind the ear drum causing pressure. Then, no matter what you do, they will keep coming back. I have found that eliminating dairy, and eggs or wheat usually brings about a rapid change and the child has much less trouble with ear infections. This is not an easy solution, but it is a good one since food allergies tend to make all kinds of other problems including bed wetting and hyperactivity. But your child has an ear- ache, no matter what the cause. Try the following:

Things That May Help an Earache

- ✓ Lots of liquids, echinecea, vitamin C hourly, and acidophilus.
- ✓ Garlic, preferably raw, on butter bread, or chopped finely on a spoon covered with honey.
- ✓ A rub with Garlic Salve (See chapter on garlic.) Especially rub around his ears and on his throat and neck.
- ✓ Garlic/mullein oil and 2 drops of lobelia in each ear.
- ✓ Microwave a cut-in-half onion until it is a bit soft, cool it until it could be put on both ears and fastened it in place.
- ✓ Heat a rice or salt sock and put it on his ears. Check it on your ears to see if it is comfortable and then wrap it around the child's neck covering both ears. Most children will cuddle up and stop crying as soon as you do that. The warmth is so comforting.

One winter our youngest had a bout with an earache. I had one myself at the time and it hurt. He was crying and so I some did the above treatment on him. It hung on stubbornly for a few days. Whenever he began to hurt he would get his sock and bring it to me and ask me to heat it for him. Then he would curl up on the couch and sometimes even go to sleep with it on his ears. It was a a real blessing for us. If I would have given him echinecea faithfully I think the duration would have been much shorter, but I was out of it.

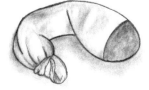

Make Your Own Mullein/Garlic Oil

Pick enough fresh mullein blossoms to partially fill an 4 oz jar.

Chop or grate one bulb of garlic and add to the jar.

Cover the herbs with olive oil and set for a week or two.

Strain and bottle.

Ear Ache Rub

Mix together:

¼ cup olive oil

1 teaspoon tea tree oil

1 teaspoon lavender essential oil

Use this oil to rub liberally around the ears when an infection starts. It is a calming, relaxing, antibacterial rub.

Swimmer's Ear

We have had good success recommending a heated onion piece inserted in each ear to help with the pain of swimmers ear. One young man of seventeen called me to ask what to do for his bad earache. He had been swimming, and the pain was intense. I had recently read about how onion draws out fluid, so I recommended that he cut an onion in half and take out the center of each side. He was to heat it a bit until very warm but not soft and insert a piece in each ear. Then he was to place moist heat, like a rice or salt sock over the ears and rest for a bit. He called me back to say that the treatment worked for him. In a short time fluid (that the onion had wicked out of his ear) was running out and the pain was greatly relieved. He repeated the process another time and the earache was gone.

It is interesting to see how the onion pulls the fluid out and relieves the pressure, thus relieving the pain. We have seen it pull out the fluid on a "goose egg" (bump) on the forehead time after time. See chapter on Garlic and Onion. This same action is so helpful in most earaches. The rice sock or salt sock also wick out moisture. Remember how your salt takes on moisture in the summer when it is humid? It will do the same for the pressure filled inner ear.

Vinegar for Ear Infection

Here is a very interesting account of how you can use a simple article in your kitchen to help where doctors were not able to help.

"My husband was suffering from an ear infection. He was in the hospital for almost 2 weeks, still nothing happened, so we decided to check out of the hospital. And then I remembered when we were still small, whenever we had throat problems or ear infections, my mom always told us to apply vinegar on the area & gargle vinegar for the throat. So I told my husband, "Why don't we try it." After one day of applying vinegar in a bit of water, his ear was dry and we continued to apply it twice a day until it was completely healed, but sadly enough he lost part of his ear bone because of the infection before we found this "vinegar wonder", but we are thankful to God, now his ear is totally healed."

Fever, Flu,
Sore Throats, and Coughs

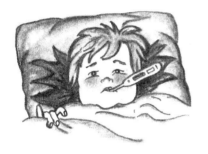

Fevers

Let's take a look at fevers. One of the first questions health care providers ask, (even I do this), is "How high is the fever?" This leads you to believe that the fever is the way to tell how sick they are. It is not.

One of the most serious children's illnesses, meningitis, does not manifest with a high fever. Fever only indicates that there is infection present. Unless there are other symptoms present such as extreme listlessness, respiratory difficulty, or abnormal behavior, high fever is not an indicator for immediate doctor visits.

A normal temperature is anywhere from 96.6 - 99.4. It may fluctuate according to the time of day. An elevation of one degree higher is normal for every evening. Fevers are not usually the dangerous things that you have been led to believe they are. They are not usually "bad" and they usually do not need to be lowered.

Your newborn should **not** run a fever. If it does check to see if you have dressed it too warmly. Overdressing is the first cause of fever in a newborn. Try unwrapping the baby and taking off a layer of clothes to see if that makes a difference. If your newborn has an infection it can be serious! Do not panic but call your midwife or doctor to get their advice.

Facts About Fevers

Most fevers are caused by viral or bacterial infections. The body will work without medical help in *most* of these cases. These infections can cause fevers up to 105 degrees. Today more and more doctors are honest enough to tell moms that even this fever is no cause for alarm.

Most of the elevated temperatures that are **serious** are a result of poisoning, toxic substances, or heat stroke after exposure to too much heat, including the jacuzzi. Temperatures from these conditions above 105 may result in lasting bodily harm. You will need help in these cases. Get it immediately. Here are a few important bits of information about fevers.

Fevers can dehydrate a sick child and you need to be aware of what needs to be done to keep the child from dehydrating. Dehydration can happen quickly from excessive perspiration, vomiting, and diarrhea. Prevent this by giving the child (a middle-sized one- 85 lbs) 6 oz. to drink every hour. A smaller child (40 lbs) will need 3 oz. every hour. A little child (20 – 30 lbs) will need at least one to two ounces every hour. Use only clear fluids, particularly water and tea, and small amounts of real fruit juice. These can be frozen into pops and sucked or blended into a slushy. Try not to give your child Tylenol or Ibuprofen to lower the fever. This will only make the illness take longer. Reserve these medicines for seldom uses! Studies are showing that they are harmful to the liver and are not the harmless pills we have thought that they are.

Fever can help most viral infections go away more quickly than medicine. There is nothing the doctor can do to dispose of a viral infection any quicker than you can. In fact, you can actually help it go more quickly and I will tell you how. Medication often interferes with the bodies attempt to get well since it suppress the fever. God has given us this way of handling and fighting disease and it is perfectly normal. When an infection develops, your body manufactures additional white blood cells and leukocytes that destroy viruses and bacterias. Fever increases the activity of these cells and they move rapidly to the site of the infection. This part of the process is called leucotaxis. It is stimulated by the release of pyrogens that raise the body temperature.

When you lower the temperature by giving Tylenol or Ibuprofen, etc., you simply make the process take longer or even hinder it. Fight off the urge that all moms have, to get rid of the fever by medicating. Where did you get that urge anyway?

Since there is no consistent relationship between the height of the child's fever and the severity of his illness, it is useless to take his temperature every hour. It only alarms you and the child.

If the child displays unusual behavior and has a high fever, check for these things:

☒ Blueness around the mouth or fingernails. This indicates an oxygen lack as in pneumonia. **Seek medical attention immediately!**

- 🕱 Dehydration - this warrants **immediate hydration and close attention. Ask someone knowledgeable to check if you are not sure.**

- 🕱 Arching the neck backward, or a seriously stiff neck along with other symptoms - possible meningitis. **Get medical help immediately.**

- 🕱 Broken capillaries all over the body, tiny pin sized dots or signs of bruising. Possible meningitis. **Immediate help is needed.**

God has placed a fever control device in our bodies that will keep them from exceeding 106. Unless, of course, there is poisoning or heat exposure. These override this mechanism.

What can you do instead to make your child comfortable?

- ✗ Nourish the child so that his body will fight the sickness off better.

- ✗ Give him lots of liquids, rest, and nourishing herbs to support his immune system.

- ✗ Do this faithfully as often as every hour, depending on the severity of the illness.

- ✗ If the fever is making the child quite uncomfortable, give him lots of love and cuddling along with your other treatments. Touching (back rubs, holding etc.) stimulate endorphins which in turn stimulate the immune system to fight back more efficiently.

- ✗ If the illness seems to be really severe and you want to hasten its demise, think about using the good, old-fashioned, ginger-bath. (See chapter on ginger.) It really helps with the aches and pains and gets the poisons speeding out of the body! Give the bath nice and hot (comfortably hot) and stay with the child (or adult) the whole time! Give him drinks of nice, warm peppermint tea. Do not overheat your patient! If he complains of a headache, put a cold wet wash cloth on his head and get him out of the bath and tucked into his bed snugly.

Convulsions

High fevers will not cause convulsions! Convulsions are **not** related to how high the fever is but to **how rapidly** it rises. Also, this kind of convulsion is seldom serious although, it is often frightening to the parents. Anything the doctor could do would be given too late to prevent the quick rise, anyway. Children over five seldom have this kind of febrile convulsion. For some reason or other, maturing bodies usually are better able to control the fever rise. Doctors are taught to prescribe Tegretol, Dilantin, and Depakote for febrile seizures, but this practice is not a good one when you consider the side effects of these drugs, the seldomness of which this type of convulsion occurs, and the age that it is usually outgrown. A seizure is the response to an abnormal electrical discharge in the brain. Anything that irritates the brain, like a fever, can produce a seizure. Two thirds of people who experience a seizure never have another.

Before you rush to the doctor in a panic for a fever seizure, use Lobelia tincture. Lobelia tincture rubbed on the spine, the soles of the feet, and dribbled slowly into the mouth - ¼ dropper, will usually stop a seizure in its tracks. Lobelia is a relaxing herb and used at that dose for a 40 pound child you should not have any problems. **Use only a few drops for a baby.** If you are worried about the fever and want to bring it down, do it without drugs. Try some of the following ideas.

Chamomile Implant

Try a lukewarm chamomile implant using a blue bulb syringe. (see chapter on chamomile) This usually has immediate results.

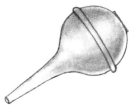

Or try the following tea.

Herbal Fever Remedy

1 ounce dried elder flowers
1 ounce dried peppermint leaves
½ pint distilled water

Mix the herbs. Place in a quart saucepan. Pour 1/2 pints of distilled boiling water over it. Cover and allow to steep in a hot place for ten to fifteen minutes (**do not boil**). Strain and sweeten if desired.

The herbal fever remedy drops high temperature associated with flu quite effectively. In some cases, the temperature has been reduced from 104 to 99 degrees within two hours! According to Dr. Edward E. Shook, a well known herbalist, "There is no remedy for colds and fevers of any description equal to this simple formula."

I would save this tea for use in the evening so that the fever can do the work that it should and you can all get a good night's rest.

Vinegar to Reduce Fever

One lady reports, "When I was an infant, the doctor told my mom I was going to die due to a particularly high fever and prolonged illness. She was told by an elderly friend to soak a wash cloth in apple cider vinegar and place one on my forehead and one on my stomach. Though it smelled a lot, it worked so well that my mom was able to check me out of the hospital. From that day onward, this remedy has been helpful to all the children in our family when they have high fevers. It takes about an hour to break the fever after you apply the vinegar." This was a well-known remedy that the old folks used. It still works today.

Dehydration

The subject of dehydration is very important. When you have a sick child or baby, particularly a small one, **you must be careful about dehydration. You must push fluids.** Nurse more often and give more drinks. Do it gently, but very often. Make it a tender, loving time, but do it.

A child that is dehydrated becomes listless, pale, and his skin is looser and kind of floppy. Check him in the plumpy areas, like his forearms and his legs, for this. Gently pinch the skin and see if it is loose or normal. Try not to get to this place, but if you do, **you must do something immediately to reverse it.**

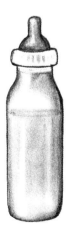

You must give fluids and/or retention enemas. If you are not successful, **you need medical help**. Use electrolyte type fluids to help balance the lost minerals and potassium that the child needs. Red Raspberry Tea, Flu Tea, or Emergen-C are good choices here. Stir the Emergen-C in juice or water and sip it slowly.

Dangers of Dehydration

Hydrating is especially important in a young child 3 or under, and DOUBLY important if you insist on giving fever medication, like Tylenol. *See A Pill for Every Ill.

I talked to a mother one day who had a toddler with a fever. If I remember correctly, he was about eighteen months old. She asked whether to take him to the doctor or not, and I explained what I believe about fevers and how to hydrate the child to make him comfortable and help him get well. I told her how to test for dehydration. She heard my advice and went on her way. The next thing I knew, her little one was critically ill in the Intensive Care Unit. What had gone wrong?

Unbeknownst to me, the mother delivered a new baby at home, the day following our phone conversation. In the excitement and busyness of the new baby, no one remembered to really hydrate the little fellow and he collapsed. He was seriously ill. It took quite a few days in Intensive Care to bring him back to where he could go home. In fact he was so ill that they nearly lost him in the hospital. I tell this story to emphasize my point. Hydration is of extreme importance in helping a sick child or baby get well, especially one with a high fever, or a fever and diarrhea. The key is a little liquid very often.

If you are nursing, nurse often. If the child drinks from a cup give him sips every fifteen minutes when he is awake. You cannot afford not to.

Flu

Influenza, commonly referred to as the flu, is an infectious disease caused by RNA virus. The name *influenza is* Italian and means "influence". The most common symptoms of the disease are chills, fever, muscle aches, severe headache, sore throat, coughing, and weakness. Sore throat, fever, and coughs are the most frequent symptoms. In more serious cases, influenza causes pneumonia which can be fatal, particularly for the young and the elderly. Although it is often confused with other flu-like illness, especially the common cold, influenza is a much more severe disease than the common cold and is caused by a different type of virus. It may produce nausea & vomiting, particularly in children, but these symptoms are more common in unrelated gastroenteritis, which is sometimes called "stomach flu" or "24-hour flu".
Typically, influenza is transmitted through the air by coughs or sneezes. Infection can

also occur through contact with body fluid or through contact with contaminated surfaces. Influenza viruses can be inactivated by sunlight, disinfectants, and detergents. Since the virus can be inactivated by soap, frequent hand washing reduces the risk of getting the infection. Here are a few things that you can do to make yourself comfortable and shorten the duration of the flu. Do not do them all but choose one or more and be diligent.

➤ Elderberry Extract – you can make your own. (See the chapter "Herbal Medicine".) In a 1995 Israeli study, <u>elderberry extract</u> was found to reduce both the severity of symptoms and the duration of flu (two to three days in the treated group versus six days in the placebo group). This herb contains two compounds that are active against flu viruses. It also prevents the virus from invading respiratory tract cells. - *Take one spoonful every two hours – adult dose*

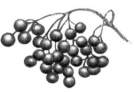

➤ Vitamin C – *take at least 1000 milligrams an hour for a day or more as needed.*

➤ Fire Water - *you can take it every fifteen minutes.* *See chapter on cayenne

➤ Echinacea – especially tincture from the fresh root. Echinacea has been a traditional favorite for colds and flu. Double blind studies in Germany show that flu-like symptoms clear more rapidly when taking echinacea. Echinacea appears to work by stimulating the immune system. *Take 2-4 droppers every hour for a few hours and then 4 times daily till better.*

➤ Garlic is known to kill influenza virus in test tubes. It also stimulates the immune system and wards off complications such as bronchitis. It contains several helpful compounds, including allicin, one of the plant kingdom's most potent, broad-spectrum antibiotics. This herb's aromatic compounds are readily released from the lungs and respiratory tract, putting garlic's active ingredients right where they can be most effective against cold viruses. Take several cloves of raw garlic per day during an infection. Aged garlic extract does not work as well. You can also use Super Duper Tonic (see Garlic chapter).

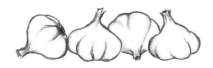

The following are guidelines on how to take your Tasty Echinacea, Hot Echinacea, and Super Duper Tonic. (You can take echinacea and Super Duper Tonic at the same time.)

> ➢ *For preventive immune boosting with no current health problems: Use two droppers, about 60 drops, five times daily until you have consumed two fluid ounces or 60 milliliters.*
>
>   *This will take about seven days. Do this if your family has been exposed to the flu.*

> ➢ *You have that "uh-oh" feeling, "No specific symptoms but I think I'm coming down with something": Use four droppers, about 120 drops, five times daily until you have consumed two fluid ounces or 60 milliliters. This will take three to four days. Start immediately.*

> ➢ *Onset of fever, chills or any of the symptoms of a cold or flu Use four droppers, about 120 drops, eight times daily (or every other waking hour) until you have consumed two fluid ounces or 60 milliliters. This will take about two days. You may continue this dosage for a week and then reduce it.*

> ➢ *High Fever, Sore Throat, Yellow Mucous, Coughing, Sneezing: Use four droppers, about 120 drops, every hour you are awake (about sixteen times a day) until you have consumed two fluid ounces or 60 milliliters. This will take about one day. You may do this for two to three days before you lower your dose.*

Make your own medicine like I recommend in "Making Medicine for your Family" and you will find that it will be cheaper and easier to get well than you ever thought.

Strep and Sore Throats

In 2003, the CDC started a program called, "*Get Smart: Know When Antibiotics Work.*" This is a $1.6 million dollar campaign to educate people about the overuse and the misuse of antibiotics. CDC warns that 90% of upper respiratory infections, including children's ear infections, are viral, and antibiotics do not treat viral infections. So before you run to the doctor, learn all you can.

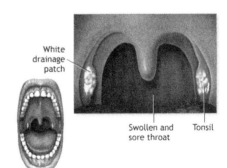

White drainage patch

Swollen and sore throat   Tonsil

Yes, most sore throats are caused by viruses! And,

once again, modern medicine has NO cure for viruses. Strep throat is a contagious disease caused by infection with *streptococcal* bacteria. Most strep throats can be identified by pus on the tonsils, swollen glands, and a temp of 103 in a child. The throat is usually red and swollen. (If there is no respiratory difficulty there is no danger of diphtheria. This disease is rare, anyway.) Some folks talk a lot about it causing rheumatic fever but this almost never happens, so do not worry. Strep throat may produce mild or severe symptoms. You can get your throat cultured for strep but the in office strep cultures are not really reliable and, lastly, the scare over getting rheumatic fever after strep throat is a fairly remote possibility.

Viral sore throats will usually respond to your home remedies very well, and in a few days everything will be fine. Bacterial strep infections respond to antibiotics in two to four days but will usually respond to home treatments in the same amount of time if you start treating promptly. Therefore the doctor is not usually needed.

Although antibiotics can shorten the course of strep, they also greatly enhance the likelihood of reoccurring strep all winter long. You see, while it kills the strep, it also works against the natural antibodies that fight disease and infection. When the body is allowed to fight by itself aided by nourishing herbs, it creates it's own antibodies that help the child to fight that disease the rest of the year.

I try to treat any sore throat **promptly,** thereby usually eliminating **serious** sore throats, though sometimes we miss it. Remember that treating a sore throat immediately often stops the infection in its tracks.

The cheapest, old fashioned remedy is to gargle with salt water.

Make a solution of 1/4 teaspoon salt to 1/4 cup of very hot tap water. Stir to dissolve the salt and then gargle the whole thing, spitting out the solution between each gargle. Do this up to every hour if needed.

Salt is very healing and really fights those germs that are growing in the throat. A few grains of cayenne in the water will aid the effectiveness.

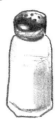 Take lots of vitamin C, *up to 1,000 mg. an hour for adults, and garlic and echinacea. For a child, remember to put their weight over 150 to determine how much to give. i.e. 50/150 = 1/3 dose. So mix up a packet of 1000 mg. in one glass of water and give them 1/3 cup every hour if needed.*

Work on the glands in the neck and the throat, massaging them with Deep Tissue Oil, Unkers or Vicks to get the lymph flow moving. Do this often (hourly) throughout the day. If the sore throat persists, my Throat and Tonsil gargle or Fire Water (*See Cayenne chapter), usually works very well. I would not be without Throat and Tonsil. We try salt water first and if that helps, we stop there. But we never let it go long before we use the Throat and Tonsil. Throat and Tonsil is a tincture made from fresh echinacea, fig syrup, cayenne, and peppermint oil, and it really works where many other things fail. *See Making Medicine chapter.

I have given it to folks who have had chronic strep throat and have had antibiotic after antibiotic. They finally came for help with throats so sore that they could hardly swallow. Two, at the most three, days of this treatment sent the sore throat away for good for that winter for most folks. Gargle and swallow two to three droppers of the liquid as often as every hour. We usually dilute the stuff in a little water so it is not too hot. You want it to be healing so do not dilute it much. Experiment. Taste it straight first. It may be hot but it will not damage you. For a smaller child, I would use one dropper with three - four droppers of water and have him gargle and swallow. The peppermint in it helps to put out the fire in your throat. The echinacea and cayenne in it help to get your immune system up and running.

Strep Throat Story

One lady came because her 19 year old son had been off work for a number of days with a seriously sore throat. It was inflamed and painful, and he was not eating; it hurt too much to swallow. She went home with a 4 oz. bottle of Throat and Tonsil and instructions to take some every hour along with 1000 mg. of vitamin C. He was to swish and swallow. If he wanted to speed the healing he could gargle with salt water in between. This morning she called to tell me that his throat is nearly healed but the tincture was gone! Should he get more? He could have but I recommended continuing with the vitamin C every hour and using an hourly salt water gargle to finish it up. That is cheaper and it usually works!

Coughs

Wild Cherry Cough Syrup

I like to make wild cherry cough syrup for anyone older than one year. It is one of the simplest ways to stop a dry, hacking cough.

Fill a quart jar with shredded wild cherry bark. Fill it again with vodka or brandy. Do not worry about the alcohol. You will distill almost, if not all of it, when you simmer this mix with honey. Anyway – most over-the-counter cough syrups have at least 5 – 7% alcohol, nighttime cough syrups have 15- 20 % and so do most asthma medicines. This will have less. Let it set for three weeks. Then strain it in a kettle and add the same amount of honey. Heat until the honey is melted and then simmer about five minutes.

Wild cherry bark makes the best syrup that I know of to quiet a cough. I make my own and try to have some to share. Do not use this for children under one because of some concern about honey and botulism.

Lemon and Honey

Another old remedy is to use equal amounts of lemon juice and honey and heat until nice and warm. Dribble this down your sore throat a spoonful at a time. If you use raw honey and do not make it too hot, it has very good antibacterial properties as well as being soothing! (Heat will kill these properties.)

An antibacterial cough syrup that you can make is lemon and honey heated together. Add one to two drops of thyme oil per tablespoonful of the mixture. Stir well and take it about three times a day. This should also help a sore throat.

I also rub the chest with Deep Tissue Oil, and if there is a congestion problem I use an onion poultice (see Onion) or Garlic Salve, rubbing the chest and between the shoulder blades on the back.

Understanding
the Immune System

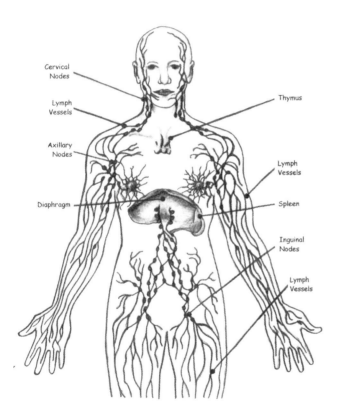

Cervical
Nodes

Lymph
Vessels

Axillary
Nodes

Diaphragm

Thymus

Lymph
Vessels

Spleen

Inguinal
Nodes

Lymph
Vessels

Take a look at this diagram to see how your lymph system serves your body. If you understand this, what I am about to say will make more sense to you.

You need to understand how the immune system works so that you are better prepared to deal with life, health, and illness. The immune system is the body's safety net. Every day potentially harmful virus, bacteria, and other pathogens enter our bodies.

We are protected from these by our bodies' marvelous defense system. Whether or not we get sick depends on our defense system. Understanding the lymphatic system is important to understanding how our immunity works. The lymph system transports lymph, a clear, colorless liquid, to all parts of the body. It resembles the circulatory system because it is composed of a network of lymphatic vessels similar to arteries. Unlike the circulatory system, it has no pump like the heart to keep the lymph flowing.

Keep the Lymphatic System Moving

Lymph nodes are collection centers located along the pathways of the lymphatic system. There are a few single nodes, but most of them are in clusters. There are clusters of them in the region of the neck below the jaw. When you have a tooth infection or a sore throat these nodes swell. This swelling is caused by an accumulation of toxins. As the lymph is filtered, special white blood cells called macrophages, remove bacteria and other foreign matter. The swollen nodes indicate that the lymph system is working to overpower the bacteria or other germs. (*No need to get alarmed! Just start treating.*) Defense against bacteria is accomplished by biological filtration. Special cells alter the content of the lymph fluid, preventing the spread of infection through the body.

Researchers are just beginning to understand and demonstrate that your ability to remain healthy and disease free is in large part related directly to how efficient your body is at circulating lymphatic fluids and dealing with the toxins and other materials that it contains. I like to do a number of things to enhance lymphatic circulation when I begin to feel a bit under the weather or when my lymph nodes are enlarged.

 - Take a brisk walk

 - Drink lots of extra liquid, especially water and herb tea.

 - Rub the swollen areas with **Sensei** or some other salve that will increase circulation.

 - Take a hot ginger bath and drink hot ginger or peppermint tea while in the bath. This increases circulation dramatically enhancing lymph flow.

In <u>Lymphing Toward Health</u> – Dr. David Williams M.D., Jan. 2006, writes: "It is important to know where the lymph nodes are located. They are most easily located in the armpits, groin, neck, under the jaw, the tonsil, and the abdomen. Watch for swelling and tenderness in the areas on the picture included. They are clues that the body may be fighting infection. When the swelling recedes, the infection has run its course. If this inflammatory response does not get rid of the toxins and the condition remains and becomes chronic then damage occurs at the cellular level and tumors and cancers may form."

One tell-tale sign of poor lymph flow is fluid retention. It results in puffiness of the hands, feet, ankles and face. This can often be eliminated by drinking more water and exercising moderately.

When your body has a toxic overload and the toxins do not move along, the body develops infection. To maintain a sound immune system the body needs water, a balanced diet, good bowel habits, and exercise to move these fluids along. About 70% of these lymph vessels are in or just under your skin. Therefore excess washing, particularly with scented soaps, and the use of lotions and perfumes leave your skin vulnerable because you have destroyed the protective bacteria that lives there. Do not use anti-bacterial soaps for this reason, and if you have to have contact with lots of soaps and detergents, use gloves.

Exercise

Exercise is so important. During exercise the muscles contract and help circulate the lymph throughout the body. You will need to do it for at least ½ hour to really get the benefit, but any exercise will help to circulate the lymph.

Deep breathing helps, along with hearty, sustained exercise. This should happen from one half to one hour daily to do its job well.

Wear Loose Clothing

Keep the lymph flowing for good breast health, too. We now know that wearing a bra 14 hours daily increases the hormone prolactin which decreases circulation to the breast area. This greatly increases the risk of breast cancer. Ladies from cultures that do not wear bras most of the time have almost no breast cancer. If you you wear a bra during the day do NOT use them to sleep at night. From <u>Shore up Immunity</u> by Dr. David Williams: Do not wear tight fitting or underwire bras at any time. They cut off lymph flow and make you more susceptible to breast cancer.

In *Dressed to Kill: The Link Between Breast Cancer and Bras*, the authors reported that women wearing a bra 24 hours daily had a 3 in 4 chance of developing breast cancer. Women who wore their bras all day but not to bed had a 1 in 7 risk, women wearing their bras less than 12 hours a day, a 1 in 152 risk and women who rarely or never wore one had a 1 out of 168 risk of developing cancer. Nursing is also one of God's ways to help a woman have good lymph flow and circulation to the breast area. In addition to that do daily breast massage if you have any breast tenderness or lumpiness. Gentle massage in a circular motion is a great aid to lymphatic flow.

Avoid Antiperspirants

Another simple thing that most folks do not think about is that of antiperspirants. Antiperspirants hinder sweating. "Of course! That's what they are supposed to do," you say. But when you hinder sweating, the lymphatic system cannot eliminate the toxins that it is supposed to in the sweating process. These toxins back up, often resulting in swollen lymph nodes. Sometimes the breasts get lumpy and tender, too. When the lymph is not circulating freely in the upper body, many difficulties result, like poor breast health, very sore areas under the arms, and even tumors in the upper body area. Instead of using antiperspirants daily, try washing well and using a baking soda rinse to make the area alkaline and discourage unfriendly bacteria that wants to grow there.

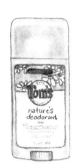

We have two interesting first hand accounts on this from close relatives. One of them was having difficulty with soreness under his arms. It was getting worse and no matter what he did it did not clear up. His wife finally suggested that it might be his anti-antiperspirant. He vigorously objected to doing without antiperspirants since he sweats so much. A short time later, however, he agreed to try since nothing else was working. He washed daily with **baking soda water** and went to work. Immediately his skin began to heal. Soon the whole thing was history and the young man decided to try and experiment. Once again he would use antiperspirants. Once again, the whole trouble came back to haunt him. He now uses a crystal based natural deodorant.

Another cousin worked hard in a very warm environment and sweated a lot. She dealt with customers and was embarrassed at the odor, so she resorted to using deodorants. In a short time she got so sore under her arms that her dresses were uncomfortable. She tried all sorts of things to heal up her skin, to no avail. When she switched to a **baking soda** wash instead of deodorant, the odor was gone and the soreness went with it.

Drink More Water

Plenty of fresh, pure water really helps the lymph flow. If you do not get enough water, your body will dehydrate and your lymph will not flow well. Toxins will back up in your system and you will begin to feel tired and weary. If you do not remedy the problem you may well become ill or manifest some chronic disease. Be sure that you get enough water to drink. Most people in America do not drink enough. What is enough? A normal person needs at least 8 – 8 oz. glasses daily. A man who works hard, a pregnant or nursing mother, or a person with health problems, needs from 12-16 or more glasses daily. Dehydration is a chronic problem in America. Many, many illnesses can be resolved and healed more quickly with increased water intake. Constipation, arthritis, asthma, chronic headaches, and bladder infections almost disappear if a person has a good water intake. Try it and see the difference. Start with 3 quarts daily and add about 3/4 teaspoon of salt to your diet or take a pinch at a time on your tongue and you will be pleasantly surprised at your success. When a nasty headache starts, head for the water. **Put a nice pinch of salt on your tongue and drink three cups of water immediately.** Your headache may well disappear within 10 minutes. The dehydrated brain shuts down and sends signals to the body to conserve energy so that it can survive. It does this effectively by sending you to the couch or your bed and making you lie very still so that you will not use up any more water than you must. Of course if you were out late last night, you may need to go and sleep for an hour or two to clear up the headache. Remember, pain is always a signal that the body is not working properly. Read the book, <u>Your Body's Many Cries For Water</u> by Dr. Batmanghandi, M.D.

Eat a Balanced Diet

A balanced diet is an aid to a healthy immune system. Not only do modern methods of producing, packaging, and distributing foods destroy many of the valuable nutrients that we need to nourish our bodies, but most packaged and processed foods contain ingredients that are harmful to us. These additives, like Monosodium Gultamate, or "MSG", actually cause us to crave the food and eat more of it. Aspartame and high fructose corn syrup are additives that actually damage our bodies. Americans have not learned to eat the foods that are really good for them. We crave the foods that suppresses our immune system and make us gain weight. This in turn affects how we plan our meals, and how we teach our children to eat. Most of us think that a day without sugar and white flour is intolerable! We are sure we need it to be happy! But what about healthy?

A good diet begins with a good meal. A good meal includes the following:

* A large green salad eaten first

*one serving of protein (meat, cheese, eggs, beans, or nuts)

*one serving of starch or carbs

(dried beans, grains, potatoes, pasta, rice)

*one green vegetable and a colored vegetable

If you fill your plate with an attractive salad, some lightly steamed vegetables, a little meat, and fruit for desert, you are not likely to miss sweet, carb-rich foods.

The following foods are not helpful to our health because they lower the immune response: sugar, white flour, white flour pasta, white rice, caffeine, and sodas. They cause us to get sick more quickly. Did you ever notice that this often happens after the holidays? That is because we often tend to overload on these items then.

Ponder what would happen if you only ate the things that built up your bodies defenses. Many years ago, the people in this country ate that way, and the incidence of heart disease was very low. Diabetes was almost unheard of, and now it has reached alarming proportions. Once diabetes was an older person's disease. Now it is affecting many children. Why? One has only to look at the TV commercials and in the fridge of most homes to understand the reason. The processed food industry of America has become the foe of good health and a strong immune system. Take a look at the normal grocery cart in front of you at the check out. It is filled with at least one case of soda, a few boxes of cereal, bags of chips, packages of cookies, instant soups and puddings, and very few fruits, vegetables, and whole grain products.

Unbiasedly evaluate the nutritional content of the food in that cart. It is not good! Worse than that it is harmful, disease causing food. Is it any wonder that a large majority of the children you see are overweight. They are not eating right and they sit at the TV instead of working and playing like children should.

Children are eating food that farmers would not feed to their livestock. One old doctor was checking out a farm family who was experiencing constant sickness that winter. He asked them what their diet consisted of. Then he asked them what they were feeding their prize cattle. When he received the answer, he said, "Go down to the barn and bring up a large amount of the corn and oats and feed them to your family. Take the food in your pantry and your fridge and feed that to your cattle." "No way," the farmer exploded. "That would kill my cattle." Then he grinned, wryly. "I get your point," he said sheepishly. That family changed their way of living and their health got better. We all believe that we are affected by what we eat, but most of us do not really take it seriously. If you ponder the above advice, and begin to live by it you may be surprised at the results!!

Get Enough Rest

To be healthy we need enough rest. Most of us do not really understand how important regular, sufficient rest is to our spiritual, mental, and physical health. Studies prove that we are more healthy if we get sleep before twelve o'clock A.M. For happy, healthy children see that they get ten hours of sleep. This is an added protection so that they do not get every bug that comes along. Studies show the importance of naps. Naps for small children and naps for busy mothers make a great difference in how smoothly the home runs. You may tell me that you do not have time to take a nap. As a homeschooling mother of 9 busy children, I will tell you that you do not have time **NOT** to take a small nap in the middle of the day when your baby and toddlers are sleeping and your older children are having quiet reading time. This rest refreshes your mind and body and spirit. It helps to give you the ability to be a sweet mother at 5:30 in the evening when supper needs to be put on the table, your children are hungry, and your husband is due home 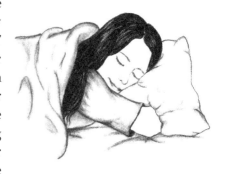 any minute. You may need to let something go, but get a bit of rest and stay well physically and emotionally.

Have a Clean Bowel

Constipation really slows lymph movement. Make sure you have at least two, easy bowel movements daily. Water, fruits and veggies and exercise really helps to accomplish this more easily.

Notes:

Understanding
Colon Health

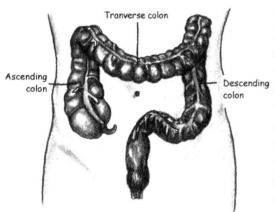

Ascending colon · Tranverse colon · Descending colon

Colon health is a very important part of being healthy. You are only as healthy as your colon. Look at it this way: Your colon is your way of eliminating all the toxins, poisons, and refuse that your body does not need and want. As long as this river keeps running and empties well, daily, you will do well. Should this river become backed up and sluggish, your whole body will suffer. When you understand how to keep your elimination working properly, you will find that many disturbing problems simply vanish and your total health is better. Think of is this way: Would you let your garbage from today set on the sink for three days without emptying it? What would happen? It would rot and smell and draw flies. It would be disgusting. The same is true of a colon that does not empty well at least once, preferably two times daily. Think about what a new baby does. It fills its diaper after every nursing. Its plumbing is not clogged yet.

Many years ago someone told me that I should be "going" ("moving my bowels"), at least twice a day, and I thought that they were extreme. I was healthy and I went, well . . . maybe every other day. Now I look back and realize that I had terrible acne, serious menstrual cramps, my feet smelled and I was always tired. I was constipated. As we have begun to teach this colon health to our children we find that acne is almost completely resolved, the teen-age smelly feet go away, and everyone is happier and in a better mood. Simply put, when you have a backup of garbage, your whole body suffers. Your head aches, you have migraines, monthly cramps, brain fog and the grumps. Try working on your "plumbing" and see what all clears up in a few weeks. Not only this, but colitis (infection in the colon), appendicitis, diverticulitis (infected polyps in the colon), and difficulties like irritable bowel syndrome, Chrohn's disease, and a whole host of other symptoms begin to resolve without any drugs at all. It is truly amazing how the whole body works together.

How do we achieve this kind of elimination so that we can become healthy?

- ☒ Go when you get the urge. Fighting the urge trains the colon not to empty when it should and it becomes sluggish. This is something that most of us need to work at.

- ☒ Drink more than eight cups of water daily.

- ☒ Eat a diet high in fiber and whole foods.

- ☒ Exercise regularly for at least thirty minutes a day.

When you do these things and you still do not go at least twice a day (once after your two main meals), then look at the next steps.

1. Start your day with two cups of water, preferably lukewarm with one tablespoon of fresh squeezed lemon juice. This stimulates the body to empty the colon.

2. Take an **herbal** laxative capsule or two (or tea) before you go to bed, increasing the amount each day, until you achieve this kind of regularity. Then, only use the herbal help if you get sluggish. Use Dr. Christopher's Lower Bowel Formula or American Botanical's Intestinal Formula #1, or Smooth Moves Tea from Traditional Medicinals.

3. Increase the amount of fresh fruits and salads in your diet. This helps tremendously and it tastes good!

Irritable Bowel Syndrome and Colitis

What if you already have IBS or colitis or rectal bleeding or any other problem related to colon health?

To heal a traumatized colon, begin by changing your diet dramatically. Cut out all sugar, white flour, and other processed foods. Take slippery elm powder, one teaspoon (not capsules),(or IBS powder – see recipe on next page) about twenty minutes before each meal and before bedtime. You can make a slippery spoonful or make it into little pellets and take it like pills. Take one fourth cup of aloe vera juice between meals and at bedtime. If that does not do the trick add two - three cups daily of comfrey tea or green drink. See this recipe in the Comfrey chapter. Sip over the period of the next hour, or drink as you like. This drink not only tastes good, it is very healing.

I worked with a man with Irritable Bowel Syndrome who was in quite a bit of pain. The pain was hindering his ability to work, what could he do? Of course there are a lot of things that one can do, like reducing the stress level and markedly increasing your fluid intake. But one of the next things on the list, simple, effective and inexpensive, is slippery elm. Slippery elm covers the inside of the intestinal tract with a smooth slippery coating that both nourishes and heals the inflamed intestinal walls. He added slippery elm to his diet four times a day, and began the road to recovery. It took him a few months to heal completely since he did not take the comfrey tea, too. But the last time I spoke with him, he was doing well, and only needed slippery elm occasionally.

Healing Powder for IBS

Mix together equal parts of powdered:

comfrey root, marshmallow root, licorice root, slippery elm powder

Add just enough water to make it into soft pie dough consistency. Roll this into large, pea-sized balls and take three every half hour, or one every five minutes if you are having serious runs. You can refrigerate these in a plastic bag to keep them from drying out so that they absorb more quickly.

This powder will help to heal things quickly. If you are bleeding, and there is fresh blood, that means you have lower bowel bleeding. If you are bleeding it will take a bit longer to heal, but you can achieve good results rather quickly if you are faithful. Add a few cups of comfrey - peppermint tea daily, and you will be surprised what it will do to heal your bowel. Comfrey will help to stop the bleeding, reduce inflammation and build new cells.

To address the cramps and pain of this difficulty, rub lobelia tincture on the area of your abdomen where the pain is. Repeat as often as necessary. Take only green drink and the slippery elm mixture for a few days to allow your bowel to heal.

I can hardly stress enough the importance of taking comfrey drink or tea, and the slippery elm mixture very faithfully, even up to every five minutes in severe cases. This will ensure rapid healing.

One gentleman that we worked with called with severe dysentery and no other symptoms but cramping, which we assumed was from the dysentery. We treated him with charcoal since we suspected food poisoning. He faithfully took the charcoal for two days but was no better. In fact, all the water he drank was running straight thru and he was visiting the bathroom every fifteen minutes or less and getting very weak. He called back and we rediscussed his case. He was in a lot of pain, he was also very weak by now. I encouraged him to go to the doctor, but he was adamant about staying home. I was at a loss, but then I thought of IBS. Was there any serious stress in the family? Yes. They were going thru a real trial. We took him a green drink, colon tea, and the slippery elm, comfrey, marshmallow powder pellets. We put him on a strict regime of no food, sips, and only sips, from one of the two drinks and a pellet of powders every five minutes. No big drinks to prevent things from going straight thru. We wanted to give his colon time to heal before he began to drink normally. We went our way after we had prayed with them.

Three hours later we checked on him by phone. He had no more hasty bathroom trips and the pain was still there. Was he taking sips every 5 minutes.? No. We put him on a timer and gave him orders to be very faithful. He was to rub on lobelia for the pain as needed. An hour and a half later we drove back to see him and found him much brighter. The pain was greatly improved and he had still not had any bathroom trips even when he had drunk a total of one and a half cups of tea and a cup of green drink (he had done this very gradually over a period of three hours) and had taken at least fifteen pellets of the powders. He was greatly encouraged.

IBS can come from stress and the above routine will help. But you must resolve your difficulty and learn to trust the Lord and rest in Him.

Most folks that I talk to about IBS say, "Oh, no, I am not constipated. I have diarrhea." Truth to tell, usually that kind of diarrhea is the result of clog higher up. So often the person is so clogged up higher that only the liquid portion of the bowel movement can come through. This is not always the case, but it often happens. So address the regular, soft, daily movements, follow the guidelines for good colon health, trust the Lord and watch your health get better.

If you need more help here is a colitis remedy that my help you.

Mix together:

4 oz. each of powdered licorice or marshmallow root, powdered comfrey root, and slippery elm.

Take one tablespoon, four times daily in juice or water. Do this for fifteen to thirty days.

For the next thirty days use one tablespoon of marshmallow root in the morning.

These herbs should not be in capsules in order to allow them to coat the stomach. If the problem is in your lower bowel, you can take it in capsules.

Also take:

1 capsule of grapefruit seed extract three times daily for fifteen days.

1 Tablespoon raw honey six times daily for thirty days.

1 teaspoon of the following tincture three times daily for fifteen days:

Mix together: 2oz. eucalyptus tincture

2 oz. goldenseal tincture

2 oz. acacia tincture

This will be bitter, so you can put it juice or in capsules. 5 caps = 1 teaspoon

Take 300 mg. Bismuth capsules three times daily for thirty days, or Pepto-Bismol in similar quantities. This facilitates faster healing time for ulcers.

Bismuth is harder to find than some things, so I have included the name that it goes by and a place to get it: Gastromycin - 150 capsules, by NutriCology.

VitaDigest.com seems to be the cheapest place to get these at this time.

Hours: 8:30AM ~ 05:00PM PST (11:30AM ~ 8:00PM EST)

Toll Free: 1-877-VITA168 (1-877-848-2168)

Constipation

Some folks have trouble with their little ones' bowel regularity, as well as their own. Understand that it is important to keep your children going regularly, too. Often a little extra water and more fiber in their diet will be all that's needed. If you have a little one that needs more help, add one fourth cup of prune juice, or three prunes, two times a day. If you still have problems, here is what you can do. Mix water into slippery elm powder. Do this slowly, like you would mix water into flour for gravy. When it is the consistency that you want, add a bit of maple syrup or honey to sweeten it. Give a tiny one (20 lbs) about one measuring teaspoon per meal and before bedtime. This should help to make the movement softer and more frequent. American Botanical's Intestinal Formula # 3 is a great help for little ones if other things do not work. It is a nice-tasting liquid formula. Use Intestinal Formula #1 (American Botanical Pharmacy p 324) or Dr. Christopher's Lower Bowel Formula to help the older ones in your family if you need it, for a little while. Chewable papaya tablets with each meal may really help to relieve this problem. You can also use a warm epsom salt bath at night to aid this.

Stay ahead of the problem and you will have happier children. I have been surprised at how few doctors understand how simple it is to get a child's bowels moving. Eating a few prunes and drinking a lot more water will often do what a doctor may suggest heavy laxatives or even surgery for. I am not exaggerating when I say that I have given the above advice in a number of cases where a doctor has suggested surgery for the bowel, and in a few weeks things were going well with the changes that the mother made with the child. Be patient, it does take time to make changes but in every case that I have worked with we have been able to achieve regularity. We will often start with Dr. Schultz Intestinal Formula #3 to get the child going and then make the other changes in his diet, while gradually cutting back on Forumla #3. It works!

If this does not work then check the diet. Unfortunately it often means the child has a gluten intolerance and you will need to cut the grains like wheat out of their diet for a bit until they are able to better digest them.

Diarrhea

Diarrhea, for little ones, can be quite disturbing and if left unchecked, even dangerous (because of dehydration). A bit of slippery elm after each bout of diarrhea will help dramatically to fix the problem. If you do not have slippery elm powder, try using a bit of cornstarch mixed with water, just like you were going to make gravy. This, too, will slow the process a bit and keep the child from dehydrating. If it does not, then look at the child's diet. Add a papaya tablet or two with each meal, and that alone may do the trick. If it does not help, then probably you are dealing with food allergies. This will take a whole new dimension of study. There is lots of information out there to help you find your way through that maze. *See baby care chapter for a quick review on food allergies. This is not as difficult as it sounds, but it does take commitment. I have had to work with my own "allergy babies" and it can be done. Adult diarrhea usually responds well to the same treatment unless the problem is the result of a bacteria or disease, and then it still does no harm. If the problem is bacteria or bad food, immediately take charcoal water. *See charcoal chapter.

Mix one tablespoon of powdered charcoal into one glass of water and drink the whole thing quickly. Follow this with another glass of water since charcoal can be constipating. Repeat the dose after each run to the bathroom and the problem is soon history.

Stomach Aches

When someone has a tummy ache you tend to reach for something to give him. Do not use over-the-counter medication for tummy aches if at all possible. Especially do not give antacids for this problem. Sodium bi-carbonate (baking soda) might help the immediate distress, but it often causes a problem because then the stomach will work overtime to replace the acid, thereby creating more than was there before.

Antacids also work against the calcium in your system, thereby depleting it. To help you know what to do for stomach aches try to determine what the problem is if you can. Ask the following questions:

1. What did you just eat?

2. When did you get the ache?

3. Do you have gas?

4. When did you last have a bowel movement?

5. Do you feel like throwing up?

6. How much water have you been drinking?

When you have determined the cause more closely, if you can, then work at the root of the problem. If it is a baby or small child and they are constipated, correct that. Also give them a good warm drink. All of these things will help to stimulate the bowels to move, often resulting in a happy tummy. If it is an older child or an adult, give him a laxative, lots of water and/or an enema, depending on the severity of the problem.

If you think the problem is gas, use very warm chamomile or peppermint tea, Digestive Tonic, or 1 drop of peppermint oil in a half glass of water. Any of these will definitely help gas. I think that Digestive Tonic works faster and better, probably because of the mix of herbs in it, but you can use whatever you have. Put two to three droppers of digestive tonic in a glass of room temperature water and sip it slowly. Usually you will begin to burp and or pass gas, and in ten minutes or less the ache will be gone! Digestive Tonic often helps an acid stomach, too. In fact it really works well to heal most acid reflux conditions.

If you use peppermint oil, do not use more than a drop diluted in ¼ glass of water, since peppermint oil is so strong, especially for a baby or small child. So while the peppermint oil helps, be sure to use it carefully and dilute it properly. If you, an adult want it stronger than that, dilute it a lot less and experiment until you find the right dose for you.

Acid Reflux Stories

I was called to check on a little one who was continually throwing up. She did not seem to be sick in any other way. Her vomit did not smell sour. I asked about her bowel habits and they were not regular, in fact they were very irregular. I gave her an enema which produced quite a bit of hard matter. Then I started her on digestive tonic for the acid reflux. As long as she took the digestive tonic in water, and some slippery elm, the problem was settled, but she needed to take the tonic for quite some months. Finally she outgrew the problem. Her smaller sister had the same problem and we used the digestive tonic to work on her acid reflux in the same way.

One day a visitor at church came up to me and asked me if I have any suggestions to help with acid reflux. A few years before, her daughter had been in a car accident. She had been seriously disemboweled and had spent a lot of time in the hospital and more time healing. Now she had serious problems with acid reflux and had been taking a strong drug so that she could live reasonably. I had just been reading about how the herbs in digestive tonic could help, so I gave her a bottle of it to experiment with. A month later she called to order another bottle and gave me a praise report! The stuff had worked! She ordered again and again. What a happy ending to a sad story!

Digestive Tonic

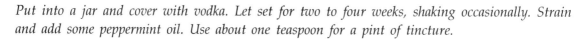

Here is the recipe for digestive tonic:

1 part ginger

1 part peppermint

1 part fennel

Put into a jar and cover with vodka. Let set for two to four weeks, shaking occasionally. Strain and add some peppermint oil. Use about one teaspoon for a pint of tincture.

Colic

A baby with gas will usually fall asleep in a few minutes after drinking an ounce or two of very warm, lightly sweetened chamomile tea. This tea will make them burp heartily or pass gas and they will feel quite comfy and sleepy. In fact, if you need to calm a restless baby just use very warm chamomile tea and your little one will soon be dozing off. Believe me, for I mothered six colicky babies who screamed far into the night, until I discovered chamomile tea. I used it with the last three, with wonderful results! I would never be without it. Even now the children who get gas pains go for a cup of hot chamomile tea!

Nausea

If you are dealing with nausea, digestive tonic may help the problem. In the case of stomach upset rather than ache, let them throw up! There is probably something in there that needs to come out! If you let them throw up, or even help them throw up, they will probably get well a lot faster. Most of that kind of stomach distress is caused by bacteria from food or flu and it needs to come out! But give them a cup a water with Digestive Tonic in it. It will help a little, and the horrible taste of throwing up will be somewhat relieved by the mint and ginger flavor of the tonic. See the recipe for

Digestive Tonic earlier in the chapter.

Sometimes just a drop or two of peppermint oil in a bit of water will help your nausea to go away. We get a good bit of help from charcoal water when we feel nauseous. *See chapter on charcoal. If you take a cup of the "gray" charcoal water at the first sign of nausea, and continue to take one every hour or so, it will often resolve a stomach "bug" before it gets you.

Another Story

Here is an interesting story that would also fit under constipation. Recently I worked (over the phone) with an older youth who was having nausea, stomach pain, and vomiting. She had been to a week-long Bible school and had eaten the diet of processed food served all week. She had little or no activity that week and not enough water. Her problem had begun a few days after Bible school was over. This led me to believe that it may be serious constipation, but to complicate matters there was also a stomach flu going around. She began to treat with lobelia rubbed on her tummy for pain, a charcoal/flax poultice for infection and pain, lots of hot tea, and some laxative capsules. Her pain level improved after a night and a morning of the routine, but she vomited again. I told the mother that I thought that she was likely very constipated (a blockage somewhere in the lower bowel). I was not sure, however, because of the vomiting, and since the mother was apprehensive, I recommended that unless she was willing to take drastic measures (a large dose of strong laxatives) immediately, she should go to the doctor. She opted to go to the doctor and called me back to tell me that yes, she did have a blockage and he had given her a strong laxative and she was feeling better. The doctor reiterated what I had told them on the phone, that with a blockage, the vomiting happens because the digested food cannot go on through so it has to come back up!

I recommended that the girl stay on a mostly liquid diet for a day or two so that her inflamed bowel could heal. Slippery elm tea or powder would help to soothe it and lots of water would help to keep her going.

Stomach Flu

The stomach flu is more difficult to work with. Be watchful so that the child does not dehydrate from continuous vomiting. Stop eating all foods and drinking other liquids immediately!

Make charcoal "gray water" (see chapter on charcoal), and administer it in small sips every five minutes. When they can keep that down for an hour switch to tea. Use only lightly sweetened yarrow tea, red raspberry, or black tea(such as Lipton). Do not give other foods or liquids. Give these liquids, by the tablespoon only, every five to ten minutes. If they can keep this down, increase the dose slowly until the person is able to tolerate more. Use toast and tea for the rest of the day if possible before you begin other solid food.

If you cannot stop the vomiting and diarrhea and your child begins to dehydrate, give small retention enemas of one of the above teas. A blue bulb syringe is very helpful for this. Use no more than two tablespoons to quarter cup of liquid, or the child will expel it and more besides, dehydrating himself even farther. When the vomiting settles, give echinacea - ½ tsp every hour depending on the size of the child. If you are nursing a baby, do not stop nursing! You can take some of these herbs and give him some droppers full of the teas if you wish!

Sometimes the upset is just diarrhea, then small amounts of slippery elm gruel or tea will help. Another simple remedy is: 1 teaspoon of cornstarch in a quarter to a half cup of water. Sip this slowly and it will usually stop the runs in short order.

Stop all dairy products and fruit, until the diarrhea is gone. Use the BRAT diet, Bananas, Rice, Applesauce and Toast. Emergen-C packets given in water help to replace the electrolytes.

Food Poisoning

We suggest that you drink straight two tablespoons of apple cider vinegar the moment you feel you might have food poisoning. Rinse your mouth out immediately so that the acid is not hard on your tooth enamel. Don't wait! Better yet, take it before going to a barbeque, or any event where the food may have been sitting around for a while.

In the case of food poisoning, we recommend unpasteurized apple cider vinegar as it is extremely strong. Grocery stores usually carry only commercial brands of ACV. Heinz apple cider vinegar will do. DO NOT DILUTE IT. However, be prepared for your throat and stomach to burn a bit! Make sure you brush your teeth with baking soda afterwards to protect your teeth. This is to protect the enamel from acid.

Or you could take a charcoal slurry if you have that. *See the chapter on charcoal. It

WILL do the trick if taken and repeated every half hour for two hours. You MUST drink LOTS of water if you do this treatment or you will become badly constipated.

Bladder Infections

Bladder infection, or cystitis, can feel like a stomach-ache or abdominal pain, or it can start with painful urination. This can usually be cleared up with immediate and careful attention. This problem can be more specific to ladies because of the way God made their anatomy. Use careful hygiene and use the bathroom often, especially before you go to sleep at night.

Drink more water! Lots and lots of water is necessary for your "plumbing" to work properly. Juice and soda are so sweet that they make the problem a lot worse. If you notice the beginning of an infection, drink and drink. Sometimes just drinking two to three cups full of nettle or lemon balm tea is all it takes. Three cups a day is very helpful, but drink a cup an hour if the problem is severe.

Cut out all sugar for a few days. Take 1000 mg. of vitamin C, acidophilus, and cranberry or blueberry concentrate or capsules every hour with the tea. I like to take about three droppers of KidneyBladder tincture which contains uva ursi, horsetail, nettles, and other herbs that are healing to the kidney and the bladder. I take this every hour for a few hours and usually in a day things are better. I keep a small squirt bottle of cranberry or blueberry concentrate in my fridge since I have one child that has trouble with cystitis. (She developed this problem after twenty-one days on antibiotics when she had Lyme disease.) When she gets the slightest burning feeling with urination she takes one teaspoon of blueberry concentrate and lots of water and she almost never has any further difficulty. Again, the key is to treat the symptoms as soon as they manifest. Do not put it off dealing with the infection and wait until it gets really severe.

Another simple, inexpensive remedy is charcoal water. Do not take it with any other thing that you are doing to help the infection or it will take that out of your system, too. Drink a quart of "gray water" daily for two days and it will usually help to resolve the infection. In fact, I find that it helps so much that I often do not need to take other things. *See charcoal chapter for gray water.

If you get a fever with this and chills you should go to the doctor. These symptoms may mean that the infection has traveled to your kidneys and you could have serious problems. If you are a person who tends to stick it out and fix it up yourself, you must be sure that you do get it fixed. This is not a thing to play with! You can land up being seriously sick!

Bladder infections often come from yeast, and although you can clear it up quickly with antibiotics, it is one thing that will tend to keep coming back to haunt you. If you do go to the doctor, do not do the regular ten-day course of antibiotic like he recommends. That will dispose you to get another one, by lowering your immune system.

Here is what Larrian Gillispie, M.D., recommends in <u>You Don't Have to Live with Cysitis.</u> Take a double dose of the antibiotic the first time and again four hours later. Then do NOT take any more.

He tells us the reason for this is to flood the bacterial pool in the bladder with the antibiotic and address the problem quickly. Then you can usually stop taking the medicine so that it will not hurt your bowel and kill all the good flora there. I have found that this really does work, and I like the idea of taking less antibiotics. It makes so much sense. But if you plan to do this be sure it is an antibiotic that you are not allergic to or you will have a problem.

If you follow my directions with herbs, you will not usually need to take antibiotics. But if you get into dire straits and do have to go for a prescription, Dr. Gillispie's way is better than assaulting your body with continued antibiotic. Drink a lot of water while you are doing this and it should cure the problem.

Appendicitis

Sometimes a tummy ache or pain is the forerunner of appendicitis. Appendicitis can happen to anyone. No one wants to have a ruptured appendix, so what are the signs? How can you know if it is appendicitis? Appendicitis is often accompanied by vomiting and fever in its later stages, but the vomiting may not be persistent and the fever may not be high.

The pain usually localizes in the lower right quadrant, meaning the bottom, lower right area of the abdomen. But this is not always true. It can be in any area. Apply deep pressure to the tender area, and let go quickly to see if the pain greatly intensifies. The doctor calls this "rebound tenderness". This is also usually accompanied by loss of appetite and sometimes vomiting. Can the person walk standing up straight, or does he double over and favor the one side? (It could be a urinary tract infection that causes this pain.)

One of the first things to do is to give the person two to three cups of hot chamomile or catnip tea *and STOP ALL FOOD*. If that does not do the trick in about fifteen minutes, use a lukewarm chamomile or catnip enema to help move his bowels. This can also be done by giving him a heavy dose of laxative. It usually takes a **heavy** dose.

Use Bowel Shot (American Botanical Pharmacy p 324), or ten - twenty capsules (adult dose) of his Intestinal Formula, five at a time over the period of two hours or until he eliminates, then stop the doses. Yes, I do mean fifteen to twenty for an adult that has not been eliminating well. If his bowels do move two times a day, use an enema instead. For a child use the child's weight/150 pounds. Example: 75/150 = ½ dose, which would be seven capsules. While they are waiting for their large bowel movement, rub the area with lobelia to relax the area and lessen the pain. The reason for the large dose of laxatives is the need to open the bowel immediately! I have tried using less for folks when they call me with appendicitis, but invariably an adult ends up needing to take that many, to my surprise. And please do use Dr. Schultz' formula because it is stronger than other formulas. **A bottle of those capsules in your medicine box might save you a hospital visit.**

Next make a charcoal/flax/castor oil poultice and warm it to lay over the sore area. *See the chapter on charcoal for poultice directions. In an hour, if the person has not had a bowel movement, give them five more capsules and another hot cup of tea. Rub them with lobelia again and reheat the poultice and reapply it. *See story in charcoal chapter. These procedures may save you thousands of dollars expense in an appendectomy and all the recuperation that follows. Please do  those things before going to the doctor. Here is the reason why: A clogged colon puts pressure on the appendix and makes it hurt, become inflamed, and sometimes swell. A clogged colon also allows toxins to leak out into the surrounding areas and these alone can inflame the appendix. A warm catnip or chamomile enema or laxatives and a poultice will relax the area and relieve the pain and allow a bowel movement to take place thereby giving some relief to the area. Do not kid yourself by saying that you do not have time. Do you know how long it takes to drive to the hospital, and how very, very long it takes in the hospital until you actually get the surgery. You have at least two - three hours, to do your work and still have a margin. Most folks find that when they do this, they can fix the problem.

Finally, do massage, gently working in from the sides to the navel and down from the navel to the pubic bone. Give more hot chamomile tea if you need to, to give the procedures time to work.

If you do all that you know how to do and the pain still persists, accompanied by fever and vomiting, then you must see the doctor. He will prescribe a blood test to check for infection and a scan to see if there is any obstruction in the bowel. This will all take at least two hours if you are fortunate. If all these tests are positive than the child will need an appendectomy.

If you can resolve the problem, the person has a large bowel movement and the pain subsides, you are on the way to recovery.

Now, give either Super Duper Tonic (two droppers every hour), or one clove chopped garlic hourly (in capsules if need be) for the next few hours to address the problem of stuff leaking from the appendix into the abdominal cavity. You do not want infection. This is important, but take it with a bit of toast or milk so that the stomach does not get upset. And keep your patient on a strictly liquid and toast diet for two days to prevent irritation to the bowel and to allow it to heal. We give slippery elm, either gruel or capsules, every three to four hours for the next two days. Use lots of fresh, unsweetened juice, preferably carrot and apple, to nourish the body and heal the colon. A few cups of comfrey tea daily will really speed up the healing too.

Let me tell you about our experience with appendicitis. This was my child who had chronic constipation problems as a small child. We did not know about the laxative capsules or the enema or charcoal poultices. We were only learning about home remedies when she got her severe belly ache. We gave her echinacea, garlic, and lobelia for a few hours, and then finally went to the hospital at 2AM, because we could not get the pain to go away, and she started throwing up and ran a fever. A blood test, yes, and a CAT scan. Yes, there was a problem. They had us wait until 7AM the next morning for surgery (five hours). And guess what – by that time all the things we had done had time to work and there was no inflamed appendix! He said, "That was the nicest appendix I ever operated on." He took the appendix out anyway, since she was cut open, but I learned a good lesson from that experience. Active treatment will often work and you usually have a few hours to do it in. *If things do not work you can still get help.*

Remember, constipation is the most common reason that people begin to have appendicitis. That is why it is important that your children have regular bowel habits.

Teach them to drink lots of water and give them a diet high in fiber. That will sometimes do the trick alone. For some children it is helpful to include a teaspoon of slippery elm in their diet three times daily. You can mix it with water and give it by the spoonful. Add a bit of maple syrup or sugar to improve the flavor. Remember to taste it yourself first, or give them three or four capsules of it daily. Prune juice or prunes usually will help this problem, too.

Steps for Resolving Appendicitis

- Do not give Tylenol or pain medication so that you can really tell if what you are doing has helped or not.

- You MUST follow these instructions very carefully or go to the hospital immediately. If you cannot resolve the pain you MUST go to the hospital.

- Stop ALL food.

- Give ONLY 100% juices and clear broth.

- Give fifteen to twenty capsules of Doctor Schultz -Intestinal Formula #1 or a bottle of Bowel Shot to empty the colon completely and take the pressure off the inflamed appendix (adult dose).

- Give a cup or two of hot chamomile tea to relax the person.

- Give an enema or two of chamomile or catnip tea, to relieve the pressure if needed.

- Put a warm castor oil, charcoal poultice (see charcoal chapter) over the area 24/7 until the pain is resolved and a good bowel movement has occurred.

- Rub the area with lobelia for pain.

- Do gentle massage on the area working in from the sides and down from the navel.

Stay on juices and clear liquids for at least two days to give the colon chance to heal.

Take 2-4 capsules of slippery elm 3-4 times for the next few days to soothe the inflamed colon.

Take some garlic with food or take Super Duper Tonic every few hours to address any infection that might have resulted from the infection.

Drink lots and lots of water and maybe take small amounts of prune juice to keep the bowel open. You need to really watch the bowel habits of this person for awhile to see that they continue to move freely. If not, they will be right back where they were before, with more pain and infection. If they learn to drink enough and keep their bowels moving they will develop habits that will help to keep them healthy for life.

If you tried the above ideas and the problem did not resolve you will definitely need other help. Do not hesitate to go for help when help is needed.

Understanding Kidney and Bladder Health

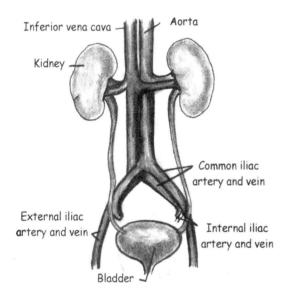

Inferior vena cava

Aorta

Kidney

Common iliac artery and vein

External iliac artery and vein

Internal iliac artery and vein

Bladder

Your urinary system is made of two kidneys, one bladder, and a series of tubes. The renal arteries bring blood to the kidneys to be filtered and cleaned. The renal vein returns cleansed blood to your body while the waste liquid leaves your body by the ureter which connects to the bladder.

The kidneys are located approximately at your waistline.

The kidneys filter the blood and regulate the acid/alkaline balance of the body. What is left in the remaining liquid is now called urine. Urine is about 95% water and 5% dissolved substances. The bladder has a normal storage capacity of about a quart or more.

Normally a person should urinate about 4-6 times a day. The average output is between 1 and 2 quarts daily. This of course, depends on how much you drink, how much you sweat, and how hot it is.

The color, transparency, and the odor of the urine tell us a lot about your kidney and bladder health. If you fail to drink enough your urine becomes darker in color and there is a stronger odor. This is hard on the kidneys and tends to give bacteria a chance to grow in the bladder and give you bladder infections.

Most of you are more aware of your kidney/ bladder health than of your liver health. You are because you can see what comes out and you can feel it very quickly if there is an infection.

Bladder Infections

Bladder infections can be very painful and cause a distinct burning sensation on urinating, or they can simply be felt as lower abdominal pain that you would not expect to be a bladder infection. Most of you will never need an antibiotic for a bladder infection if you learn to live with good kidney/bladder health in mind. Drink two quarts of water daily. If you are exercising, nursing, or if you are sick, then you need to drink more. When a person consumes too much sugar or processed foods, the acid/alkaline balance shifts, predisposing you to infections, and you need more water to help your body get well. Most people drink less than this at any given time. Coffee and sodas dehydrate the body by causing it to lose fluid. So if you have a caffeine or soft drink habit you are going to need to drink more water!

If you do get an infection in spite of careful living, what should you do? Treat it immediately. The more quickly that you treat any infection the more quickly you can resolve it. Here are some things that you can do. Start with the first one and add others if needed.

- ☒ Take 1000 mg of vitamin C every 2 hours. Emergen-C works quickly.

- ☒ Drink a cup of water every 15 minutes.

- ☒ Rub 3-4 drops of Frankincense oil over the pubic bone as soon as there is burning.

  Repeat every time you use the restroom. This is so easy. Carry it in your purse.

- ☒ Empty your bladder frequently to keep the bacteria at a minimum.

- ☒ Take 1-2 droppers of Kidney/Bladder Formula every hour (or 10 minutes) till the burning or pain stops.

- ☒ Take acidophilus.

- ☒ Take D-Mannose like it says on the bottle. (You can take it more often if needed.)

- ☒ Take cranberry or blueberry concentrate by the spoonful. You can do this every half hour followed by a full cup of water.

- ☒ To the above list, add 2 droppers of echinacea and 2 droppers of Super Duper Tonic every hour.

- ☒ Stop and rest and concentrate on allowing your body to get well.

- ☒ If needed, drink 2-3 cups of water with 5 capsules of charcoal – take another 5 capsules with 1 full cup of water each hour till the problem is resolved. (A full cup of water is a must so that you do not get constipated from the charcoal.)

Usually this will resolve an infection in a few hours. If you wait until you have a lot of pain or blood in the urine, this routine will still work but it will take longer and you must be more aggressive. This is almost a sure-fire cure. You can do it for two to three days if you need to without any problem. When you do stop taking the herbs and vitamins, still continue to drink more water than usual for a few days.

Poultice for Infection

You can also use a charcoal poultice over the kidney or bladder area at night.

Make the poultice by mixing together equal parts of charcoal and ground flax seed. Add only enough castor oil or water to make a nice smooth moist mix that stays together. Spread it on plastic wrap about ¼ inch thick. Heat it to cozy warm and lay it on the area (you should grease the area with olive oil first to make the cleanup easier).

Cover the poultice with another rag (it may get black), and then keep it cozy with a heating pad or a warm rice sock.

This will help to get rid of the bacteria that is there by actually pulling it through the skin. It will also really help to relieve any pain that you have in the area. Repeat as often as desired, and you can reuse the poultice if you wish.

You can make a few poultices at a time. Roll up the ones you do not need right away, put them in a bag and store them in the fridge. When you need one take it out and warm it.

Eight Hours to Clear an Infection

Here is an idea of what you could do in an 8 hour day. Get aggressive about clearing up the infection if the above information did not work.

- ☒ Hour 1 - 1 teaspoon of baking soda in an 8 oz. glass of water. Drink immediately. This makes the bladder environment alkaline. Take 1 tablespoon of blueberry concentrate every 15 minutes for 1 hour. Drink a full glass of water with each spoonful.

- ☒ Hour 2 - Drink 1 cup of parsley tea every 15 minutes. 4 teaspoons of dried leaf to 1 quart of boiling water. Steep 10 minutes. Take the tea with 5 capsules of charcoal every 15 minutes. Fresh parsley is best but dried works as well.

- ☒ Hour 3 – Take 1 tablespoon blueberry concentrate with 1 cup water, 2 acidophilus capsules and 1 finely chopped clove of garlic. Repeat in a half hour.

- ☒ Hour 4 – 8 oz. of water with 5 more capsules of charcoal. Repeat in 30 min.

- ☒ Hour 5 - 1 tablespoon Apple cider vinegar in 4 oz. water.

- ☒ Hour 6 – 1 chopped garlic. Take 1 glass of water with it and 5 more capsules of charcoal. Repeat in 30 minutes.

- ☒ Hour 7 – Take 1 tablespoon blueberry or cranberry concentrate with 1 cup water, take 2 acidophilus capsules, and 1 finely chopped clove of garlic. Repeat in a half hour.

- ☒ Hour 8 - 1 Tablespoon apple cider vinegar in 1 glass of water.

This should clear you up. If you are not quite over it, simply repeat the steps starting again at 1. Do not do it during the night unless you are in serious trouble. Sleep is important too.

If you spike a **high(103)** fever while treating yourself, you need to get checked by a doctor because bladder infections can turn into serious kidney infections. These can be very serious if not paid attention to promptly.

But while you are making your appointment and waiting to get to the doctor, take 5 charcoal capsules by mouth with two cups of water and place a warm charcoal poultice over the kidney area. Keep drinking water and take more capsules every hour. Reheat the poultice every hour and keep the area warm. You may be able to get rid of it that way, before he can even see you.

An Answer to my Urinary Track Infections- A Story

Used by permission of the Bulk Herb Store

"I suffer from many urinary tract infections related to abnormalities from birth. These infections have been getting worse over the years and the last two were extremely painful. Within 2 hours of the first symptoms I could barely walk. Over the last 18 months, I began developing allergies to the antibiotics.

On the last infection I decided to try herbs and was astounded at the results. No more antibiotics for me.

I took 1 tsp. of raw apple cider vinegar every 15 minutes, 2 homemade garlic pills every 6 hours, 2 homemade cayenne pepper pills every hour, a dropper full of "Immune Booster" (*I would use 2 droppers*) every 8 hours *(every 2-3)* and the infection was gone faster than the antibiotic usually relieves it. Since antibiotics usually take 5-10 days, I decided to follow up the above regimen with 1 tsp of apple cider vinegar, 2 garlic pills, 2 cayenne pills and Immune Booster, 3-4 times a day for a week. That was October 1st and I haven't had a problem. No re-occurrence, no side effects."

This lady did well on her little plan, but she could have taken the pills every 2 hours if she had wanted to, without any bad effect.

Immune Tea

Use 4 oz. Each of: nettle leaf, alfalfa leaf, peppermint leaf, chopped echinacea root, echinacea herb, and dried elderberries.

You can mix these herbs and put them in a glass jar, ready for a cup of tea when you need it. This will make about a gallon jar of mixed herbs, more or less. For ease, purchase empty tea bags from Bulk Herb Store. Fill them and staple or iron shut and, presto, you have nice cup of tea. They carry them in lots of 50 or 100. They also carry Double -E Immune Booster Tea mixed and ready to use.

Or you can make a glycerin tincture out of that tea mix. Using the above herbs follow the glycerin tincture recipes in the medicine making chapter. If you make a gallon – you will get about two quarts of finished tincture that will see you and your friends through the winter. We like to make half of our tincture with alcohol and half with glycerin. When we are done we usually pour out a small amount of the glycerin tincture and reserve it for any little children. Then we mix the alcohol and the glycerin together half and half so that you have a nicer tasting product. I think that straight glycerin is way too sweet and straight alcohol is rather sharp though it does do a better job with extracting the medicinal part, especially for roots and seeds and bark!

Adult dose for this: ½ – 1 teaspoon every hour at the first sign of a cold or flu or infection. Take it until your symptoms disappear. Give the children about half that dose and the babies just a few drops each nursing.

Causes of Bladder Infections

1. Not drinking enough water.

2. Being a newly-wed and accustoming yourself to new bacteria.

3. Holding off going to the bathroom when you need to go.

4. Not going to the bathroom after making love (bacteria needs to be washed out).

5. Pregnancy, which increases your need for water drastically and changes your acid balance.

6. A high sugar intake and a low water intake; acid balance is off.

7. Improper wiping after bowel movement. Always wipe front to back.

8. Poor emptying of the bladder. If you are prone to infection and you covered the above points, try to sit on the toilet and lean forward while urinating to get a nice strong stream of urine. This empties the bladder better and insures that you will have less chance for bacteria to grow.

9. Antibiotics and spermicides WILL imbalance your intestinal and vaginal flora, causing bacteria to grow.

This covers most common reasons. If you are prone to reoccurring infections there are a few things that you can do.

1. Do the opposite of the above problems and you should see immediate improvement.

2. Drink one cup of lemon balm (Melissa officianalis) and peppermint tea morning and evening. Lemon balm is a natural antiseptic and helps to keep the bacteria from growing. This is especially helpful for pregnant women who are more susceptible to bacteria growth.

3. Take 2 capsules of cranberry extract or D-Mannose a day to keep your bladder acidic.

4. Drink 1 cup of charcoal water daily. This helps to "get" the bacteria before it begins making a problem. To do this put ¼ cup of charcoal in a quart of

water and shake it up. Let it set overnight and in the morning do not shake but pour off a cup of water to drink and put it back in the fridge. You can keep adding water until the charcoal is used up. Shake each time and let the charcoal settle for at least ½ hr. before drinking. The grit will not hurt you, but it is less pleasant.

5. Do not take antibiotics if at all possible.

What happens when you do take antibiotics? The antibiotic does clear up the problem but it messes up your immune system and kills the friendly flora in your body. This makes you prone to another infection sooner or later, which requires another antibiotic. After awhile the medicine does not work very well anymore because your body is accustomed to it. Then you need a bigger, stronger, and more expensive medicine. The recent medical discovery that women who take frequent antibiotics have a much higher incidence of breast cancer makes this kind of decision a poor choice. So learn all you can so that you do not usually need antibiotics.

Kidney Infections

Small kidney infections that result in kidney tenderness in the lower back area and a low grade fever can be treated the same way as a bladder infection without the cranberry added. Be faithful to drink enough water if you want to treat these infections.

Kidney Stones

Kidney stones are another difficulty that you can deal with yourself if you are well informed. There is a simple routine that will dissolve kidney stones efficiently so that you can pass them without a lot of pain.

Kidney stones can cause terrific pain. I had been told that folks would rather have a baby than have kidney stones. I was doubtful, until the day I had a kidney stone attack that left me on the floor in great pain. I did not know how I was going to make it until I remembered that lobelia is a strong muscle relaxant. My husband brought me a bottle of lobelia and I took two droppers by mouth and then rubbed my kidney area liberally with lobelia. Within 5 minutes I was able to get up off the floor and sit in a chair. The pain was going away and I was so relieved. Apparently the lobelia had relaxed the area where the stone had lodged and it had moved.

But I knew that my job was not done. It would take a bit of faithful work to dissolve those stones or they would bother me again. I was very sure that I did not want to go through that pain again.

The routine that I used was from American Botanical Pharmacies. It is not a fly-by-night routine. This has been done for many, many people successfully. You can go to Herbdoc.com to see it or order through the mail or over the phone. *See Medicine chapter for American Botanical Pharmacy's address.

Purchase lobelia at Nature's Warehouse.   1-800-215-4372

Information About Kidney Stones

"Kidney stones, also called renal calculi, are solid concretions (crystal aggregations) of dissolved minerals in urine; calculi typically form inside the kidneys or bladder.

Renal calculi can vary in size from as small as grains of sand to as large as a golf ball. Kidney stones typically leave the body by passage in the urine stream, and many stones are formed and passed without causing symptoms. If stones grow to sufficient size before passage - on the order of at least 2-3 millimeters - they can cause obstruction of the ureter. The resulting obstruction with dilation or stretching of the upper ureter and renal pelvis as well as spasm of muscle, trying to move the stone, can cause severe episodic pain, most commonly felt in the flank, lower abdomen and groin (a condition called renal colic). Renal colic can be associated with nausea and vomiting due to the embryological association of the kidneys with the intestinal tract. Hematuria (bloody urine) is commonly present due to damage to the lining of the urinary tract.

Kidney Stone Flush

Mix 2 oz. of olive oil and 2 oz .of lemon juice, drink it down. (Putting this in the blender makes it foamy and easier to get down.) This is also effective as a gall bladder flush. Follow with a large glass of water at the first sign of stone pain. The stone(s) will pass within 24 hours.

This is the routine that many people use. It seems to work for them. However, I like to use American Botanicals stone dissolving method better. To me it makes more sense to dissolve them before you do a flush since I would not want a stone stuck stubbornly in the ureter causing me a lot of pain. If you want that information you need to go online to Herbdoc.com to his 5 Day Kidney detox program and see his quick start directions, or order his Kidney detox kit. *See making medicine chapter for the phone number. Following is a cheaper way of dissolving the stones that seems to also work.

Dissolve Your Kidney Stones

Dissolve kidney stones in a few days with no pain.
Day 1
6 limes
4 liters water (16 cups)
alfalfa tablets
Mix limes w/water, drink throughout the day. Every waking hour take 2 alfalfa tablets.
Days 2 & 3
Throughout the day drink the same amount of water and take same amount of tablets but do not take the limes. This time add 2 teaspoons of vinegar and 2 teaspoons of honey to every 2 cups of water. The vinegar relaxes your urinary tract and also helps to dissolve the stones. Avoid all caffeine products and chocolate during this cleanse.

Banaba Leaf for Stones

Melissa writes: "I wanted to add another remedy to your list for kidney stones. I'm still not sure why this one is not getting out there to the people as quick as it should, since it is such a fast and reliable fix. I would like to suggest Banaba Tea (crepe myrtle). I buy mine from overseas, though I have seen herbal shops online in the US carry it as well. It's fast, thankfully! Not only do I use it, but my friends and family use it too. It's much better than the regretful look doctors give you as they hand you pain pills and pat you on the back to say good luck when they send you home to pass a stone the old fashioned way!

Not only does it dissolve the problem stone but anyone that was sent home from the doctor with a strainer will be shocked at just how much other potential stone minerals they had in their kidneys as well, when they begin seeing what looks like clumps of wet sugar in their strainer!

Try this to break up your kidney stones.

1 dropper of **Stone Breaker** in 8 oz. water every 4 hours.

3 tablets every 4 hours - **Stone Free**.

Do this faithfully until the stones are dissolved.

"Stone Free" from Planetary Herbal contains: turmeric root, gravel root, dandelion root extract (4:1), ginger root, lemon balm leaf, marshmallow root, parsley root, dandelion root, and licorice root.

You can buy this online at vitacost.com or call 1-800-383-0759 to order Stone Free – 180 tablets (Planetary Herbal) for $11.99. You can also purchase Herb Pharm's Stone Breaker (chanca piedra) through VitaCost at $7.09 an ounce.

Kidney Detox Routine

If you have been having infections and/or kidney stones try Dr. Schultz' kidney detox program for a week and see how much better you feel. I have not had any more infections since I have been doing this at least two times a year. The steps are simple. Purchase your supplies from American Botanical Pharmacy. See suppliers in the medicine making chapter. You can also go online to herbdoc.com to his five day kidney detox program and see his quick start directions.

Note: I am not connected with any of the companies that I suggest, nor do I get remuneration from them. I am only passing on to you information that I hope may be helpful to you and may result in your improved health without a doctor visit.

Kidney/Bladder Formula

2 parts Juniper Berries
1 part each: Cornsilk (fresh is best), Uva Ursi leave, Horsetail herb, Burdock Root,
Pipsissiwa leaf, Goldenrod flowers, Hydrangea root, parsley leaf and root
Cover with vodka and let set for 4 - 6 weeks shaking often. Strain, bottle and use. It is very effective for most kidney and bladder problems. Use as often as needed unless pregnant.

I need it to use this often because of my weak kidneys, especially when I am on trips.

Understanding Liver
and Gall Bladder Health

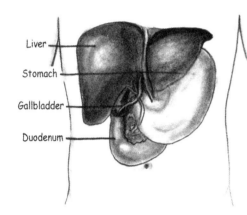

Liver
Stomach
Gallbladder
Duodenum

Although you cannot see it and seldom even think about it, your liver is a very important part of your body. It is the largest glandular organ in your body. It receives one and one-half quarts of blood every minute. It cleans your blood nonstop twenty four hours a day, seven days a week, three hundred and sixty-five days a year. It is the liver's job to trap and clean out anything that you have consumed or breathed in that is harmful to you.

The liver serves many important functions:

- it regulates carbohydrate metabolism and turns glucose into glycogen to regulate your blood sugar. Glycogen is actually energy for you and your brain.

- It regulates protein metabolism and manufactures clotting factors and sex hormones. If you are having a difficulty in that area it just may be that your liver needs a housecleaning.

- Performs the synthesis of urea - a waste product of protein for elimination through the kidneys.

- It modifies fats for cell use (filtering out cholesterol) and manufactures bile for digesting fats.

- It detoxifies harmful substances (drugs, etc.) for your whole system.

- It stores vitamins like vitamin B-12, and vitamin A, glycogen, and iron to be used any time you need a charge of energy.

Your liver plays a very vital role in your well being. It is your blood cleaning filter. Without the liver your blood would be full of toxic chemicals and poisons from the water, food, and air around you. If your liver failed to do its job continually you would be dead in a very short time.

Poor digestion, bloating, weight gain around the abdomen, constipation, reflux, and irritable bowel syndrome are due to a sluggish liver. A sluggish liver allows toxic metabolites to enter the blood stream and affect brain function. This can lead to a foggy brain, depression, and mood swings. If your liver is not functioning well your concentration and memory will be affected. Poor liver function really affects the condition of the skin. When the liver is not working well you can be afflicted by all manner of skin rashes and conditions. Many times headaches are triggered by a toxic liver. If you have been on many drugs of any kind, including Tylenol and Ibuprofen, antibiotics, alcohol, or coffee you tend to have more headaches, especially migraines.

High blood pressure and fluid retention are often directly related to a chemical problem with the liver. Excessive amounts of aldosterone in the liver raise the sodium and lower the potassium and this in turn can raise the blood pressure. A malfunctioning liver also does not filter out the fatty substances, causing cholesterol deposits on the arteries. This raises the blood pressure, too. Hypoglycemia is directly related to liver difficulties, since the liver controls the glycogen which converts into blood sugar. Hypoglycemics really benefit from extra liver care. Constipation and bowel difficulties often stem from a liver that does not work properly.

Hepatitis, jaundice, gall stones, obesity, heart attack, stroke, hormone problems, diabetes, and cancer all have a direct relationship to the state of your liver. The medical texts say there is no specific treatment for hepatitis. The only remedy for gall stones they offer is surgery. Liver cancer is treated by radiation and chemotherapy. Hormone problems, diabetes, and high cholesterol are all treated with drugs. If you think about it, this does not really address the problem. It simply stresses the already overtaxed liver by challenging it to detoxify all the chemicals that you are loading into your body.

Gall stones and gall attacks are directly related to a poorly functioning liver. Fatty bile flows into the gall bladder which causes attacks and gall stones in many people. What does the gall bladder do? It stores the bile for the liver. When the bile contains too many fats, especially from animal products and hydrogenated oils, stones form in the gall bladder and in the bile duct causing acute pain. These stones must be dissolved and passed and the liver made healthy to eliminate the problem from reoccurring.

What is the Answer?

God has provided a number of things for man to live healthily and to heal the body when it becomes sick. The best thing is to live preventively and not wait until your system becomes overloaded and fails to work properly. It is far better to understand what is helpful to good health and to begin to practice it. This is like putting a fence at the edge of the cliff to prevent someone from falling over it, rather than putting an ambulance at the bottom to pick up the folks that fall over the edge.

Water

The first and simplest thing that you can do to keep you body healthy is to drink LOTS of pure water daily! You need 10-12 glasses a day and more if you are nursing, doing strenuous work, or it is very hot. This water thins the blood and makes it easier for the liver to filter out the toxins and waste matter from our blood. Raised cholesterol is a sign that the body has provided a defense mechanism to prevent further dehydration of the cells. Cholesterol acts like a clay-type barrier to prevent this osmosis from happening. Knowing this, it makes sense to drink plenty of water so that your liver does not have to filter out excess cholesterol. Water is available and free. Be sure to drink at least one cup before each meal and quite a few between meals and you will find out that you feel much better. It is a simple protection.

Eliminate Bad Fats

Another thing you can do is to cut back on the amount of bad fats that you use in your diet. These fats do not break down easily in the liver and contribute to liver sickness. Use real butter sparingly and use oils like olive oil for many of your cooking needs. This oil is handled more easily by your liver. You do need some fats but pure plant oils, like almonds, flax seeds, coconut oil, and olive oil are easier for your body to assimilate. (Watch out for highly processed vegetable oils, particularly corn and soy. Unless they are organic, they are almost certainly genetically modified.)

Eat Right

Fresh fruits and vegetables provide the anti-oxidants that help your liver to work more efficiently. Eat lots of them and enjoy better all around health. Cut back on the amount of sugar, white flour, and processed food that you eat. Over-consumption of processed food really loads the system with things that your liver has to filter out for your body to work efficiently. As the liver becomes overloaded and sluggish your whole body becomes sluggish. You never have energy. You need more sleep. You tend to gain weight, especially around the middle. To change this, your diet must change.

Exercise

Exercise is also very helpful because it increase the circulation to all parts of your body, including your liver. It stimulates the flow of blood and lymph to every part of your brain and body. This is necessary for good health.

Sleep

Sleep enough. Every adult needs about 8 good, restful hours of sleep. Without that, your body does not have time to rebuild and detoxify. I read someplace that about two AM, in the middle of your night is when the liver is rebuilding. If you shortcut and do not get enough sleep this process is greatly hindered.

Helpful Hints

Following are some helpful hints on how to care for your liver every day.

1. Do not eat when you are not hungry. Overfeeding overtaxes the liver.

2. Do not eat large amounts of sugar. If you crave something sweet, have fresh fruit, dried fruit, or a bit of honey.

3. Do not overuse animal protein. Use grains, nuts, seeds and legumes for most of your protein. These provide good sources of protein. And while we are on the subject of meat, milk, and eggs, remember to try to obtain these products without hormones or antibiotics, which further stress your liver. There are plenty of delicious bean (legume) dishes that you can prepare and enjoy. The trick here is to plan ahead because it does take soaking or pre-cooking to make tasty meals. Nuts make great pick-me-up snacks and provide good protein. Get creative and have fun experimenting. We love Haitian rice and black beans, tortillas made with our own re-fried beans, Mexican lasagna made with beans, honey-baked lentils with cheese, and many, many more bean dishes. Actually these are quite economical as well as tasty. If a pound of beans costs little more than a dollar and feeds eight people for one meal, that adds up to less than sixteen cents per person for protein, when beef costs $2.89 a pound and costs $.36 a person and makes a smaller helping per person at that. One pound of beef will not go as far for eight people as one pound of beans! Beans are great

for the budget!

4. Eat lots of fresh fruits and vegetables. They are cell rebuilders and vitalizers. They help the liver and the rest of the body work properly.

5. Be careful what fats you use. Bad fats choke up the fat-burning organ of the body and your metabolism slows down. As a result you gain weight, especially around the middle. A healthy liver provides lipoprotein which coats the fat and allows it to travel though the blood stream properly. If there is not enough of lipoprotein in your blood, your risk of stroke, high blood pressure, and cholesterol greatly increases.

Your body needs some fats. These essential and non essential fatty acids are necessary for good cell health. You can find them in seeds, raw nuts, legumes, leafy greens, primrose oil, lecithin, and spirulina. There are some in fresh fish like mackerel, tuna, sardines and salmon.

Hydrogenated or partially hydrogenated oils (margarine and shortening) are not easy for your body to use. They impair the liver function of breaking down and eliminating toxins. They are also stickier, and tend to result in increased blood clots. Doctors recognize this fact, too. In 1990 The New England Journal of Medicine published a study that showed that trans-fatty acids (hydrogenated oils) greatly increased the risk factors for heart disease. Hence, margarine, potato chips, french fries, and packaged cookies are very hard on your liver. Check the labels on your food for hydrogenated or partially hydrogenated oils. Avoid them whenever possible.

Helpful Herbs

1. **Milk thistle** is first on the list. It is an all around liver protector and regenerator. It is anti-inflammatory and antioxidant. Milk thistle improves the enzyme cytochrome P450 that breaks down toxic substances. Studies that followed patients with chronic hepatitis, liver disease, and liver damage showed that milk thistle greatly helped their liver disease.

2. **Dandelion** is also a great aid in stimulating good liver function and bile flow. It is a great help in purifying the blood. It is a great detoxifying herb. Dandelion has been used successfully to heal hepatitis and other liver diseases.

3. **Yellow dock and burdock** are great herbs to clean up the liver and the bloodstream.

4. **Chaparral** is also an excellent detoxing herb. It is best taken as a tea, although it tastes and smells a bit like band-aids. If you add peppermint you may not mind the flavor.

There are other good liver teas and tonics that you can also take to aid your liver's health if you are ailing.

Detox and Cleanse

Dr. Schultz' 5 Day liver cleansing and detoxifying program is a very helpful one. I have used it often and recommended it to others with good results. You can call for his products at 1-800-HERB-DOC, or go online to herbdoc.com to see his liver cleansing products. You can even look at his **quick start directions** online, to see what it involves, since I am not allowed to give you the directions here.

If you are experiencing any liver difficulties, nausea, gall bladder attacks or gall stones, stop and take a week to nourish and cleanse your liver. But before you start and while you are cleansing your liver, be sure that you are having at least two to three good bowel movements a day. Why? Because as the liver detoxifies, the bile flows into the intestines carrying waste products. If you are not, going well, you will feel foggy, you will have a headache and you may even get ill for the detoxing that you are doing. When the bowels are moving well, then the wastes flow right on thru and do not make you sick.

Hepatitis

Hepatitis is an inflammation of the liver, usually from a viral infection. The liver becomes tender and enlarged and does not function normally so toxins build up and hence the jaundice that is prevalent in hepatitis. There are many different types of hepatitis.Hepatitis may be caused from:

• Infections from parasites, bacteria, or viruses (includes hepatitis A, B, C).
• Liver damage from alcohol, drugs, or poisonous mushrooms.
• Overdose of acetaminophen, high blood pressure medication, antibiotics.
• Immune cells in the body attacking the liver and causing autoimmune hepatitis.

Whatever the cause, the liver, the one organ responsible for filtering and removing most toxins from the body, is temporarily or chronically incapable of fully doing its job. Symptoms include:
• Dark urine and pale or clay-colored stools
• Loss of appetite
• Fatigue
• Abdominal pain or distention
• General itching
• Jaundice (yellowing of the skin or eyes)
• Nausea and vomiting
• Low grade fever
• Weight loss
• Depending on the cause, hepatitis may become chronic, leading to liver failure (cirrhosis) or liver cancer.

What You Can Do to Help

Do American Botanical Pharmacy's Cleansing Routine. Then do the liver detox program. Drink lots of pure water - at least 12 cups daily to help the system flush out the poisons. Use apple cider vinegar - to help flush out the liver. Take 1 tablespoon in one cup water with 1 teaspoon of honey. Take four times daily. This is cheap but very very helpful. Try to get the health food store brand or any non-pasteurized brand if possible. Eat a diet of fresh fruits and veggies for four weeks to give the liver a rest.

Take These Supplements
Milk thistle(silymarin) - liver healer and rebuilder - 300mg – three times daily
Alpha lipoic acid - 300 mg. Twice daily (depletes some vitamin B so you must take a B complex with this)
Selenium - 400 mg. daily
Vitamin E - 800 IU daily
Vitamin C - 1000 mg. three to four times daily
Charcoal water or capsules

Use a Castor Oil Pack

A double-blind study, described by Harvey Grady in a report entitled *Immuno-modulation through Castor Oil Packs* published in a recent issue of the *Journal of Naturopathic Medicine,* examined lymphocyte values of thirty-six healthy subjects before and after topical castor oil application.

This study identified castor oil as an anti-toxin, and as having impact on the lymphatic system, enhancing immunological function. The study found that castor oil pack therapy of a minimal two-hour duration produced an increase in the number of T-11 cells within a twenty-four hour period following treatment, with a concomitant increase in the number of total lymphocytes. This T-11 cell increase represents a general boost in the body's specific defense status, since lymphocytes actively defend the health of the body by forming antibodies against pathogens and their toxins. T-cells identify and kill viruses, fungi, bacteria, and cancer cells.

Castor oil packs are therefor a simple home therapy which often produces astounding results. * See Castor Oil chapter for instructions on how to make a pack.

In hepatitis, neonatal jaundice, cirrhosis, and liver cancer, the liver is unable to filter certain poisons and waste products from the blood. The build-up of these toxins in the blood pose a major health risk. Activated charcoal, taken internally or applied externally, is well known to adsorb these poisons and to support the liver in its work of detoxifying the blood. Use it often in capsules or by drinking the "gray" water. *See charcoal chapter.

Growing Girls and Changing Hormones

We have marvelous bodies that God created. These changing bodies of ours take wisdom and understanding to live with. If we understand how we are made, what the functions of our bodies are, and how to nourish them carefully, a lot of our health problems can be resolved.

There are many areas of health affected by our hormones. Perhaps that is why women (who generally experience more fluctuation in hormone levels) are so interested in health issues. We deal with health on a day to day basis with our families. We are responsible to maintain our own health as well as our family's health.

As our daughters begin to grow up, we need to teach them how to live with themselves "according to knowledge". This means that they must understand their cyclic nature and how God created a woman. We need to teach them to get enough rest, drink more water, and keep their elimination regular. This is especially important at the time of the month when their period comes, because all of our body works together to make our cycle. If one part of our body is not functioning properly, our cycle will be much more difficult. Acne, cramps, and PMS are often difficulties that our growing girls face that they would not need to experience if they understood their bodies. Teenage acne has one very simple answer for many girls. It is often related to constipation and dehydration. Why? The answer is evident. If you have a garbage can, you have flies. If your lower bowel does not clean out at least once a day and preferably twice, the fecal material does not flow through like it is intended to and it begins to putrefy and give off gases and bacteria. These poisons, called toxins, need to leave the body promptly or you will become sick. If you do not eliminate properly through the digestive canal like God has planned, you will eliminate these poisons through your skin. They must go somewhere or you will become very ill. Since your skin is your body's largest elimination organ it begins to break out in pimples, some of which can become very infected and make life difficult for you. Hormones trigger these outbreaks since a large amount of hormones are flowing in the body system in an adolescent. Drinking more water dilutes the hormones flowing through the system and really helps lessen hormonal acne outbreaks as does a healthy lower bowel.

Why is constipation a problem today when it was not a problem long ago? The answer lies in our changing lifestyle and diet. Two hundred years ago, in this country, women worked in the gardens and fields. They hoed by hand, carried water, and scrubbed the family's laundry on a scrub board. All this exercise made their elimination work better. There were no processed foods and no sugary drinks. All the wheat had its brown covering and fiber intact, and they ate mostly fruits and vegetables that came from their gardens. Each of these had all of its fiber intact. In 1880, steel roller mills were introduced. These mills enabled the millers to easily separate the flour from the germ and the bran. That made the product whiter and finer and greatly retarded spoilage. The result? A product that sold well but was greatly inferior in nutritional value and fiber. The health change that went along with the processed flour was dramatic! By 1931, heart attacks, appendicitis, and colon difficulties had all drastically increased. Today most foods have all the roughage and fiber eliminated and we are suffering the consequences in health difficulties. But the answer is not complicated. The colon should be a moving stream, but for many of us it is a stagnant holding tank. Most of you eat fruits and vegetables and some whole grains, but they do NOT make up the majority of your diet! *British Journal of Nutrition* (2000), **83**, Suppl. 1, S157–S163 Dietary fibre, lente carbohydrates and the insulin-resistant diseases.

Check your diet for a week. You will be very surprised that a very large part of your diet is composed of starches that have been refined, like noodles, crackers, sugary cereals, breads, white rice, and deserts. Experiment and see what happens when you take any one of these, and moisten it well, and then let it set for a day or two on the counter. It gets hard and dry like paste. When you do not drink enough water (2 quarts minimum) and do not exercise daily, your waste products tend to dry out as your colon absorbs the fluids from them. This makes them move very slowly through your colon and produces very poor elimination and a build-up of poisons in your system, resulting in acne and other disorders like cramps and headaches. This is not only a teenage problem but one that worsens as you go through pregnancy and becomes a major difficulty when you reach your older years, often resulting in colon disease and cancer. A person with a high roughage diet, who drinks enough water, will store their food in their colon for less than eighteen hours as opposed to many of us who do not eliminate it for two to three days. This additional storage time allows the colon to be irritated by the bacteria in the waste and over a period of time it becomes weakened and infected and a myriad of colon diseases result, including appendicitis.

Add more fresh fruits, vegetables and whole grains into your diet. These items should make up the bulk of your diet! Whenever you can, eat your veggies raw. They add more nutrients and fiber to your diet than you can imagine. Steam your vegetables lightly, until they turn a bright color and are still crisp. Or stir fry them lightly and serve them with a plate of brown rice and a small bit of chicken for a satisfying meal. Eat lots of fiber and drink lots of water and you will be surprised at how quickly your skin problems will clear up and your headaches go away.

A tablespoon of blackstrap molasses mixed into a cup or two of water and drunk first thing every morning will also really help the elimination, as will a few prunes daily. Two or three teaspoons of apple cider vinegar added to the blackstrap water will double the effect and will really help to get rid of the acne faster. You may be surprised to note that this may also clear up the cramps and diminish the flow if you have a heavy one. Are you lacking in energy? Add a pinch of cayenne to the blackstrap drink and you will have increased energy. Do you need to lose weight? Have the drink about twenty minutes before your meal and you will find that it not only curbs your appetite but it helps you digest your food better. This in turn, should make a difference in fat burning.

Pure water is a crucial factor. It washes the toxins into your colon and keeps the waste soft enough that you can eliminate freely. I always thought that the fuss about toxins was just that, a fuss, until the last few years. Even medical doctors are recognizing this, because poor colon health is becoming a major epidemic. Quoting a medical text that I have been studying, "The kidneys are also involved in excretion of unwanted substances such as waste products from cell metabolism, excess salts and toxins. These toxins, if not eliminated by the kidneys and the bowel, begin to make health difficulties for us." All growing girls need at least eight cups of water a day. Milk, juice, iced tea and soft drinks will not do the same for you as pure water. Start the habit of drinking more water!

Exercise daily and you will increase your circulation and your elimination and your skin will begin to clear up! Your cramps will markedly decrease, too, since increased circulation takes place when you exercise and this often eliminates cramps.

If you suffer from cramps and PMS, doing the above things may be the answer you were looking for. If not, drinking 2 - 4 cups of red raspberry tea daily will usually cure most of your problems, if you started with the first suggestions of elimination, diet, and water. Red raspberry tea is high in calcium and minerals. We find that it really makes a difference with cramps when our girls drink it faithfully and exercise. I combine red raspberry with nettles and alfalfa for increased mineral content and add peppermint for flavor. It tastes almost like the flu tea that we make for colds in the winter. We all like to drink it and it is really good for everyone. The vitamin and mineral content in these herbs is very high and easily absorbed. Teach your girls to respect their bodies and not plan huge jobs over their monthly period. If they learn to chart their cycle and know when it is coming, they will understand their changes in emotions and be able to cope with them better. It is a known fact that when a number of women live together they tend to begin to cycle close to the same time. This has a unique difficulty. If you all are going through your difficult time of the month at the same time, it takes extra love and patience to live with each other. This is a good learning experience for all of us.

If your teenager has an especially difficult time, give her a little extra space. Make it a day for her to read a little more, or sew if she enjoys that. Be patient with her and teach her how to be gracious even when she is not quite feeling like herself. She will need this developed character when she is a wife and a mother later on. Severe cramps can usually be avoided if you follow the above routines. But what can you do if they still happen? *Take a large mug of clove tea, (1 tablespoon clove buds in two cups of boiling water, boil for twenty minutes strain and sweeten) as hot as you can drink it. Sip it slowly, place a warm rice bag or a heating pad on your tummy over the cramping area. This often works.*

You can rub the area with lobelia tincture, and take some extra cal/mag capsules. Cramp bark capsules (taken two every fifteen minutes for an hour) should also help this problem. A common, low growing herb with red berries that grows on the forest floor, is called squaw vine and makes a tea that really relaxes the body and stops cramping. (Do not use a plant you have collected yourself unless you are SURE what it is!)

Make two or three cups of red raspberry tea daily with a small amount of squaw vine for cramps. It may be just "what the doctor ordered" in case of bad cramps!

This is the time of life, when girls need to think about getting their bodies into optimum shape for coming motherhood. Help them learn about nutrition and get what they need. Teach them to exercise, eat well, and drink the water that they need now, and motherhood will be so much healthier and easier for them. How I wish that someone had taught me all these things.

Girls in the United States are reaching puberty at very early ages, increasing their risk of breast cancer, social problems, and emotional problems. While the biological signs of female puberty -- menstruation, breast development, and growth of pubic and underarm hair -- typically occurred around thirteen years of age or older just decades ago, today girls as young as eight are increasingly showing these signs. Aside from the social and emotional implications, early puberty exposes girls to more estrogen, which increases their risk of breast cancer because this disease thrives on estrogen.

According to biologist Sandra Steingraber, the author of the report titled "*The Falling Age of Puberty in U.S. Girls: What We Know, What We Need to Know*, "The data indicates that if you get your first period before age twelve, your risk of breast cancer is fifty percent higher than if you get it at age sixteen. For every year we could delay a girl's first menstrual period," she says, "we could prevent thousands of breast cancers."

Theories behind what is causing the early-puberty trend abound, but the actual causes are not known. Potential causes noted in the paper include:

- ☒ Rising childhood obesity rates and inactivity
- ☒ Formula-feeding of infants
- ☒ Excessive TV viewing and media use
- ☒ Family stress
- ☒ Exposure to environmental chemicals
- ☒ Fluoride in drinking water

Early puberty is likely an "ecological disorder," according to Steingraber, that's being caused by a number of environmental factors. *"The Falling Age of Puberty in U.S. Girls: What We Know, What We Need to Know" Chicago Tribune Sept. 16, 07*

Hormone Help

I find that if the simpler things that we have discussed do not work quickly, Ladies Formula works wonders for your growing girls. Usually a few weeks of taking that will cure the irregular cycles, the depression or the irritability that can develop when the hormones are out of whack.

A number of mothers have called me, badly distressed about daughters who have begun to show signs of obsessive, compulsive behavior and this amazing formula cleared up the difficulty in a short time. We were all thankful because behavior-altering drugs are so harmful to the body and yet no one can live well with the difficulties that they were experiencing. We have also used it successfully for irregular cycles and the moodiness that this brings. Usually one bottle will do the job and you will have a bright, sunny daughter back. Very occasionally I find someone who says it did not work, but I always wonder if they followed the instructions and used it for three months. I have never seen it fail for the young girls that I was working with personally.

One of the more recent experiences involved a youth that was uncharacteristically talkative and yet very depressed. Her family was at their wits end and ready to take her to a mental health unit but they did not want the drugs that would be used. They called me and I suggested *very* strong doses of Ladies Formula in combination with Dr. Schultz' Nerve Formula, (American Botanical Pharmacy) also in large amounts and presto they had their girl back until her next cycle when she was worse for the time of the cycle. They will need to be very faithful in using the two formulas until things get evened out and it may take at least three or four months of consistent use. Usually you can cut back the dose when the symptoms are alleviated. * This recipe is not in my first editions but folks kept asking for it. So here it is. Or you can order it from **Elysiumnaturals.com 616-965-1549.**

Ladies Formula or Hormone Health

75% Mix - use a separate jar for this and cover with vodka. Use equal parts of:
   3 ½ cups Angelica (Don Quai)
   3 ½ cups Mexican Wild Yam
   3 ½ cups Chaste Tree Berry (Vitex berry)
   Put these herbs in a gallon jar and fill it with vodka. Let it set for 6 weeks.
25% Mix – use a separate jar and cover this with vodka.
   1 ½ cups Damniana
   ¼ cup each
   Licorice Root, Hops, Passion Flower, Valerian Root, Uva Ursi, Juniper Berries
Put the 25% herb mix into a quart jar and then fill it up with vodka. Let this set for 6 wks. Strain both jars out and measure the finished product. You want to have 75% (1 ½ qts) to 25% (½ qt.) to make the right mix. This is a bit more figuring than for the other tinctures and makes more finished product so it may be something you will want to do with a few families. The finished tincture will be good for at least ten years since you use only vodka to make it. You may want to take it in juice to make it taste nicer. Experiment! Remember – you can use it for ladies, too.

Take this formula on days 14 – 28.   Always stop when bleeding starts. Take a dropper AM and PM.   For older ladies with PMS, hormonal, or menopausal symptoms, fibroids, endometriosis, or other lady problems, take a droppers three times daily.   If symptoms or pain is severe, you can safely double or triple the amount for a month or two.   If you are having trouble with missed periods and you know you are not pregnant, take it all the time until you get a normal cycle. Stop as soon as bleeding begins.   We have had some rather good success with it for endometrial pain, using double or triple the amount. Do not use while pregnant.

We have also been able to use it to get some women off antidepressants after taking it in double doses for a few months.   They then cut back to a normal dose for awhile.

Never take it if you do not need it.

Pregnancy
and Motherhood

Good Habits

Pregnancy is a wonderful time with a new, little life forming. It is a time of excitement and anticipation. But unfortunately, sometimes it is a time filled with nausea and unnecessary aches and pains. Attention to good health habits will go a long way toward easing these difficulties. If you start with these habits before getting pregnant you will probably not experience most of the usual difficulties that women today go through. There are some good habits that you should form.

- ✓ Drink 1-2 quarts of pure water daily.
- ✓ Drink 1 quart of pregnancy tea daily:

    2 parts red raspberry, 1 part nettles, 1 part alfalfa

- ✓ Eat fresh fruits, vegetables, beans, whole grains, nuts and seeds. These should make up most of the diet.
- ✓ Walk at least one mile daily.

Add these supplements:

5 super food tablets three times daily (1-800-437-2362) for extra minerals

2 capsules wheat germ oil - AM & PM or vitamin E for oxygen for the baby

1 Tablespoon chlorophyll - AM & PM to build the iron

1 Tablespoon blackstrap molasses – AM for iron and elimination help

Do the following -

- ✓ 50 Kegel exercises broken up into five intervals (every time you answer the phone, or 5 times a day)

- ✓ 25 pelvic rocks before bed
- ✓ No soda or caffeine
- ✓ Cut out most white sugar and flour
- ✓ No meat, eggs, or milk that has antibiotics or hormones in it.
- ✓ Use free range meats and eggs or lots of dried beans for protein.

This will minimize the hormonal imbalance after birth like postpartum blues.

Infertility

If you have trouble conceiving, there are a number of things that you can do together as a couple to help increase fertility. Follow all the above habits, with a few additions.

- ✓ Start with the water, more if your husband works out in the heat! Add in Lower Bowel Formula and do that until you both have 2 or 3 regular movements daily.

- ✓ Work on changing your diet if you do not already eat like this. Pay special attention to the last suggestions, above. From what I can read and hear from the folks that I work with eliminating the hormone sources is of major importance.

- ✓ Take Ladies Formula and Male Formula (American Botanical Pharmacy) respectively -regularly for about three months. These products have been a tremendous help for many infertile couples who also followed the above guidelines. A few of them found that when they changed their source of meat, milk, and eggs, that that was all that it took to change their fertility levels.

- ✓ Husband should take extra zinc daily.

- ✓ Use castor oil packs. (See Castor Oil chapter.) This increases circulation to the area.

The benefits of castor oil are many. First of all, it removes the waste products from the cells and tissues where it is applied, enhancing detoxification of the organs. Then, it decreases inflammation and assists the body in the removal of inflammatory components like prostaglandins. One of the main castor oil benefits is its ability to assist the liver eliminate excess hormones.

The most important function of the liver, as far as fertility is concerned, is to regulate blood sugar and take part in hormone metabolism. Castor oil is also easily absorbed into the lymphatic circulation. There, it stimulates the relaxation of the smooth muscle of the blood vessels allowing the free flow of oxygen and nutritional substances to reach the tissues more efficiently. Furthermore, the relaxation of the smooth muscle of internal organs, such as the stomach, intestines, gall bladder and liver, and uterus is highly effective for pain relief as castor oil therapy reduces inflammation and excess congestion.

When to Use a Castor Oil Pack

Duration of castor oil therapy: 45-90 minutes, 3-5 times a week for at least 8-16 weeks. During the first two menstrual cycles the ovarian pain and menstrual discomfort should decrease. Taper off slowly by decreasing the number of sessions per week. Sometimes a longer period of time is required.

Safety Precautions

Do not apply a castor oil pack on broken skin, during menses, and after ovulation if you are trying to conceive. If you are suffering from any serious or chronic condition, consult a natural health practitioner before applying castor oil. Do not use a castor oil pack if you are pregnant or suspect to be pregnant. It is best to avoid castor oil treatments if you have uterine bleeding. Castor oil should not be taken internally because it causes severe abdominal spasms.

Try castor oil packs for a few months before trying to conceive, just to be on the safe side, because castor oil has a detox effect which moves all the toxins away from your organs. After that you can apply castor oil packs only until ovulation, while trying to get pregnant. **Do not do an herbal detox while doing castor oil treatments because the detox effect can be too strong.** If you are on an herbal liver or bowel cleanse, do castor oil packs only once or twice a week. It is not harmful to your body but you may experience detox symptoms that may make you feel unwell. These symptoms are transient and their duration depends on the level of toxicity of your body. If you do experience them, ease off on the frequency of the castor oil therapy sessions.

Morning Sickness

Why are some mothers plagued with morning sickness? What causes it?

There are three main reasons and probably some minor ones. Many mothers who have morning sickness have low blood sugar, hormone imbalances, or digestive challenges. If the mother has all three she will probably end up in the hospital on I-V because of dehydration unless she or someone who loves her can guide her toward healthy alternatives.

No food or supplement will be effective for her if she is not digesting it. A person can have a B vitamin deficiency even while taking B vitamins if there is not enough hydrochloric acid in the stomach. Without HCL acid, B vitamins are not utilized, and neither are minerals or proteins. Without properly digested proteins blood glucose cannot be stabilized, thus creating a hypoglycemic, or "low blood sugar" problem. Apple cider vinegar (a tablespoon in water after meals) can substitute HCL acid to make a big difference in the utilization of B vitamins, minerals, vitamin C, and proteins. This alone often works toward curing morning sickness and aids in the problem of digesting B-6.

Digested protein aids in the stabilization of blood sugar or blood glucose. Basically HCL acid is responsible for this factor. Without stable blood sugar a mother can experience nausea, dry mouth, craving for sweets, ravenous hunger between meals, nervousness, chronic indigestion, mental confusion, crying spells, headache, irritability, depression, insomnia, poor appetite and forgetfulness. Besides using the apple cider vinegar remedy, adding GTF chromium will help regulate the pancreas output of insulin, preventing gestational diabetes and extremely large birth-weight babies.

Nausea is a really difficult thing. No one feels good when they are throwing up. There is a lot of speculation as to why this happens. No one knows for sure. Some of us have come up with some plausible ideas. Hormone levels, blood sugar levels, and the condition of your liver (your blood purifying organ), all seem to affect how ill you feel. If your body is toxic with chemicals that you have been taking, or if you have not been feeding it well, it will surely react adversely.

If your body is really deficient in vitamins and minerals that it needs, and your diet is mostly macaroni and cheese and hot dogs, spaghetti or pizza, or even noodle or rice casseroles, you will be much more nauseous.

Lemon Water Fasting

Some folks have had very good success with water or lemon water fasting for a few days.

The reason seems to be that this cleanses the body. I would not do this until I was sure that my elimination was working very well or you may become even sicker since you will not be able to eliminate the waste that you are cleansing. Then I would definitely try it. It will not hurt you. How many ladies throw up all they eat for days and weeks on end? To do this successfully you will need to drink lots of water. Lots and lots. Sip it slowly. No gulps, so that you do not throw up. If you need to sweeten the water with a small amount of maple syrup that is OK. Do not make it too sweet and DO NOT USE SUGAR to sweeten the lemon water! It will negate the effect of the cleanse and you will still have an upset stomach.

To make lemon water, squeeze the juice of one half a lemon into a 12-18 oz glass of water. Try to avoid unnecessary contact with the teeth because of its acidity.

When the three days are up, begin immediately to take ginger tea. For many women this tea is a great help. If you still have problems, sip it, only one tablespoon at a time. Ginger is also an excellent stomach calmer. You can take ginger capsules, ginger tea, or a preparation called digestive tonic. This helps to calm the stomach. Most woman find that a cup of ginger tea sipped throughout the morning makes a great difference. Make a cup of boiling water. Stir in ¼ - ½ teaspoon of powdered ginger. Sweeten with honey and add a bit of milk if you wish. *See Ginger chapter. Eat small, frequent meals, and eat even before you get up. One lady who had extreme sickness was able to get ahead of it by putting a tiny cooler by her bed with a cup of yogurt. When she got up in the middle of the night to go to the bathroom, she ate half of it. Immediately upon waking before even getting up, she ate the other half. That brought her blood sugar up and she was much less sick.

Using B6

Using B-6 and B-12 helps some ladies.

Take 25 mg. B-6, 1 mg. of B-12 and 1 mg. folic acid in the morning.

Take another at lunch and another late afternoon. Do not take it after supper.

This tends to calm and quiet everything. Many Certified Nurse Midwives add Unisom, but I do not believe that that is a good thing. The chemical load on the liver is already too great. I would try progesterone crème first. (from Nature's Sunshine)

Progesterone Cream

As a last ditch effort, there is progesterone creme to fall back on. I would not use it unless the other things do not work. It does change the amount of progesterone that your own body will put out. But, if you are facing a possible hospital stay and you just cannot get ahead, try it. Rub some over your uterus and into your breasts a couple times a day. Do this and sip ginger water or digestive tonic water every few minutes.

A young Amish dad-to-be called a nutritionist wondering what to do. His wife had been in the hospital a number of days on IV and he had no insurance. He wanted her to come home and the doctor was reluctant because she was doing so poorly. My friend told him about progesterone creme (from Nature's Sunshine) and suggested that he try that for her. A few days later, he called back jubilantly. "Guess what?" My wife is up cooking for the harvest crew that is at our house today. That Progest really worked!"

"How much did you use?" queried my surprised friend.

"Half a bottle!" was his enthusiastic response.

We do not suggest that you use that much creme, but in her case it did the trick and saved them a hospital bill and she had no more problems. We suspect that along with low blood sugar, the other main cause for extreme nausea is low progesterone levels. That is why this treatment was so effective.

Some mothers like to use it a half hour prior to preparing a meal. They rub it over the stomach area. Actually the application sites should be rotated each usage. Under upper arms, inner thighs, neck, and tummy are possible sites.

Meat and Hormone problems

We are seeing more and more severe nausea, and I am suspicious that the reason is whacky hormones, especially low thyroid levels. Why are more women having hormone problems? Medical doctors across America are doing studies and coming up with some unusual facts. But the facts make a lot of sense. In fact, they make so much sense that they are becoming the answer to some heretofore unanswerable problems.

Quoting Dr. Julian Whitaker M.D.: "Perhaps the most insidious residue in milk and meat, comes from the two hormones called "bovine somatropin" (BST) and bovine growth hormone (rBGH). These are given to increase milk production, which they do, by 10 - 25%. Treated animals, however, have a significantly increased incidence of mastitis and infections, so they are given antibiotics more often and their milk contains " antibiotic traces."

Studies are linking the relationship of the growth of tumors, fibroids, increased nausea in the first trimester, PMS, and severe menopausal difficulties to this high level of hormones in the meat, milk, and eggs that we eat. They have also linked antibiotic filled milk, meat, and eggs to the development of stronger strains of virus and bacteria that are resistant to the original antibiotics. Europe and Canada have put a ban on these hormones for animals for health reasons! America is behind the times!

Female hormones fed to cattle are the possible culprits behind the increase in female disorders like severe hot flashes, painful periods, and breast lumps.

This excess estrogen tends to override the progesterone needed to have an easy first trimester in pregnancy. Can you see why so many ladies are needing to add progesterone to overcome nausea?

Miscarriage

When you begin to spot with bright, red bleeding, you often start to cramp. It is normal to worry about a miscarriage. We usually advise mothers to stop what they are doing, rest, drink lots of water, and eat well.

One of the biggest reasons, outside of implantation problems or hormone problems, is a bladder infection or a urinary tract infection. These infections tend to trigger cramping. So drink lots of water, take some blueberry or cranberry concentrate (*see kidney bladder chapter), and drink some charcoal water. (*See charcoal chapter.) If this is not the reason for your cramping or spotting, you may want to call Wish Garden Herbs (*see suppliers) and order their wonderful product called Welcome Womb. They will send it to you overnight, and it may be worth it. It contains: wild yam root, black haw bark, and false unicorn root. Suggested use: two to three droppers in water, two to three times per day.

I find that that in many cases this product is very helpful and the cramping and spotting stops completely as long as the mother is careful with her amount of activity and stops if she needs to. Here is a testimony from a Welcome Womb user.

"We conceived easily but I miscarried twice in a row around the 7th week of pregnancy. I have a friend who strongly believes in herbs so I asked her if she had any recommendations.

She advised that I take Welcome Womb the next time I got pregnant. Again, we got pregnant very easily and as soon as I found out, I started taking Welcome Womb. I am now in my 13th week of pregnancy and have seen and heard the baby's heart beat.

We are not completely out of the woods yet, but I firmly believe that Welcome Womb has gotten me through the first trimester of pregnancy with no miscarriage, and I am further along than I ever have been in the past. I will definitely use Welcome Womb with another pregnancy because of my age and my history for miscarriage."

Constipation

Sometimes constipation is a problem because of changing hormones. When blackstrap molasses and extra water is incorporated into the diet the problem is usually eliminated. If it is not, check what you are eating. Do you have fresh fruit and whole grains for breakfast, a big salad for lunch, and lots of veggies and salad with your supper? Or are you filling up on pasta, bread, and cookies? If all else fails try a good, natural, bowel tonic, like Dr. Christopher's Lower Bowel Tonic. This one does not contain habit-forming herbs, but rather nourishing ones that will help your bowel begin to work again. This formula is harmless enough that it would not hurt a baby, and it should help you. Always start with only one dose AM and PM and then if that does not do the trick, add another one until it begins to work. When your bowels are moving at least twice a day with nice, easy consistency, than begin to back off on the formula, one at a time making sure that your bowels continue to move easily.

This is important information because most women with varicose veins are also constipated. Constipation of the lower bowel puts extra pressure on all those veins and they begin to swell and sting and hurt. Sure, you can take vitamin E or wheat germ oil, but if you do not get rid of the constipation you are fighting a losing battle. If you clear up the constipation and you still have varicosities that hurt, buy white oak bark capsules and butcher's broom capsules and take three of each, three times daily. You can also make a strong tea out of white oak bark, dip long stockings into the tea, pull them over your legs and cover with another set of stockings to keep the moisture more contained and leave them on till morning.

White oak bark will absorb through the skin and begin to contract and pull those veins back to their normal state. It is an astringent herb that has no harmful side affects. Order it in bulk. *See supplies and suppliers.

Yeast Infection

It is not uncommon for women to get yeast infections in pregnancy. The hormonal changes and the moist environment foster its growth. You can usually clear up yeast infections if you treat them intensively for a few days. Most times these treatments work as well as a doctor visit or over-the-counter medications like Monistat.

Here is one lady's experience. It may help you. She writes, " I took acidophilus on the first day I noticed the infection, twice the normal doses (in the morning and evening). I also inserted two acidophilus capsules vaginally in the morning and again before I went to bed. I took about 3000 mg. of vitamin C each day. The last thing I did was put hydrogen peroxide on my labia to relieve the itching. It stings for a minute, but afterwards it is sweet relief. After the first night of this regimen there was about 90% less discharge and much less itching. I was amazed that I was almost completely cured in just one day. That is what I did."

> a double dose of more than one brand of acidophilus

> Insert acidophilus twice daily, in the morning and before bed. But I think the gel capsules are best for inserting into the vagina.

> 3000 mg. of vitamin C each day. Do not take more than this in early pregnancy as it may cause miscarriage.

> Hydrogen peroxide on a cotton ball swiped over all the itchy parts. I used it whenever I itched and after each time I used the bathroom.

You can also dip a tampon into plain yogurt and insert it vaginally morning and evening to help with killing the yeast. Some ladies report good success in swabbing the area with apple cider vinegar diluted by half with water. Others use ACV straight but this tends to burn a bit. Still others report that when they swabbed with the vinegar and drank the ACV tonic that we recommend in the apple cider vinegar chapter, their troubles were over in just a few days. This is worth trying. It is cheap and it is in your kitchen.

Some ladies find that they need to take major amounts of acidophilus to really get rid of vaginal yeast. (perhaps 5 times the amount)

Gall Bladder

Sometimes gallbladder symptoms show up during a pregnancy for the very first time. If the symptoms are not too severe, using lots of lecithin and milk thistle may get you through the pregnancy. (Lecithin is important anyway to prevent stretch marks, the need for an episiotomy, or to prevent a tear that could cause heavy bleeding.) Here is my friend's pregnancy/gallbladder story that was severe enough to need attention.

"At age forty-two during the fourth and fifth month of my last pregnancy, I began to get very nauseated. After each meal I wondered why I had eaten anything at all. I had pain under my right rib cage, front and back. I had a bad taste in my mouth and a bad feeling in my stomach. Eventually it got so that the pain was there all the time. I could not lie on my right side to sleep. I couldn't lay on my back or stomach either. That gave me a panicky feeling. I called it morning or all day sickness. My husband disagreed and said it was too late for that to start. He was sure it was my gallbladder. (He'd had his own attacks to deal with before.) Not a bit eager to deal with surgery during my pregnancy and feeling the following would be safer for our baby I decided to do the gallbladder flush. I did it, and my pain went completely away.

Gallbladder Flush

Take a mild bowel cleanser at night. Next morning have tea and toast for breakfast. No more food all day. Drink up to a gallon of apple juice (NOT APPLE CIDER) throughout the day.

At bedtime, Put 3-4 ounces of fresh squeezed lemon juice and 3-4 ounces of cold-pressed virgin olive oil, (at room temperature) in the blender and mix them together. Drink immediately.

Take 4-6 capsules of slippery elm following the oil mix. Follow these with another glass of apple juice.

Go to bed and lay on the right side until you fall asleep. In the morning take a water enema, first thing.

My friend got rid of five or six gallstones about the size of small, baby-lima beans. She has never had an attack since. Doing this cleanse between pregnancies may prevent further nausea in future pregnancies

Rash and Itching

One lady had what I think was PUPPP (Pruritic Urticarial Papules and Plaques of Pregnancy). Violently itchy, she said she felt like she was going to go crazy, it itched so much. Online pictures I found seemed to fit her rash. She tried dandelion root tinctured in cider vinegar. After eight days on it, her itchiness and rash went completely away!

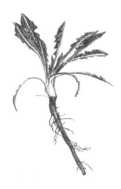

She is thrilled and I am thrilled. Especially because the cases I've heard of with PUPPP, don't go away until after delivery. It would be wonderful if women could take dandelion tincture instead of cortisone creams (occasionally prednisone is prescribed) for this condition.

Fall-dug dandelion root, tinctured in cider vinegar has a tonifying effect on the liver and kidneys, spring root has more of a cleansing action. She took a dropper three times a day, noticed the rash lessening after day three or four, and the rash and itching were all gone on day eight. - selected

Pre-term Labor

Red raspberry tea will give you the calcium / magnesium you need and you should not get muscle cramps if you are faithful to get nice, green salads, and drink your two quarts of water a day. However, if you have been so mineral deficient that you still get leg cramps, try "Natural CALM", from Natural Vitality, a powdered magnesium formula available in most health food stores. Mix a spoonful into a bit of warm water to dissolve it and then add it to eight ounces of juice and you will find that the cramps leave quickly.

Many woman find that if they take this regularly before they go to bed, they sleep much better, too. Magnesium is a smooth muscle relaxer. Did you know that this is what they give women who go into the hospital in pre-term labor? They give them mag-sulfate and magnesium is part of that formula.

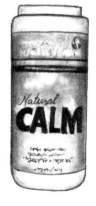

So if preterm labor begins to be a problem, consider slowing down, drinking more tea and water, and taking Natural CALM every few hours until the danger is past. False unicorn tincture also really helps preterm labor to quiet down when coupled with bed rest. Order it from Wish Garden Herbs. *See suppliers.

False unicorn tincture helped our daughter who went into preterm labor eight weeks early to wait until two weeks before her due date to have the baby. The mag-sulfate in the hospital stopped her labor but when they discharged her and sent her home, she started up again so we put her to bed and gave her doses of false unicorn whenever the contractions would pick up. (order from Wish Garden Herbs - see suppliers)

We also gave her Natural CALM. This was very effective and we continued it until four weeks before her date when we allowed her to get up and resume normal activity, without the false unicorn. She began contracting again and had a nice, healthy, six and one half pound baby at thirty-eight weeks. We were blessed.

Some women cannot drink red raspberry tea. In their cases red raspberry stimulates their uteruses and causes contractions. You will need to experiment and if you decide that that is what is happening to you, do NOT drink the tea.

Braxton Hicks or Preterm Labor

So how do you know the difference? First of all, if you are worried, take this feeling very seriously. Second of all, if your midwife or OB diagnoses preterm labor, take this information very seriously. If you are less than thirty-seven completed weeks, it is too early for your baby to come. Such a baby if born would be "preterm". A baby born at less than thirty-five to thirty-six weeks would almost invariably be considered "premature" (their body organs are not mature yet). For example, if you are thirty-four weeks pregnant and experiencing intense or frequent contractions, please do not assume all is well and the baby is just "done a little early". Call your care giver for help.

I think some of the confusion comes because when some of us use the term "preterm-" or "prodromal labor", what we really mean are just normal contractions or Braxton-Hicks that are part of any healthy pregnancy, or a very prolonged early labor (but for a full term baby). If you are contracting six times an hour and your cervix isn't doing much, you're not in labor. Labor = contractions that produce cervical change. But if you're like any number of other mamas who had real preterm labor (contractions plus cervical change long before the baby/ies should be born), you should take serious action to stop the contractions as soon as possible. That's different from someone who has contractions but makes it to full term, and that's just how their body does it. What if you think you are contracting too much? For those who are at risk of developing or are currently experiencing true (as in bad) preterm labor, here are some things you can do:

☒ Take a lukewarm water (not hot!) bath loaded with epsom salt. Use two to three cups of epsom salts. Epson salt is magnesium sulfate which is what they actually use to stop preterm labor in a hospital. Do it every day if you need, to keep strong contractions from coming back. Especially do it at bedtime to relax you so that you can sleep better.

☒ Drink AT LEAST 12 - 14 8-oz. glasses of water a day. More if you can take it. Dehydration (even mild) is a leading cause of contractions. But when you do, you also need to take at least ½ teaspoon of salt to keep your minerals in balance so that you do not feel dizzy from flushing them all out with water.

☒ Eat a nice amount of good protein. Protein foods include milk, eggs, cheese, meat, nuts, and peanut butter.

☒Stop drinking all tea and coffee, whether caffeinated or not. Tannins in these beverages can be very irritating to the uterus.

☒ Stop drinking red raspberry leaf tea or eating anything with raspberries at all. Yes, I know this is controversial, but I've read a lot of research saying while it's safe and beneficial for most women, for some women (women with "irritable uteruses") it can bring on preterm labor.

☒ **Avoid all herbs in the mint family,** including any mint and also basil. Again, these can be irritating to the uterus in large quantities (mint tea, large helpings of pesto, and so on).

☒ Lie on your left side as much as possible. It improves blood flow and calms contractions.

☒ 5 – 10 drops of false unicorn tincture every fifteen minutes for an hour and then hourly for a few hours if needed (while lying down). Order overnight from WishGarden herbs. *See suppliers. This works well and is much cheaper than the hospital.

☒ Start taking at least 1000 mg. vitamin C per day, immediately and throughout your pregnancy, and two to three grams of alfalfa per day, or two to three cups of alfalfa tea, which will help prevent premature rupture of membranes (PROM) and prevent bleeding.

Talk to your doctor/midwife to see if you should be on full bed rest.

To recap... To stop contractions as quickly as possible and buy yourself some time, do this ASAP:

- ☒ Lie down (completely horizontal) on your left side.

- ☒ Drink 4 huge glasses of water and take some Natural CALM. Repeat in an hour if needed.

- ☒ Drink a large protein drink.

- ☒ Take false unicorn .

- ☒ Call your OB or midwife.

- ☒ When your contractions settle a little, take a bath loaded with epson salt.

A Good Protein Shake

1 egg

1 cup of milk

1 tablespoon powdered milk (extra protein)

1 tablespoon peanut butter

1 tablespoon instant chocolate powder or carob if you wish

Blend in the blender. Add a bit of ice and blend. This will give you two or more cups of drink. Drink two cups immediately. This will give you a quick bit of protein that your baby needs. I often say, "The baby wants to come out because he is hungry." This is more true than many mamas realize. See the story at the end of this section.

Supplemental Progesterone for Preterm Labor

There is a lot of cutting edge research going on now about the benefits of supplementing with progesterone throughout pregnancy for women with a history of preterm labor. Progesterone has always been known to "quiet" the uterus and prevent the uterus from contracting during early pregnancy and harming the fetus, and it looks like it is needed throughout pregnancy too. Women with low progesterone are now thought to be at higher risk for premature labor and delivery.

Anemia

Anemia, or low hemoglobin, is sometimes a problem. This is usually remedied by taking the supplements that we recommended above, consistently. If that does not work try the following hemoglobin booster diet. It also helps to reverse toxemic symptoms.

Add:

- ☒ 4 cups dark greens daily taken in salads and/or as a smoothie (See the recipe below)

- ☒ 30 mg. chelated iron taken three times daily after meals with 8 oz. citrus juice

- ☒ 250 mg. vitamin C

- ☒ 400 IU of vitamin E daily with prenatal vitamins (or wheat germ oil)

- ☒ 15 – 20 min. brisk exercise daily (walking or biking)

Dark Green Smoothie

You might think this sounds strange but it really works and it actually tastes good if you put enough fruit in it. You will need

4 cups of spinach (stuff the blender full)

1 or 2 bananas (used to sweeten it)

1-3 tablespoons of pineapple concentrate

3 cups of water

Put all of the ingredients into the blender (a hi-powered one is helpful but not necessary) and blend on high speed until the contents are <u>completely</u> liquid. Taste your mix. Is it sweet enough? I usually start with one banana and one heaping spoon of pineapple and then if I need it sweeter I add another banana/or more pineapple. When it tastes good I like to whiz a few ice cubes into it to make it really cold. Then sit down and drink two cups if you can.

Refrigerate the rest in a jar and drink the remainder throughout the day. This will bring up your iron and give you energy. (You will need to drink **all** of the smoothie to do this. Start with one in the morning and one in the afternoon to get adjusted to the taste. Do not leave the rest for the next day as it loses its value when setting overnight. If you cannot drink that much make half the recipe at a time or share it with your little ones. This is a great way to get leafy greens into your little ones.

Most small children love the way this tastes and beg for more. Change the way this tastes by adding other dark greens like kale. You can use any fruit you wish in place of the ones I recommended. Frozen strawberries work nicely and taste good but be warned that the resulting color is NOT the lovely green of the first recipe. These turn a muddy, sludgy brown, but they will still do the same job and the taste is good.

Bleeding

Bleeding during pregnancy is NOT considered normal. If it does happen and you are doing all the above things, and the bleeding is only slight, take two extra, wheat germ oil capsules and two cups of red raspberry tea and go to bed. If the bleeding continues call your midwife.

Red raspberry also seems to work for tears in the placenta in first trimester. My niece was bleeding in the first trimester and had an ultrasound to see what was the problem. Her OB said she had a 7 cm tear in the placenta, and put her on bed rest but the bleeding did not stop. She still had bright-red bleeding daily. Her mother-in-law came to visit and suggested that she drink red raspberry tea. Yvonne drank six cups the first day and a quart, daily, thereafter. The bleeding slowed and stopped in two days. She continued drinking it and when the OB took an ultrasound two weeks later the tear was completely healed. Her OB was amazed. She said that she had never seen a case where tears that big had healed. God is good. He has made herbs for our use and our healing.

Labor Preparation

Nature's Sunshine Five Week Formula is good to take for a quicker, smoother, easier birth. Begin to take them five weeks before delivery taking one three times daily for the first two weeks. The third and fourth week take 2 - 3 x's daily. The rest of the time take 3 - 3x's daily.

Give your body a rest on Sunday and do not take any supplements that day. Figuring that amount you would need almost three bottles of this formula. Finish taking them 2 - 3x's daily after the birth. They will help with the after pains and postpartum bleeding. You should also continue your tea until the bleeding stops.

Two weeks before your date, begin to take evening primrose oil capsules, one in the morning and one in the evening. Take them for a week, then change the dose to 2 - 3x's daily and cut the tops off two more and insert them vaginally before you go to bed. This will help stimulate the production of prostaglandins to soften your cervix and make it easier to dilate. Do NOT use this if you already have fast labors! You might have to deliver the baby by yourself!

Overdue?

If you tend to <u>always</u> go overdue, order some capsules of Master Gland from Nature's Sunshine. Two to four weeks before your date begin taking 2 capsules, 3 x's a day. Take them until you have your baby.

There are a few other herbs that can be taken to stimulate labor if you are overdue. Ask your midwife if you need help on this one. **The following formula will NOT do you any good unless the cervix is soft and ready to go. Do not even try it.** You will just waste your money and time. You **cannot** find most of these in a health food store but they can be ordered by calling Wish Garden Herbs from Colorado. (Phone number is in Making Medicine chapter.) Start the tinctures early in the morning when you are rested. They seem to work better then and that way you will not need to do the hard work late at night when you should be sleeping. **You must not use this formula without the consent of your midwife, I only included this to keep a few women from having the inductions they hate!** The recipe includes three herbal tinctures and they must be used together to be effective.

blue cohosh - black cohosh - ginger root

Take 1 dropper of each (together) every 15 minutes for an hour along with massage and nipple stimulation.

Then take one dropper of each every half hour for the next two hours.

*If a good labor pattern is developed you can keep on for another hour or two. But do **stop them** when labor is really kicked in. **These herbs could cause bleeding if used just before delivery.***

Otherwise, if they are ineffective, after three hours, stop for that day and try again, later. Baby is not ready yet. I have had really good success in getting overdue mamas going with this little formula and avoiding a number of planned inductions for moms who have called, desperate for advice. I have also tried it myself on a baby that was due (we thought) and had no success, only to birth him two weeks later when we thought he was three weeks overdue. He was NOT overdue at all. He was right on time and he was the size all my babies are at term. We were wrong with the dates and the tinctures did not work.

I specifically remember the mother who dropped in to see our daughter's brand-new baby. She was on the way home from a check up and already overdue. Her midwife was planning to induce her the next day since this had always been necessary in her previous births. The lady was not anxious for the induction since they had always been difficult experiences for her. My daughter suggested that I might be able to help her get going in a natural way, thus avoiding the hated Pitocin and it's difficult contraction. I pulled out my herb case and mixed up the first batch in a bit of juice. She drank it and took the next doses along ready to drink as she went to finish a bit of shopping. The next morning she called to say that she had gone into labor and delivered her baby and everything was going well. Needless to say, her midwife called for my little formula. Miss Midwife was really impressed since she had always had to take this lady to the hospital for an induction. I do not know who to thank for the formula since I found it about seventeen years ago. But it really works for most, truly, overdue ladies! And even though it does contain cohosh it does NOT cause extra bleeding at the birth if you stop using it as soon as you have a good labor pattern established.

Blood Loss

You should not experience much bleeding if you follow the guidelines at the beginning. But if, for some reason, you do experience severe blood loss during the birth, you can quickly build up your blood by drinking one half bottle of chlorophyll in a day, for four days if needed. Then use another bottle over the next four days. Three half glasses of grape juice with as much cayenne as you can tolerate, mixed in, will really help things too. Use at least one fourth teaspoon of cayenne in each half cup of juice. This adds a great amount of oxygen into the blood and will increase the hemoglobin levels steadily.

Post Partum Sitz Baths

An herbal sitz bath is one of the most wonderful and healing things you can do for yourself to aid your healing after giving birth. A sitz bath is basically a small bath that you sit in to ease the swollen, stretched muscles and tissues around your vagina after giving birth. Sitz baths will also help heal perineal tears. You can use a small basin or plastic tub that will fit right into your toilet seat (when the lid is up) or you can buy one at your medical supply store for about twenty dollars. You can buy one at Walgreens. Medline Sitz Bath - $14.99

Call: 1-877-250-5823 Walgreens Co. 200 Wilmot Road. Deerfield, IL 60015

There are different sitz bath herbal recipes available prepackaged at health food stores, online or from your midwife.

Or you fill the tub and add a gallon of herbal tea made from the recipe below.

Sitz mix:

1 oz. of each of the following herbs:

calendula flower	*rosemary leaf*
lavender flower	*shepherd's purse*
witch hazel	*uva ursi*

Add 2 oz. of sea salt to the mixed herbs. Put the mix in glass jar until ready to use. This amount should make you enough for a week of sitz baths, 3 x's daily. You could add others or delete the last two if you cannot find them.

Soak in soothing sitz bath one to three times a day after delivery for up to two weeks. Place a handful (approx. ½ cup) into a quart of boiling water. Simmer for five to ten minutes on low heat. Strain out herbs and add remaining liquid to warm water in sitz bath tub, available in most pharmacies. You will need to use a two cups of mix to four quarts of water for a full bathtub. This is a good way to go if you do not have a sitz bath and it is really relaxing. Do not be afraid to take baby in with you. Soak in the tub for fifteen to twenty minutes as often as you feel a need to.

Peri-pad

You can soak sanitary pads in the fresh tea and refrigerate them for seriously soothing and healing cold. In heat-proof container, add one-fourth cup tea mix to one-half gallon of boiling water and allow to cool.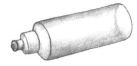

Strain and pour the cooled tea into a peri bottle and keep refrigerated (cool tea is very soothing and provides additional swelling reduction) until ready to use. Rinse vaginal/perineal area after urination and gently pat dry.

Breast Infections

Breast infections should not happen if you are well hydrated but sometimes they do. If you do get one, treat it IMMEDIATELY. This kind of infection gets bad very rapidly, and you can get very sick.

- ✓ **Go to bed immediately and stay there** unless you are in the shower or the bathroom.
- ✓ Drink two glasses of water every hour.
- ✓ Take 1000 mg. of vitamin C every hour.
- ✓ Take Super Duper Tonic or Hot Echinacea if you wish.
- ✓ Put a cabbage leaf in your bra over the sore area to draw out the infection and rub well with poke root oil, to get the lymph flowing again.
- ✓ Get in the shower and massage the sore area well under very warm running water twice daily.
- ✓ Try a charcoal poultice over the area. See charcoal chapter.
- ✓ RUNNING A FEVER? Step up the above routine. Do step two to three every half hour for three hours.
- ✓ **Always nurse the baby. The breast must stay empty even if nursing is painful.**
- ✓ Rub the area with a bit of peppermint oil diluted in olive oil.

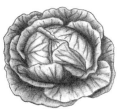

Caring for
Your New Baby

Colic

Colic is not just a word. It is an experience! If you have never lived through days of walking a very fussy, screaming baby, you can count your blessings. Doctors who rub their hands and smile and say, "It is just colic and he will outgrow it," have obviously never lived with a baby like that. As I have had nine babies, eight of whom had severe food intolerances and colic from three weeks on until various maturities, I have much sympathy for others in the same shoes. Most of what I know comes from my own trial and error and from my studies in the last eight years.

It seems that most food intolerances have their roots in the mother's digestive system and in the health of her own liver. This is difficult to address properly when already nursing a tiny baby. The liver must be cleansed and nourished to help to change this and detoxing is not recommended with a small baby. So, in a way, you will have to live with the difficulty that you have until this baby is older and then you can work seriously on it before another pregnancy. But there are some things that you can do that may make a difference.

Begin by strengthening the digestive system as much as possible. It seems that the undigested protein molecules that pass through into your milk, really make most of the problems. Following are a few suggestions that I have.

First - take a very good digestive enzymes before each meal. I recommend Maximizer from R Gardens. *See medicine chapter, if you do not know where to find this product. Other good quality digestive enzymes may work equally as well. Try them.

Second - give a digestive enzymes to your baby. Do this by opening a capsule of the digestive aid you are taking and putting it into a contact lens case or some similar thing. Before each nursing dip a damp finger into the powder and let the baby suck it off. Do this two or three times and then nurse the baby. Do it faithfully before each nursing. This will give your baby a better chance of digesting the offending proteins.

Third- take acidophilus or probiotics yourself and give the baby some, the same way you did the digestive aid.

These three things may help but you might still need to do more. If you do not find enough relief read on.

☒ Make sure that your own bowels move at least two times a day and that you drink at least three quarts of water (and take ¼ teaspoon salt to replace minerals so you do not get dizzy) This will help more than you can ever know.

☒ Take 2-3 capsules of milk thistle or Thistlyn three times daily to gently detox your liver in a way that will not harm your baby.

☒ Use aloe vera juice three or four times daily with nursings. See information on following pages.

☒ If you still have trouble with a screaming baby, give an ounce or two of very warm chamomile or catnip tea to your baby to quiet him and relieve the gas that he is having. The bottle must be very warm and must be given after nursing so that you do not lose your milk. We have had a very good success with this bottle of tea. I hate to recommend it because some women cannot give tea after a nursing and keep up their milk supply. They need all the sucking stimulation that they can get and any bottle is detrimental to their supply. You need to know your own body, but usually this is not a problem if you only do it AFTER nursing is completed. I usually waited until the already nursed baby became fussy and did not want to settle down and sleep.

After the baby is three weeks old, make sure that you do not nurse oftener than every two hours. My babies cried so much that I would nurse them to soothe them and then they seemed to cry because their stomachs were too full. When I learned to only nurse every two hours and then give a hot chamomile bottle if the baby was in discomfort, we made some progress. When the little one is at the place where she should be able to go three hours between nursing, do the same thing, only wait three hours instead of two.

We would make a pint of chamomile tea (unsweetened) and keep it on the counter for the day. When the baby began screaming one of the children would heat it and we would give it to her. Often she would pass gas, always she would visibly relax and many times she would fall asleep. That chamomile tea bottle was a real nerve saver for all of us. A screaming baby can do quite a bit to upset the peace of the home.

We found that mama's diet did, indeed, make a big difference in the way our babies felt.

How will you know whether this is true or not? Here are the top common offenders: Coffee, chocolate, milk, eggs, wheat, corn, oats, potatoes, and tomatoes (in that order) are the most common offenders.

Take the first three foods and eliminate them for at least a week. **Have none in any form whatever.** If baby improves you are on the right track.

But you must eliminate the offending food for at least a week and often for two whole weeks so that you can tell if you are on the right track. It usually takes that long for the offending food to leave your system completely. Then if baby seems to be a bit better, have a "milk day". Have cereal for breakfast, pudding for lunch and milk to drink. If the baby immediately gets worse these things are very likely offenders that need to be eliminated from your diet and NOT fed to the little one until he is at least two. If not, sorry, you will have to try the next thing on the list. There was a time in my life that I said, " I can only eat grass." Of course that was not true but it certainly felt like it and I was having a pity party for me. As I learned the above things about acidophilus and digestive aids and being **very consistent** with my diet our life went more smoothly, even though baby still was restless.

Above all, trust in your heavenly Father and stay very close to Him. Through my many sleepless nights I learned one thing; I must be content and happy even in my trials. When I could pray and meditate in the night even though I could not sleep, I had a much better day the next day. When I felt all uptight and was distressed because I had missed so much sleep, I had a terrible day. So as I went, I learned to rest in the Lord and accept my baby the way he was and be thankful that he was not blind or otherwise handicapped. Each baby outgrew his difficulties and went on to be a normal child, though some took longer than others. A thankful heart is good medicine and a happy mother, though tired, is a good mother.

Eat carefully. Cut out the sugar. For some people sugar ferments in the stomach giving rise to more gas, even in your baby. I think that that may be the reason that so many babies have serious gas. Mountain Meadow Herbs has a colic relief tincture. Some of my friends have used it and found it to work very well. It was not around when I had my little ones.

You can make your own colic relief tincture using the following recipe and it really works. If you are really in a hurry use the crock pot method given in the medicine chapter. That only takes short time.

Colic Relief Tincture

Mix:

1 part - chamomile flower

1 part - catnip leaf & flower

½ - part fennel seed

½ - part dill seed

½ - part fenugreek seed

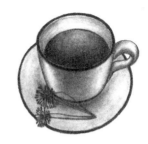

Fill your pint jar half full of the herb mix. Pour one-fourth cup of boiling water over the herbs. Fill the jar with glycerin. Stir well to mix thoroughly. Let set for two weeks or so and strain out the herbs. Bottle and keep in a cool dark place. Give your baby a dropper full whenever he has tummy ache or colic. You may repeat the dose a number of times in a day or night. The only problem resulting from this could be diarrhea if you give too much glycerin to your baby. So be watchful and if your child develops diarrhea cut back on the amount that you give.

Colic Relief Tea

Use the same mix of and add a teaspoon to a cup of boiling water. Let steep for ten minutes. Strain, sweeten just a little bit, and cool awhile. Give as warm as your baby will tolerate. This will relax your baby and help him to move the gas that is causing the belly ache. (Don't sweeten with honey for babies under one.)

Papaya Tablets

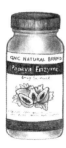

I needed to watch my diet for more than a year for most of my babies. But when I discovered the digestive enzymes and gave them to both of us, things went better, although I still could not use any milk or eggs without lots of crying, rashes, and diarrhea. If I gave my twelve month-old papaya tablets whenever he ate table food, his chronic diarrhea disappeared immediately. He began to gain weight normally and his color really improved. If we ran out of the tablets or forgot to use them for a bit, our problems returned. You will need to experiment and see what works for you.

Aloe Vera Juice for Colic and Infant Constipation

If your newborn is having trouble with colic you might find that adding a dropper of aloe vera juice to three or four nursings a day will help. Take a dropper of aloe vera juice and insert it by your nipple allowing baby to get the juice while nursing. This seems to improve digestion enough that for some babies it completely clears the colic. For others, you may need to look further.

If your newborn has infrequent bowel movements or misses going every day, the aloe vera juice treatment will often resolve this difficulty. It improves the digestion and the bowel function and eliminates the gas that sometimes troubles a new baby.

Bathing Baby

Infant bathing may be one case where less is actually more. According to Loyola University researchers, the average one-month-old baby is bathed four times each week and shampooed three times in the same period. Most babies need only an occasional bath in warm water with no soap or shampoo, unless you are treating a condition such as cradle cap. Following a bath, a gentle rubdown with a quality baby oil (preferably herbal) helps to replace lost skin oils.

The *vernix caseosa,* a whitish protective coating that covers the skin after birth, can have long-term beneficial properties: Natural childbirth advocates believe that if this coating is rubbed into the child's skin instead of being washed off (as is the practice at most hospitals), the child's chances of developing skin problems in the future will be reduced.

They have also discovered that too frequent bathing with lots of shampoo and baby wash actually lowers your child's immune system by depleting the vitamin D on the skin.

A new study brings out the fact that America's babies and children are so clean that have less immunity to germs. We all know that we build up immunity on contact with germs and although we want to be clean, this over-emphasis on cleanliness is resulting in poor immune health and more cases of eczema and dermatitis than ever before.

Cradle Cap

Herbs can be used to heal cradle cap, a thick, yellowish, crusty rash that forms on the scalp and sometimes the face of newborns. This rash is caused partly by an overproduction of oil. The standard medical treatment is cortisone cream, but most pediatricians would rather not use such strong steroids on babies. Instead, wash the scalp with a gentle baby shampoo to reduce excess oils, and treat daily with antiseptic and skin-healing lavender, tea tree, and aloe vera. After washing use a fine tooth comb to comb all the crust out.

Cradle Cap Remedy

¼ cup aloe vera - 3 drops each lavender and tea tree essential oils

Combine ingredients in a bottle and shake well to blend. Apply directly onto the skin a few times daily.

Thrush

This nasty problem can usually be resolved with consistent applications of the following remedy before and after nursing. You must also swab your nipples with the same solution before and after nursing.

¼ tsp. Baking soda in ¼ cup water. If that does not work in a few days switch to

¼ tsp lemon juice in ¼ cup of water and repeat the treatment. Usually one of these will do it.

Here are a few recipes that you can use to make your own baby products that will have no chemical additives to irritate baby's skin.

Chamomile Spray

This spray is very convenient for diaper rash or other skin ailments. You can make it easily.

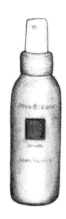

Our daughter says that it works better for diaper rash than anything she has found. And there is no greasy salve to rub on. Just spray it and you are finished. It seems to do a great job with yeast rashes, too.

¼ cup of chamomile infused oil

2 tablespoons of witch hazel (from drugstore)

15 drops of lavender essential oil

¼ teaspoon tea tree essential oil

Mix well and put in a spray bottle. Use after diaper changes and wherever or whenever the skin needs soothing and healing. One operating room in Germany is using chamomile spray after operations to heal the incisions faster and without infection.

Baby Powder

Use:

½ pound cornstarch

¼ teaspoon lavender essential oil

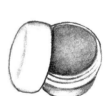

Place cornstarch in a sealing plastic bag and add the oil drop by drop. Tightly close the bag and shake it to distribute the oil, breaking up any clumps through the bag. Let stand four days to distribute the essential oil.

Use with every diaper change, or as needed. Potato starch or arrowroot powder can be used instead of cornstarch. Spice or salt shakers with large perforations in their lids make good powder containers. If your baby has a **yeast** rash this will not help him, in fact it may make it worse.

Diaper Rash Salve

1 cup baby flower oil (see below)

½ ounce beeswax

½ teaspoon lanolin (optional)

6 -400 IU vitamin E capsules

25,000 units of vitamin E with added vitamin D

Heat the baby flower oil just enough so that you can melt the beeswax and lanolin in it. Pop the vitamin capsules with a pin and squeeze their contents into the oil. Stir well. While the mixture is still hot and liquid, pour it into wide-mouthed jars (baby food jars) and let cool.

Apply with every diaper change, or as needed. Be aware, though, that lanolin causes a reaction on some people's skin. If you wish, you can test your baby beforehand by rubbing a tiny amount of pure lanolin on her skin. This salve can be used to treat abrasions anywhere on the body and to combat diaper rash. Or you can use black walnut tincture on the area.

Baby flower oil

Mix ½ cup each of: lavender flowers, calendula flowers. elder flowers

½ cup comfrey leaf

3 cups almond oil

Chop dried herbs and place them in a clean glass jar. Cover with almond oil and stir to remove air bubbles. Put in a warm place (near a radiator or in the sun) for two to three days, then strain out herbs. If necessary, strain again using a cheese cloth or fine strainer to remove the tiniest particles. Store in a cool place.

Teething Oil

Mix together:

1 handful of chamomile flowers

½ handful willow bark shredded

6 drops clove bud essential oil

1 drop of peppermint oil

almond oil

Combine ingredients and fill pint jar. Cover with almond oil. Set the jar in your crock pot and fill the pot with hot water to the neck of your jar. Heat on lowest heat for two days. Make sure your crock pot really does have low heat. Strain and add one tablespoon vitamin E oil to keep this from spoiling. This is alcohol-free and should help to stop the pain and soothe your baby's gums.

The Mature Woman
and Changing Hormones

Peri-menopause

Peri-menopause is another unique time in a woman's life. Just when you think you are going to keep on having babies and nursing until you are a grandmother, you start to experience changes. You may have irregular periods, heavier periods, hot flashes, insomnia, and major mood swings. You may experience difficulty in hitherto good marital relations. There is vaginal dryness, lack of interest, and general mood difficulties. You may feel mood swings like you did as a teenager and you do NOT understand yourself. Is it any wonder that your husband does not always understand you?

Peri-menopause can begin as early as thirty-two if your hormones are out of whack. This can be reversed by the suggestions below and you can go on to live more comfortably for quite a few more years. The average age of menopause is somewhere between forty-five and fifty-five for most ladies. It tends to occur later in well nourished women.

In most ladies the onset is gradual, with things changing over a period of years. Even when the menstrual cycle is still occurring, ovulation tends to slow down as the hormone levels change, resulting in less chance of pregnancy and greater chance of miscarriages. This is normal. You can have a baby after forty-three years of age, but most ladies do not!

This is a time where the periods become different. They may be closer together or farther apart. You may experience heavier bleeding or scanty flow. You may have severe PMS for the first time in your life. There may be vaginal dryness. Your hair may begin to thin. All in all, you may have difficulty accepting who you are and who you are becoming. Your emotions will likely be on a roller coaster. This is due to changing hormones.

What can be done to ease this stressful time of life and make it more livable? After all, some of us still have home-school to teach and some of us have toddlers to cope with, too, if we have had large families. I have been extremely interested in this because I just came through this stage myself, and I talk to so many women who are experiencing these symptoms. For years I have been looking for answers and I found quite a few for myself.

First, accept who you are and who you are becoming. You may not look or feel like you would like too. But a sweet acceptance of yourself and God's plan for you to change and grow older will make this transition somewhat easier. If you understand that this phase is not for long and that others walk this way too, you will navigate these waters more easily.

A closer walk with God will ease these difficult years. God is our refuge and strength and a very present help in trouble. He is our loving Father and our tender Shepherd. Without Him, we would fall apart and our marriages would be under severe stress. But He does help us and we need Him! Let us not forget that fact!

There are a number of things that you can do to make life more bearable and enjoyable during this time. Let me share a bit of my journey with you.

After spending twenty-three years pregnant or nursing (we had 9 children), I began having difficulties sleeping. I mean big time difficulties! For nights on end, I would not fall asleep until twelve or two AM. My difficulty was Restless Leg Syndrome, and while it was not painful, it was incredibly annoying and distressing. The sleep deprivation that followed brought about a variety of other symptoms that were equally distressing. Try as I would, nothing seemed to have a lasting benefit. I suffered through days and weeks and years of the problem, sometimes better and sometimes worse. Then my cycle began to change. I began to flood and bleed for a full week. I would stop for a week and then bleed for the next one. This took a real toll on me physically, so I tried the expensive hormone testing and it's subsequent "natural"? hormone drops. They helped some, but soon I was back to the same problem and they had to increase my dose. The doctor visits were expensive and I did not have that kind of money. I also was concerned about what the drops might be doing to my body. I began to study and see what I could learn about the whole process.

Female Formula – Ladies Formula

Then I found Female Formula from Dr. Schultz and began to take it and it really worked! But it did cost more than I liked. Next I made my own tincture following his idea, and my own Ladies Formula worked just as well! My restless leg problem diminished and I could sleep most of the time. But my periods were way too heavy. So far so good. I found that taking Evening Primrose Oil in substantial amounts helped too. But there still had to be more answers. Finally I stumbled onto an interesting fact. Here is how it happened.

As a family, we went on a grocery fast for about two months to be able to share more with our missionaries. We decided to empty out our freezers and pantry and live on what we had and try not to go to the store if possible, excepting one gallon of milk a week, a few eggs, and a bit of fresh produce. The challenge was fun. But what was even better was the way it affected me. My subsequent periods were not heavy. I was not flooding and clotting and cramping. My mood swings were less severe. I felt better all around. And I began to sleep well again, finally! Why?

I guessed that it was the meat and dairy hormones that I cut out when we were not buying meat at the store, but I was not sure. I began to read about the medical debate and discoveries in that field. I was fascinated to say the least, but not completely convinced. As my phone began to ring, interesting stories began to collect, and my interest grew. Let me tell you a few.

One lady who had been trying and trying to get pregnant for at least five years, even with medical help, was counseled to eliminate all meat, milk, and eggs from her diet for three months and see if that made a difference. In desperation she tried it and at the end of the three months she was pregnant and very happy! Her sister, on hearing that said, "If it helped her, maybe it will help me." She had been having repeated miscarriages at nine to twelve weeks, and was very discouraged. She was not willing to eliminate the meat, milk and eggs from her diet, but she switched to all organic meat without hormones and antibiotics and used much less of it than before. She used free-range eggs and unpasteurized milk from a hormone-free source. In three months, she was pregnant and she did not have a miscarriage. She went on to have a healthy baby. The third, a sister-in-law, was very impressed! Her own PMS and monthly periods were making life miserable for her and her family. She decided to do an experiment and see what would happen to her. She followed the second sister's routine and the first month she noticed improvement. The second month was better and the third month everything was fine. Now that is impressive, and these were real people whom we knew!

When the books say so you sometimes wonder, but when real people you have met find this kind of answer it is truly amazing! There are other ladies that have called about their success, too. But let me tell you the ending to my own story. I finally experienced normal, trouble-free cycles after three years of major problems. This came about after I was doing some experimental food changes like the last two sisters had made and taking Ladies Formula. I am not a vegetarian, nor am I teaching you to be vegetarian. As I see it, the Bible puts teaching abstaining from meat in the same category as forbidding to marry (unnecessary). And I agree! However, if you are having severe health problems or cannot find decent meat, milk, and egg sources, you may need to learn how to eat a whole lot less hormone containing foods, or suffer the consequences. If you are really suffering through change of life, the following information may be valuable to you.

Quoting Dr. Julian Whitaker M.D.: "Perhaps the most insidious residue in milk and meat, comes from the two hormones called "bovine somatropin" (rBST) and bovine growth hormone, (BGH) These are given to increase milk production, which they do, by 10 - 25%. Treated animals however have a significantly increased incidence of mastitis and infections, so they are given antibiotics more often and their milk contains " antibiotic traces."

Studies are linking tumors, fibroids, increased nausea in the first trimester, PMS, and severe menopausal difficulties to this high level of hormones in our meat and milk. They have also linked antibiotic filled milk, meat, and eggs to the development of stronger strains of virus and bacteria that are resistant to the original antibiotics. **Europe and Canada has put a ban on these hormones for animals for health reasons!** America is behind the times! We live in a farming community and more folks do their own cooking, so the quality of meats in general is better. But our meat sources still are not that good. Animals today are given a high load of hormones to speed their growth so that they are ready to be food much more quickly than they used to be. This overload is what is giving us the problem.

Quoting another source: "The FDA's own 1990 screening tests indicate that 46% of all milk samples contain more than one sulfa drug. Female hormones fed to cattle are the possible culprits behind the increase in female disorders like severe hot-flashes, painful periods, and breast lumps." This excess estrogen tends to override the progesterone needed to have an easy transition into menopause. Since most of us are aware of our need for progesterone wouldn't it seem more sensible to go to the root of the problem and cut back on our estrogen intake instead of adding progesterone to our skin and budget?

If you understand that all meat and milk has the normal animal hormones in it, this makes more sense. That is the way God made animals and they do not loose their hormones just because we turned them into meat to eat. Therefore if you are having hormone difficulties it only makes sense to cut back on the amount of extra estrogen that you put into your body until things settle down.

My advice to you is not to be radical but experiment yourself and see what happens. Do not force your family to make the changes. Work at the changes you need, yourself, if you need it, and then if you find that it does indeed make a difference, present the idea to your husband. Most men find the idea of no meat very unsatisfactory. If so, find sources of free-range cattle and chicken that have not been fed extra antibiotics and growth hormones. They are around. The meat is more expensive but it is worth the difference. Locally there are a number of free-range farmers who will raise you chicken or beef and sell it at a fair price. There are other options to the serious looker including a simpler diet more of the time. Use many more bean dishes and whole grains for your protein and use meat sparingly like I suggested before and you will be able to afford it. This kind of diet, along with Ladies Formula, can make a major difference for you. *See recipe on page 242

Research has shown that herbs can help a good bit. Vitex (also called chaste tree berry), dong quai (also called angelica), and wild yam are phyto (plant) hormones that help a good deal. Motherwort is also great for alleviating the stressed out feeling. Midwives recommend it in the tincture form for panic attacks that tend to come (especially at night), at this time in your life. Ladies Formula or Dr. Schultz' Female Formula, contain all of these and has been successful in helping quite a few ladies that I know with severe PMS, and heavy bleeding. It often helps clear up fibroids, that are a cause of heavy bleeding.

We worked with one lady who was facing surgery for fibroids, and in three months of using the formula, without diet changes, she was able to cancel the surgery. This alone will not help everyone. Interestingly, estrogen dominance is a major cause for any uterine growth and puts you at risk for uterine cancer. To cure this you may need to combine the Ladies Formula with less meat, milk, and eggs, especially those without growth hormones.

Ladies Formula (get it at 616-965-1549) also helps for PMS and heavy bleeding. It is not always a sure-fire cure, especially if you are eating lots of estrogen filled meats and milk, and are struggling with constipation. Low thyroid levels will really contribute to heavy bleeding, too. You can eliminate this problem by taking iodine drops. Research the help that magnascent iodine can give for hormonal problems. *See www.magnascent.com. It is very interesting but I will not go into it here. Most of the time you will need to take the formula for three months until you find full relief. It is helpful to incorporate the rest of the healthy living tips at the beginning to assist you. I always hate to see a person take expensive medicine if they are not willing to help it work by making other changes.

The estrogen/progesterone difficulty is usually addressed by giving "natural" progesterone creme or drops to a woman. I feel strongly that this should be a later resort. It is a bigger gun. Use it only if necessary. Try to work on these areas first.

1. Eat a better diet

2. Drink more water

3. Exercise - 30 minutes or more brisk walking four times a week

4. Supplements

    A. Beta carotene / A

    B. Vitamin E

    C. **Evening primrose oil - 1000 - 1300 mg. daily**

    D. A good B vitamin

    E. Calcium/magnesium (liquid is easier to absorb)

    F. Zinc

    G. Iron builder - chlorophyll, floridex, or dandelion root

    H. **3 Tablespoons of fresh ground flaxseed daily.**

5. Daily relaxation (naps) including prayer and meditation

Most ladies who have PMS and hot flashes are also deficient in B6. 100 milligrams daily will often dramatically alleviate these symptoms, as will adequate water intake (8-12 cups daily). If you are interested, you can read the book "You're Not Sick, You're Thirsty!" by F. Batmanghelidj M.D. One reason that water makes a difference is that it helps to dilute the many hormones in the blood stream, making it easier for us to live with ourselves. It also helps the lymph flow tremendously. Evening primrose oil is often beneficial for this difficulty as well. If I begin to have even the slightest hot flash I reach for my evening primrose oil and take a few capsules for a day or two and I am fine again. I began to do this after reading a unique book by a woman who had been going crazy with hot flashes. She had tried her doctor's medicine but it did not work. When she began taking evening primrose oil, the change was dramatic.

Breast Lumps

Breast lumps will often resolve when hormone problems are addressed, but **do not** wear tight garments and do drink enough to keep the lymph flowing. If you do notice lumps, do frequent, gentle massage and dry skin brushing to get the congestion broken up and help the lymph to flow again. This is a must, since these lumps can be a harbinger for cancer. I really think that good diet, water, and exercise will eliminate many of the problems, but massage makes a marvelous difference and if done frequently may help you to avoid a serious outcome. Evening primrose oil taken internally is often a great help for breast tenderness and the anxiety and mood swings that accompany this time of your life. I and many other ladies find that taking evening primrose oil regularly helps a lot with hot flashes. And check on what magnascent iodine could do for you.

Do NOT take regular mammograms. Listen to Dr. Gofman, M.D. who has his PhD. in nuclear and physical chemistry. He has been studying the effects of radiation on human health for 45 years and he reports in his book *Preventing Breast Cancer*, that breast cancer is the leading cause of death among American women between the ages of forty-four and fifty-five. Because breast tissue is highly radiation-sensitive, **mammograms can cause cancer**. Like we've said before, the lymph system must be up and running well, too. But yearly mammograms make NO sense. Learn to check your own breasts and be healthy. It may also shock you to learn that scientists first suggested there might be an antibiotic/breast cancer link more than 25 years ago. With all that in mind, be wise.

A new study (2009) just presented at the annual meeting of the Radiological Society of North America (RSNA), concludes **the low-dose radiation from annual** mammography **screening significantly increases breast cancer risk in women with a genetic or familial predisposition to breast** cancer. This is particularly worrisome because women who are at high risk for breast cancer are regularly pushed to start mammograms at a younger age -- as early as 25 -- and that means they are exposed to more radiation from mammography earlier and for more years than women who don't have breast cancer in their family trees. "For women at high risk for breast cancer, screening is important, but a careful approach should be taken when considering mammography for screening young women, particularly under age 30," Marijke C. Jansen-van der Weide, Ph.D., an epidemiologist in the Department of Epidemiology and Radiology at University Medical Center Groningen in the Netherlands, said in a statement to the media. "Further, repeated exposure to low-dose radiation should be avoided."

If you are concerned about your risks for breast cancer, study what can be done naturally. There is a lot of information out there about what diet and lifestyle can do to heal breast cancer, if you are willing to make some changes.

I know two ladies, right now, who have made those changes a part of their daily lives and they have beaten their breast cancers. One of the ladies is in her 70's. The other lady is in her late 50's. I met the latter one at the place where I get my produce, and I was amazed. She looked so well. Her eyes were bright, her skin looked good, and yet she had unhooked from the system and refused to do chemo and radiation. After a lumpectomy she radically changed her diet and lifestyle. I asked her how her two teenaged daughters were responding to her new way of serving food. "They love it," she said. "They say that it clears up their skin and eliminates their cramps and PMS." I was impressed. I am still learning all I can about this. I do believe that God made food to feed, nourish, and heal our bodies and it still works. It may be at a price. We might need to cut out the salty snacks, the rich food and the sweets that we love. But who cares if the result is a much better quality of life!

Finally, if you do find that you have a serous health disorder like diabetes, heart disease, or cancer, you can do something about it. It does not have to be a drugged out, terrible time of your life. Drugs do not address the root of the problem. They only try to fix the symptoms.

If you are to regain your health, you will need to take responsibility yourself. No doctor can do that for you. If you do not, you will end up taking many different types of medicine, each to compensate for the side effect of the other. Your health will go into a rapid decline and you will spend the later years of your life seriously compromised, unable to be a blessing to anyone. Here is how it usually goes. You are given blood pressure meds for high-blood pressure and heart meds for the heart problems that come with the B/P meds. Then you need diuretics to accompany the b/p meds and potassium to replace what the diuretics took out. Finally you get laxatives to keep your bowels moving since the drugs slowed down your system. You are now on five different medicines daily and that is just the expensive beginning.

The list goes on. In fact it is endless. Many people over fifty are buying into this system and their health is leaving as they bring bottle after bottle of drugs into their kitchen to be taken daily. This type of chemical dependance does only one thing. It compromises your health. Drugs are drugs, whether they are sold on the street or in the pharmacy. They are more harmful than helpful in most cases. Take responsibility for your health. Study your problem and learn about how change of diet and exercise can change most of these problems. Read some of these books.

Eat to Live – Joel Fhurham

Reversing Heart Disease –Julian Whitaker M.D.

Reversing Diabetes – Julian Whitaker M.D.

The Liver Cleansing Diet – Dr. Sandra Cabot

TREATING BURNS
AT HOME

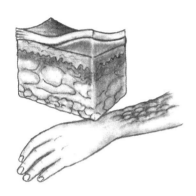

I was studying about burns, one of my most-feared accidents. I was fascinated by how rapidly burns healed using natural remedies and old-fashioned common sense. No more debriding, and no skin grafting. No more infection, very little scarring, and much, much less pain. I was inspired, when I read the success stories of other burn patients, to have the things on hand that I needed to treat burns. I knew that the inside of the aloe plant would soothe the burn and make it heal faster. I kept a small plant in my house to use for small kitchen burns, but it would not do for larger burns. How was I going to have enough aloe to heal a larger burn? One day in the health food store I noticed a quart of 99% pure aloe gel and I brought it home, along with a pint of wheat germ oil, just in case. You know, emergencies tend to happen on Saturday night when all the stores are closed.

Then my phone rang! Since I believe in a God who knows everything, I know that He made sure that I had the information and ingredients that I needed before He sent me my first burn call. My friend was in tears. She had burned her whole hand badly from a fire in her kettle.

"Can you come quickly?" she pleaded.

"Keep it in cold water. I will be there in twenty minutes," I answered. I threw my things into a basket and left in a hurry. When I arrived, I found an angry, red hand that was painfully blistered. A classic second degree burn! We immediately immersed her hand in cold aloe gel to take out more of the heat and begin the healing process. She sighed with relief. Her hand felt so much better. The only way we could keep her

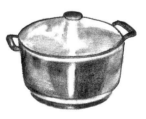

279

comfortable was to keep the aloe gel cold. We did this by rotating bowls, one to soak in and one in the freezing compartment. I left for home an hour and a half later leaving instructions to cover it with vitamin E oil and wrap it when she took her hand out of the soak. The next morning she called me jubilantly. Her hand was doing so well that she was able to go about her duties without pain.

Aloe vera has amazing healing properties and soaking it immediately eliminated the dehydration of the cells that occurs in burns. This is extremely important for all burns. The heat must be taken out and the cells re-hydrated if you want to take away the pain and speed healing.

About the same time a friend of mine who was working on the mission field in Africa was called to attend a two-year old who had rolled into a cooking fire while he was sleeping at night. She had none of the supplies that I have. All she had was honey and a few herbs in a powdered mix, that I call People's Paste. She took pity on the helpless little one who looked like he would not make it. He was in severe pain and badly dehydrated. She did what she could. She applied honey to the whole area (his whole back) and heavily sprinkled it with the herbal powder, and bandaged it. Every morning she went back and added more honey and more powder. These were deep second degree burns, but they healed in three weeks, in a poor native hut with a dirt floor, and there was very little scarring. Impressive?!

A few months later a child in our area stepped into a pan of very, very hot water that had been set off the wood stove onto the floor while his brother went for water to refill it. His whole foot blistered badly with second-degree burns. We immediately soaked his foot in cold aloe gel/juice until the heat was gone and he was able to tolerate having it out of the soak with not too much pain. At that time I did not know how important it was to keep a dressing of herbal burn salve on the burn at all times to keep the pain down, to keep it hydrated, and speed the healing. His parents covered it with vitamin E oil and wrapped it and went to bed. They had a good night but the next few days he was in a lot of pain. Twice a day they soaked his foot in strong comfrey tea (infusion). They gave him Tylenol for pain, daily. This would not have been necessary if I had understood how to dress his burn. Even so, his burn progressed much better than I ever expected. About day 6 they brought him to me because they were concerned about how the burn looked. There was some bleeding and gray- white strips of skin were hanging off the foot. I was concerned about the possibility of his toes growing together as they healed (this is a concern and it is good to bandage the toes separately so that this does not happen). Altogether, the area looked awful to the inexperienced eye. There was redness that I was not sure about. Was it infection? Since I had never treated this serious a burn, I felt very insecure and sent them to his doctor to see what should be done. When the mother called me a few hours later, I received a nice surprise. "Keep doing whatever you are doing, I couldn't do any better," was the doctor's response. "There is no infection. The new skin is growing nicely. It looks great!" (The redness is a normal thing since there is increased circulation to the damaged area to make new skin cells.)

Day 1 – lots of blisters

Day 3 – blisters popped - pain

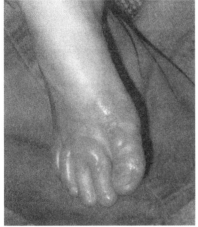

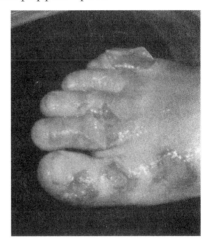

Day 6 - some bleeding, no infection

2 weeks – at 2 ½ he wore his shoe!

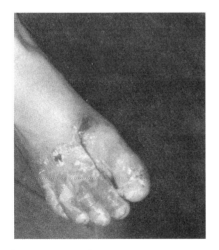

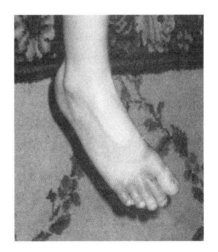

This was all the encouragement I needed to keep on going. The parents continued to do what they had been doing. In two weeks he had nice, pink new skin. He was able to put his shoe on and walk in two and a half weeks. Knowing what I do now, I know

281

that we could have controlled his pain and sped up the healing process.

I continued to study and found a very interesting book called *Help for the Burned and the Wounded* by John Keim. This man had explored the possibility of treating burns in a non-conventional way. He knew what I knew about comfrey, aloe, and honey. He understood about taking out the heat of a burn and hydrating a burn victim. He even made a wonderful salve called B & W salve. But he took the treatment one step farther. He introduced the idea of using green leaves as part of the wound dressing. He did this because of all the problems that he was having with the burn dressings sticking to the wound and causing pain and tissue damage when they changed the dressings twice daily. John Keim began by using plantain leaves over the burn salve that he had developed, and then wrapping the whole thing with gauze. He explained the procedure and his successes with various patients. I was still skeptical. As usual, I had to see for myself. And I did.

One day I burned myself with hot oil, not a big burn, but a painful, second-degree blister the size of my largest finger. I applied what I knew, cooling the burn and then applying the B & W salve that I purchased from John Keim. I did not use the plantain leaf on the salve because I wanted to see if what he said was true. After enduring forty-five minutes of pain, I gladly went to find a plantain leaf in the yard. John was right. I placed the leaf over a fresh application of burn salve, bandaged it, and in less than five minutes I was pain-free. I was convinced. My burn healed quickly and painlessly. But that was not the end of my journey.

My phone rang again and this time it was a two-year old who laid his hands on a red-hot flat-topped stove. *See the comfrey chapter. He healed so well and without a scar. I was becoming more and more comfortable with the body's ability to heal. The Lord had given me lesson after lesson in burn healing and I was beginning to wish that there was a way I could learn more. Then I saw "Burn Classes" advertised in our local health food store. John Keim, who was skilled in caring for serious burns was coming to teach us how to do it ourselves. My husband and I enrolled in the class and it was an extremely informative day. We are continually thankful that we took the class. Time and again I fall back on the information that I learned.

Our teacher explained that burns of any kind should not be exposed to air. This dries them out and causes pain. He showed us how to dress a burn and wrap it to cushion it and keep the moisture in. He taught us how to determine whether there was infection or not. He taught us what supplies to use, where to get them, and what problems to look for. This information was so helpful to me. I would like to pass it along to you so that if you ever have a serious burn, you will know what to do or where to find help to do what you need to do. I will tell you why a hospital experience should be avoided unless you are dealing with third degree burns or an extensive burned areas. I will tell you where you can order your supplies in a hurry when you need them. I will even give you a phone number that you can call if you need a bit of information when you are at your wit's end and you want to talk to someone.

At the end of this information I will tell you the story of Seth, a two-year old who sustained deep 2nd and 3rd degree burns to at least twenty-five percent of his body. We learned so many things treating this child that you need to know. I will tell you the story from the perspective of the burn caretakers. Seth is still healing today as I write this and I continue to be amazed at how God works. We all made mistakes as we worked with this burn. But we learned from our mistakes. We hope that you will learn from them, too.

Burn Percentage Chart

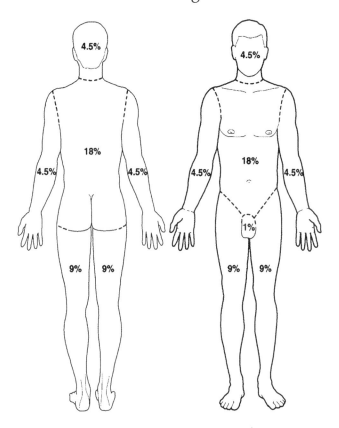

This chart shows you how to determine what percentage of the body is burned. It is important that you learn to recognize the percentage of the body that is burned. You will probably not want to treat more than ten percent body burn at 2nd degree unless you have supervision. This is because the body tends to go into shock because of tissue damage and fluid loss and must be carefully monitored, especially in a smaller child. Loss of fluid puts a severe strain on the heart and blood vessels. This coupled with the emotional trauma and serious physical pain makes a person vulnerable to shock when there is more than ten percent of the body burned. Perhaps you can find a person in your area who is skilled in dealing with larger burns. Become familiar with the following list of symptoms of shock so that you can recognize it before you have problems. You should also get at least 24 ounces of B & W salve for any emergency.

Diagnosing Shock

The most common symptoms of shock include:

- An extremely low blood pressure
- Fast but weak pulse
- Dizziness, faintness, or light-headedness
- Feeling weak or nauseous
- Moist, clammy skin
- Profuse sweating
- Unconsciousness or extreme sleepiness
- Rapid, shallow breathing
- Feeling anxious, agitated, or confused
- Chest pain

What To Do in Case of Shock

- Immediately give cayenne tincture by mouth if the person is not unconscious.
- If they are unconscious, rub a few drops of cayenne tincture on their tongue or on their gums.
- Repeat in five minutes.

Call 911 for immediate medical help. Shock can develop rapidly. You will need help.

While waiting for help do the following:

☒ Check the person's airway, breathing, and circulation. If necessary, begin rescue breathing and CPR. Even if the person is able to breathe on his or her own, continue to check rate of breathing at least every five minutes until help arrives.

☒ If the person is conscious, place the person in the shock position. Lay the person on the back and elevate the legs about twelve inches. DO NOT elevate the head. If raising the legs will cause pain or potential harm, leave the person lying flat.

☒ Keep the person warm and comfortable. Loosen tight clothing.

☒ Give more cayenne if the person is still conscious.

IF HE VOMITS OR DROOLS

DO NOT give the person anything by mouth, including anything to eat or drink.

Rub cayenne tincture or powder into his gums.

Do NOT give him liquid that will choke him.

DO NOT wait for milder shock symptoms to worsen before calling for emergency

medical help.

Here are some reasons that you may consider treating **some** burns yourself or with qualified help.

1. A hospital is very expensive, and burns done the medical way usually take longer to heal.

2. Hospitals are scary places for a child who has been experiencing the pain of a burn.

3. Hospitals today are trained to look for child abuse and often suspect it in burns, even when the whole thing was an accident. This can lead to investigation and all that Social Services involves.

4. Hospitals are germ filled places since there are so many different kinds of virus and bacteria there from all the sick folks that they are treating. A burn patient tends to contract staph and other bacteria since many burns are open and unprotected.

5. Burn treatment today is very painful and very antiquated. Let me tell you what

they often do. This procedure varies from place to place but most of it happens regularly.

a. The burn is scrubbed with some antibacterial solution. This is very painful and the burn is already hurting.

b. The burn is then covered with antibacterial salve or cream and bandaged. Since burns seep fluid, this fluid dries onto the bandage. Two times a day these bandages are ripped or stripped off the burn to change them. This causes severe pain as the burn is pulled and torn during the procedure. Many nurses refuse to do this and it is often hard to find nurses that will do burn care as the patients usually scream and cry.

c. As the new skin cells develop, if they even get the chance with the above procedure, the wound is debrided. This happens daily in an effort to keep bacteria away. Debridment is the process of taking away all the old tissue and dead skin. It usually involves scraping or water pressure. This process is extremely painful.

d. The patient is then taken to the burn tank where they are soaked in an antibacterial soak. This is in an effort to keep the burn from growing bacteria on the treated areas. Burn patients tell us that this part of the treatment is excruciating. I am sure that they are correct since I have watched children with bad brush burns react violently to soaking in water.

e. Lastly, there is skin grafting on deep 2nd degree and 3rd degree burns to help new skin grow. Grafting is another very painful process and often the skin grafts do not take well. Sometimes the body refuses them and the graft must be redone numerous times. These grafts have problems even when they do well. Many times the skin graft does not grow at the same rate as the normal skin. Then there must be numerous surgeries to cut and release the skin so that the fingers do not curl or the skin does not become too tight.

f. Often there is severe scarring resulting in keloids which are unsightly bumps of hard, whitish tissue over the burn area.

Let me review each of these points and tell you what the herbalist would do to treat serious burns. I will use John Keim's success again. He has treated burn patients for over 20 years. He has had an incredible opportunity to see what his method will do and where its weaknesses are as compared with the normal medical route.

1. Home burn care is far less expensive, with the majority of the cost being the bandages and the salve. Most burns heal in less than half the time it takes using burn center methods.

2. You are the child's familiar caretaker and the trauma is greatly reduced.

3. Child abuse investigations could still be an issue if you run into problems and need medical help.

4. Germs are present in the home, but not more than in the hospital, and you must take very good care that you use sterile material and wear gloves or have your hands scrupulously clean when doing burn care.

5. There should be much less pain dressing the burn the way I will show you. If it does occur, there are many things that you can do to alleviate it. Check the dressing, add more salve, change the salve and dressing, rewrap, etc.

6. Treating the burn:

   a. With this method we never, never scrub the burn. We almost always leave the old skin in place until the new skin begins to form under it, and then we pat it off with gauze or clip it off carefully, never pulling or ripping. Occasionally a deep 2nd degree burn will have a blister that will need a little help later on. If it does not come off,infection could begin.

   b. The bandages do NOT stick to the wound since we have used the burn salve topped with the scalded leaf/s. This dressing peels off like a ripe banana skin.

   c. We do debridement by patting the gauze against the wound and picking it up gently. If that is not enough, we use another gauze and pat again, repeating this process to gently lift off all old, dead material. This allows all fragile, new skin cells to grow rapidly, especially since we are nourishing them with the herbs and oils that are in the burn salve. When you feed the skin it will regrow at a rapid rate. We do not use the painful burn tank at all. We simply redress the wound again.

   d. Mr. Keim has never had a need for any of his patients to have skin grafting. He has even treated many serious 3rd degree burns that covered up to 30 percent of the body. **We do not recommend that you treat 3rd degree burns yourself.** Perhaps in your community there is someone who is able to do it the natural way. Your local health food store may know who would be available. The herbal way seems to grow skin in a way that is miraculous to the doctors looking on. They do not have the same results.

e. Scarring happens much less since we have nourished the tissues and provided the necessary ingredients to help the body form new, flexible skin. This skin has all the sweat glands and hair follicles just like the rest of the body. Grafts never have sweat glands and hair follicles. Folks that have skin grafts say that this area is very uncomfortable in the heat of summer.

This way of treating burns is so much more humane and provides gentler results than the other way. If the patient is well nourished, it provides faster results, too.

Is it any wonder to you that we recommend finding someone who can help you save your child the agony and long term trial of living in a hospital's burn unit somewhere, only to spend the rest of their life disfigured by the scars that most burn patients have?

We realize that you will be appalled with the damage that has been done, unnerved by the awful thing that has happened, and distressed by the pain your child is going through. It is good to think about it beforehand and be ready with a game plan if this was to face you.

What to Do if You Have a Burn

- Immediately **cool the area** in water, aloe vera juice, or milk (whatever is handy).

- Cool **until the pain is gone,** if possible.

- It usually takes at least ½ hour and can take as long as 4 hours if the burn is over a large area, like a whole leg or a whole arm.

- **Immerse that part** in a bowl or pan of water or whatever it takes to thoroughly cool that area. It can take a few hours to cool the burn.

- **Assess burn damage.** Is it 1st, 2nd, or 3rd degree? Assess percentage of body burned.

- 1st is just red and not blistered. 2nd is blistered. 3rd degree usually has the skin burned or sloughed away. Occasionally it is still there and looks white or gray since it is dead. This burn is very serious and you will probably need someone to help you do this, after you have done the first steps. These burns are treatable, but it is more important to really know what you are doing.

☒ **Dress wound -** apply B & W burn salve very carefully at least 1/8 inch thick.

☒ Cover the salve with a scalded plantain, burdock, or grape leaf. The leaf should be scalded in almost boiling water until it is wilted and then cooled. Scald it while you are cooling the burn and allow the leaves to cool while you are getting your other things together. If you need burdock leaves, or any other dressing supplies, you can call in an order to the address below and they will overnight them to you.

☒ Over the leaves, place an ABD pad. This pad will trap in the moisture so that the burn will not dry out. It will also provide a cushion to protect the wounded area. If you do not have an ABD pad, fold up part of a blue bed pad and use that to cushion it.

☒ Now wrap this all carefully with a 4″ gauze wrap. Tape it a small bit with paper tape. Only use paper tape.

☒ If you have a large area that you have dressed, you will need to get a package of blue bed pads (Chux or something similar) and wrap the area completely with that, tape it in place, securely wrapping the tape several times to hold the whole dressing in place. If the dressing slides, it will cause pain.

☒ **Change dressing every 12 hours**

Gently pat the unwrapped wound with as many gauze squares as you need to pick up loose bits of skin and dead material. Never rub or scrape. The whitish jelly-like material is new skin growing. Do not disturb it.

If there is pain, unwrap and check to see what is causing the pain. Perhaps there is an area of burn that is not covered well enough. Perhaps the salve is not on thickly enough. It should be "1/8" thick . Perhaps the dressing slid. Did you wrap it too tightly?

Maybe you need to use a different salve for a few days if you have been treating the burn for a week or more. Ask a trained burn care person for ideas.

☒ See that the patient drinks enough fluid in a day

20 lbs. - 2 cups or more

40 lbs. – 4 cups or more

60 lbs. – 5 cups or more

80 lbs. – 6 cups or more

100 lbs. – 8 cups or more

120 lbs. – 10 cups or more

140 and up - 12 cups or more

This is **very important** since burns really dehydrate a person and to rebuild healthy cells quickly, you need lots of water or other electrolyte fluid. Use Emergen-C or Pedialite, or make your own. THIS IS IMPORTANT!!! If the person does not feel like drinking, give them small sips every 15 minutes. Divide your dosage of cups up into 12 hours and see that they get enough to finish the desired amount in that time. If they do not get this fluid, they may dehydrate so badly that you will need emergency medical help. Almost always, small sips very often, will work better than big drinks occasionally.

Another thing that you must think about is physical therapy for bad burns. The healing skin may constrict movement and motion if the person is not forced to exercise the area. THIS IS EXTREMELY IMPORTANT. I spoke with a care giver recently who did not see to it that this was done for a small child with serious burns on the chest and under the arms. The child was from a home where there were other little children and the mother was the care taker and she either did not understand the need for physical therapy or because she was so busy, she never got around to it. Today the burn is healed with scarring and the child's range of arm movement is restricted. If we want the doctors and the hospitals to recognize that we are knowledgeable and able to provide the needed help for our burn cases, we must be faithful in helping our burn cases to do physical therapy.

Burn Supplies – B & W Salve

The address for supplies is: Holistic Acre – 15526 St. Rd. 258, Newcomerstown, OH 43832

Write for their catalog. **They supply B & W salve and bandages** at a good price but **you cannot call them** so order in advance so you have B&W on hand for emergencies. I would order at least 16 – 24 oz.

If you cannot find B & W salve and you have an emergency, call Miller's Natural Foods to order it. Phone – 717-768-7582 or order it from ElysiumNaturals.com – 616-965-1549.

Call Moore Medical Supplies for a catalog for bandage supplies: 800-234-1464. Our favorite: Moore conforming gauze 4" non- sterile.

Another Burn Story

We treated a serious burn using part of the method that our Amish friend recommends. I really think that if we had used his method for the whole time the duration of the treatment would have been shorter.

The child, a seventeen month old boy, was seriously burned on more than twenty-five percent of his body when he tipped over a kettle of boiling water his mother had prepared to use for steam inhalation with his sick baby brother. He tipped the kettle then slipped and fell on his back in the scalding puddle. This resulted in deep 3rd degree burns over most of his back, under his arms and on his thigh (about 20%). There were other burns of 2nd degree nature on about one quarter of his head, his arms and elbows and his shoulders (10%).

His mother immediately immersed him in a tub of cold water and when we got there we used aloe-vera juice and gel over the whole burn. He screamed seriously through the whole ordeal. Finally we applied B&W ointment and wrapped him with gauze, but it was too early in the year for the Burdock leaves and none were available. When he was wrapped he immediately quieted and lay resting peacefully. The change was both dramatic and convincing. I had seen it before and it never ceases to amaze me. I assessed the burn as 30% of his body and when I called another person who has been treating burns, he highly recommended that we take him to the hospital since the burns were extensive and the child was so young.

We arrived at the hospital and like they usually do, they stripped his dressings to assess his burns and felt unable to treat him themselves, which we were not asking them to do anyway. All we wanted was for them to keep him stable and we would take care of the burns. But this hospital had never treated a baby that was burned that badly before and they were terrified. They left his burns undressed for the next four hours while they waited for a transport to the nearest burn center. This children's hospital is accustomed to treating a child with extensive burns. By midnight the baby was on its way and we were promised a chance to dress him in the morning. Morning found us there at ten AM, ready to do our job. But we waited and waited on the doctor. We were accompanied by another man who had been trained in a different method of dressing burns. He had been allowed to help dress another child in this hospital the year before and the doctors there knew him.   All this delay made the burn worse in the long run.

Finally at 1 PM the doctor came and graciously allowed us to dress the burn while he watched. When we were finished he told us that we can keep on doing what we were doing and discharged us, asking us to wait a bit so that they can see if the little one will eat before he goes home. He did, and by seven PM we were on our way home. Knowing what I do now, if that were ever to happen again, I would ask them to keep the child for a few days for hydration. But they did not know, and neither did we, how badly the child was really burned.

The first dressing of B&W ointment and the aloe-vera had done such a good job of already helping that we were fooled into thinking that the burn was less severe than it really was. To make the story shorter, we landed back in the hospital for many days, because of our first mistake of going home too quickly. The burns progressed nicely but the child was seriously compromised and we needed the hospital's help to stabilize him because of dramatic fluid loss and trauma to his little body.

The man who had connection with the burn center and helped them to allow us to dress the burns uses union salve. The hospital was comfortable with his method because that was all they had seen done before. Since I am an herbalist, I would have rather used the B&W ointment, but I feel so strongly that the body will heal if allowed to take its course that I went along with them. We switched to B&W ointment after about two weeks of using the union salve, when I felt that the staff was comfortable enough with us that I dared to try it. This change was a hurdle but their top specialist had just come back from a burn seminar where they had introduced the idea of using honey and they were interested in the fact that the B&W salve had honey in it. They also liked the look and the smell of the B&W ointment better. We ran into a snag with them when the skin began to come off and they saw that it was really 3rd degree burns on most of his back, thigh and arm pit.

The doctor strongly recommended the use of a chemical debridement (colaginase patches), not trusting that his body would be able to do the job efficiently. The parents, already traumatized and unsure, went along with his suggestion and we suffered a real set-back, that has affected the burns even until now. This debridement seriously affected the new skin growth and sloughed it off and we had to begin over again. Never-the-less, the staff never ceased to be amazed at how well he did at dressing change time. He sat and allowed us to change his dressing with a minimum of discomfort, although they continued to insist on giving him some pain medications. You must understand that most burn patients have severe pain at changing time and this causes everyone a lot of distress. But the B&W ointment way truly takes most of that pain away.

Because of the severity of the burn, which the doctors finally acknowledged was mostly 3rd degree, we spent a lot of time in the hospital with him on a feeding tube and IV's. But always they allowed us to do the dressing and were very impressed with the results. It took longer for the burn to heal than I expected it to, partly because we were not really allowed to do the burdock leaves with the dressing in the hospital until the end when we had won their confidence. Since we could not use the leaves he was on way too much pain medication which definitely slows the healing. He also was on very poor nutrition in the hospital which is another set back. Burn patients need optimum nutrition. He should have had lots of fresh carrot juice and fruits instead of hamburgers and french fries. But, no matter how we "cut the cake" the boy is healing well from large 3rd degree burns, without grafting. This, in my estimation, is well worth the effort that I spent in the weeks of dressing the burns. He is at home now, still healing the worst areas and he is a very happy little boy.

From time to time we had to give his body a break from the B&W and use another cream for a day or two. But the staff admitted to us that they also have to change dressings when they have used one for awhile. We did get some very unusual blisters all over his third degree areas that were extremely disheartening, just as we thought we were coming along really well. No one that we could talk to knew what they were and our mentor, himself, was in the hospital at the time. We kept on doing what we were doing and gradually they deflated and disappeared. I am still in search of information on those blisters and if anyone else has seen them, and what they have done to shorten their duration.

One lesson I learned from all this is that to be really effective in the hospital, the parents and the care giver must be on the same page. If I were to do this again with parents that did not know about the natural way to heal burns, I would sit them down and carefully share how it is done so that we would completely agree in the presence of the doctors and thus prevent the use of the medication where possible. This alone would speed the healing time. I would also teach them about the value of good nutrition in speeding up the healing time. I am convinced that freshly juiced veggies and greens would have been far better in the feeding tube than the sugary stuff the hospital used, and the fast food that they sent up for him to eat almost daily. If we had been able to do it the optimum way, we would have used burdock leaves, no medication, and better nutrition. This should have hurried the healing time. But life is generally not optimum and this is a testimony that the body heals if you nourish it and work with what you have and trust the Lord to help you as you go.

Notes:

"A Pill For Every Ill"

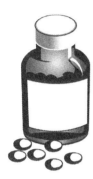

Adult onset diabetes is reversible with diet, exercise, and a few supplements. Doctors know this, but they seldom tell you, since diet counseling is both time consuming and unsatisfactory to most consumers. You see, most people do NOT want to make the strict changes necessary to change the onset of a disease.

Only you can make that difference in your own life. Heart disease and diabetes usually go hand in hand. Heart health is possible using the diet outlined in the previous pages and some added nutrients like hawthorne berry syrup, cayenne, and exercise. If you take the time to learn how, you can combat most diseases like colitis, osteoporosis, heart problems, and even cancer. The challenge is yours! Begin today.

America uses lots of pills. We use them for fever, headache, and tummy ache, with almost no caution. Many people take over-the-counter medicine with as little thought as if they were eating candy. "Surely," they reason, "These pills will not hurt us. If they could, they would be prescription drugs."

Yet this is not true. Over the counter medication can do a lot of harm. It should seldom be used, and then used carefully. I used this line of thought myself when our children were small. I had very fussy babies and I learned that if I gave them some Benadryl when they were extremely fussy, I might get a few extra hours of sleep. What a terrible thing to do to a six month old baby, but I did not know better. I did not know any of the information that I am giving you. The more informed I have become, the less I have used drugs. They are a great blessing when we need them, but mostly, we can do much better things to relieve headaches and get rid of pain. After all, pain is a signal that something is wrong. Learn to look for the cause of the pain and deal with that instead of popping a pain pill.

Look at the following newspaper clipping. Even at advised doses, Tylenol may harm the liver.

R_X

"Though overdoses have been linked to organ damage, this study is the first to suggest trouble in healthy people taking the drug as directed."

By Denise Gellene, Times Staff Writer
July 5, 2006

"The highest recommended dose of Extra Strength Tylenol sharply increased liver enzymes in healthy adults in a clinical study — an early sign of possible organ damage. Although overdoses of Tylenol have been found to harm the liver, this study published today in **the Journal of the American Medical Association,** is the first to spot hints of trouble in healthy people taking the pain reliever as directed."

Even the medical world is beginning to tell us **to pay attention to what we take.** Incidents abound, where over-the-counter meds are responsible for liver and kidney failure in children and adults alike. I cringe when I hear a mother say, "You can take Motrin and Tylenol alternately if your child has a fever." That is what she may have been told, but here is a story about what can happen even when medicating your child exactly as you have been told to do.

This present day story is reprinted by permission of the author.

"Let me tell you about an adventure my family had a few weeks ago," says author Andy Kaiser. " I should also say that I'm not a doctor, and nothing you read here is official medical advice. This is my understanding of what happened in this specific case. I have to lead with this information because, while the story starts out fun, it ends in the hospital.

My family went on vacation. Unfortunately, after just a few days, my daughter, Ally, got the flu. She's four years old, and this was a bad flu, the kind that really wipes you out. My wife and I had to take care of her full-time. We decided to ditch the vacation and come home, but not before stopping off at the local hospital to see if Ally was okay. And she was, the doctor told us. Just a standard flu. *Keep her hydrated*, wait it out, and she'll be fine soon. For controlling her fever, we also got a prescription for Motrin (that's a brand name ibuprofen used for fever and various aches and pains).

On the ride home, I called Ally's pediatrician, and he agreed with the other doctor.

But after five days, Ally was still wiped out. She hadn't eaten in that entire time. She couldn't eat anything without having to give it back within the hour. She could barely keep down water.

The fever was gone. She just had continual nausea. While she was really weak, every once in a while she would move on her own. She'd burst into tears and say that her back hurt. She'd then flop around to change position, and that seemed to help. My wife and I thought this was just because she'd been laying in that position for so long, her muscles were cramping up. I get backaches after sleeping the wrong way overnight – my daughter had been laying in the same position for almost a week. We brought Ally to her pediatrician's office, and were reassured that – again – it was just a regular flu.

Then we found blood in Ally's urine. We drove to the emergency room.

When we got to the E.R., the doctors, thankfully, were excellent. When we described all that had happened, one of the first things they said was, "We think she's having problems with her kidneys. Has she mentioned having any back pain?" That was one of those times where I felt like a complete failure as a parent.

"Yes," we said, "She has complained of back pain. " The doc was right: Ally was in the process of kidney failure.

From there, they moved very quickly. I'll keep most of the details to myself because, well, I want them private. But here's one to give you an idea of what the parents and child had to go through: Ally went into surgery to have an IV inserted into her neck. Minutes after she woke up from the anesthesia, they started kidney dialysis. The neck IV was hooked up to a big machine that looked like a giant clothes washer. It took the blood out of her body, cleaned it, and put it back in.

That was day nine. Nine days of no food, little water, bad sleep, the physical trauma of a bad flu and, as we found out, kidney failure.

Luckily, that was the worst of it. Things turned around very shortly after the dialysis. It was just what her body needed, and having a machine clean her blood gave her kidneys a chance to recover.

Things are fine now. The rest of the story is just recovery. After a week in the hospital's intensive care, we got to go home. Ally needed help walking again, but after a few wobbly trips to the hospital's children's activity room, she recovered with a speed I can only envy. We're now home and we're healthy.

I told you the whole story so you can understand how we got to the point we did. I tell you this so you can prevent something similar from happening to someone you know.

Remember earlier, when I mentioned that Ally was given Motrin for fever control? According to the kidney specialist, the Motrin was probably a contributing factor to Ally's kidney failure. Even if she had just one dose.

Motrin, ibuprofen, aspirin, and similar drugs are part of the same class. This class is called *"non-steroidal anti-inflammatory drugs"*, or NSAIDs.

NSAIDs are used for fever control, pain reduction and a few other things. However, they have bad side effects when used in the wrong way, or when used under the wrong conditions. They also work the kidneys overtime.

Based on our conversations with the hospital doctors and Ally's kidney specialists, here's what we think happened:

Ally got the flu. At the beginning of the flu, she may have also had a small existing infection that didn't show any symptoms. (This happens, and often the body can fight off such a thing without having the infected person realize there's a problem.) This weakened her kidneys.

She got some Motrin for fever control. This NSAID drug did its job, but it stressed her kidneys. She was dehydrated from the flu. This weakened her kidneys even more. After a few days of this, Ally's kidneys couldn't take any more. They started bleeding and shut down.

When the doctors realized this, they gave her tons of liquids and electrolytes through an IV, gave her some other drugs to reduce the kidney damage and jump-start her metabolism, and they also did the dialysis.

This is one of those situations where – not too many years ago – this problem would kill someone. Fortunately for us, today's medical technology is advanced enough that we can monitor what's going on, and replace the function of the kidneys so that they can take a break and recover.

My wife and I spoke with the kidney specialist for quite a while. There were four interesting points the specialist made that I want to make clear:

She said, "Don't use Motrin or any Ibuprofen on children if that child has a chance of being dehydrated. You're better off giving the child acetaminophen. A brand name acetaminophen is Tylenol. Its effects on fever and pain are similar to those of ibuprofen, but acetaminophen is processed by the liver.

Ibuprofen is processed by the kidneys. The short version:

(1) If a person is dehydrated, that person should not take any ibuprofen (like Motrin).

Author's note*(I believe that they should not take Tylenol either, in similar situations. Tylenol is just as hazardous as it depletes glutathione in the liver, which is a VITAL factor for proper immune function. In other words, if a child gets sick and is given Tylenol, right when that child needs a hard working body, you knock it to the ground and disable the immune system.

This is currently causing a lot of controversy within the medical community as Tylenol has been the prize choice by doctors (despite no scientific foundation). Given in conjunction with vaccines, studies show it can cause mitochondrial dysfunction, predisposition to autism and a lowered response to the vaccines themselves. The parenthesis are mine, inserted into the story for clarity and warning.

(2) For adults and children, if you must take an ibuprofen like Motrin, take it with a lot of water. Let's examine my own favorite headache medicine – a bottle of Motrin (Andy Kaiser writing again). Nowhere on that bottle does it say anything about water intake or dehydration. I also have the original prescription detail sheet from Ally's hospital-assigned Motrin. (It does give warnings. They're buried in the small print, but they're there. It says, "TAKE THIS MEDICINE with a full glass of water." It also says, "DO NOT lie down for 30 minutes after taking this medicine." …do those sound like reasonable instructions to give to a kid who's been vomiting all day, and is so weak she can't even sit up on her own? What's also strange is that the Motrin prescription with the "take with water" warning was for 100 milligrams. The Motrin bottle with no such warnings was 200 milligrams – twice the strength of the prescription! I would think the larger dosage would have more warnings, but the opposite is true.

3) She said that if Motrin was brand-new and released into the marketplace today, there's no way it would qualify as an over-the-counter medication. It would be prescription only. It's a powerful drug. In fact, the specialist said that they sometimes need to intentionally shut down people's kidneys for certain kinds of treatments, and the drugs they use to make this happen are indeed drugs like Motrin and others in the NSAID class.

4) There's small print on a lot of medicines that says, "Only take the smallest effective dose." Heed this warning. Sure, if I have a headache, it's tempting to just take a double dose of Motrin. But I'm potentially damaging my kidneys when I do so. And if I'm really dehydrated, I could really damage my kidneys. For the record, the specialist also said that you need to be more careful with children than adults – NSAIDs don't affect adults as much as children.

"Got all that," says Andy? "Let me cut to the chase:"

If Tylenol or any acetaminophen will do the job, don't give children Motrin or any Ibuprofen. If you do give a child Ibuprofen, make sure they're well-hydrated. That's my story, and what I learned from it. It's easy to think certain medicines are safe, and the prevalence of Motrin in every pharmacy, grocery store and doctor's office gives a false sense of safety. In Ally's case, it wasn't just the Motrin that hurt her kidneys. It was a combination of problems, of which the Motrin was a large part. - Reprinted by permission of Andy Kaiser

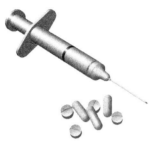

I have included this story to help you understand that simple, available medicines can do great damage. You may have often used them and had no *noticeable* side effects, but you do need to understand the risks. **Always read the fine print on the bottles and always use them sparingly.** Many times a cup of hot tea or a back rub and some herbal remedy will help your child to do without potentially harmful drugs.

Quoting *Washington Post,* February 10, 2004, *Making Us Nearly Sick,* "Working with doctors and our federal government, the drug industry has succeeded in creating a new medical category called "pre-disease." It's no surprise that a majority of Americans now fall within the guidelines of this "nearly sick" classification for at least one pre-disease. Many people will meet the criteria for several." This new classification allows for more room to take more drugs.

From *Prescription of Fear* by Dr. Julian Whitaker, Whitaker Clinic, CA

By lowering the cut-off for healthy cholesterol from 220 to200, the number of people in the US who qualified for medication TRIPLED. Because of the changed guidelines, 104 million, or 50 percent of all adults are now considered to have unhealthy cholesterol levels. In just two years, cholesterol-drug sales **increased** by a whopping 32.5 percent! . . . Yet every medical study ever done on people with borderline conditions shows that they benefit most from simple lifestyle changes before considering treatment. **Drug treatment at this point is premature, unnecessary, expensive, and potentially dangerous.**

But ask the average M.D. and he'll tell you "lifestyle changes don't work." That's because most doctors aren't well educated about these changes. They have little or no interest in helping people make behavioral changes. And really they are not interested because the healthcare system won't reimburse them for this approach, and most folks do not really want to change. (*Most Americans want a pill, not a lifestyle change) parenthesis mine.*

Quoting U.S. News and World Report *"Risks of pain medication.*

"Studies as to the safety of many of the available prescription drugs are doubtful and even sometimes downright misleading, as was proven in the Vioxx outrage. Many people were harmed before the company made their $2 billion and pulled the drug. What is more alarming, a cousin to Vioxx was developed when Vioxx seemed to be coming under fire. Now the FDA is taking a closer look at other NSAID's (non-steroidal anti-inflammatory drugs). This list includes Ibuprofen, Motrin and Advil. Actually, none of these over the counter meds are without difficulties. In fact most of them have not been tested for their safety. They were grandfathered in when the drug safety act was passed in 1938. It has been said that many of the over-the-counter drugs would need to be pulled, including Ibuprofen, if they would be under present scrutiny."

Here is more information that helps me arrive at the idea that we MUST take responsibility back for our own health.

Breast cancer risk linked to over-the-counter pills - By Betsy Querna 6/1/05

"What the researchers wanted to know: Is there a connection between use of aspirin and ibuprofen and breast cancer risk?

What they did: The researchers followed more than 114,000 California women between the ages of 22 and 85 for at least five years. All of the women were cancer-free at the beginning of the study and completed a questionnaire that asked them how often they took over-the-counter pain relievers and for how long they had been taking them. The researchers asked about all pain relievers, including acetaminophen (such as Tylenol), but they concentrated their analysis on ibuprofen (such as Motrin or Advil) and aspirin, which belong to a class of pain relievers called non steroidal anti-inflammatories (NSAIDS). They used the California Cancer Registry to determine if and when the participants were diagnosed with breast cancer, as well as characteristics of the cancer.

What they found: Regular use of aspirin or ibuprofen did not change breast cancer risk until the pills had been taken for more than five years. Long-term ibuprofen users had a 51 percent greater risk of developing breast cancer."

The researchers were puzzled because they *said* the drugs did not contain cancer causing agents. What they forget is that any drug or chemical needs to be filtered out by the liver so that the bloodstream remains pure. The liver becomes more and more toxic, predisposing the body to allow cancer to grow. It is that simple. It does not take a million dollar study to figure it out.

Doctors are often only the middle-men between the drug company and you, with the pharmaceuticals offering them cruises, bonuses, and trips to Vegas as incentive for the use of their drugs. There is not enough of time for your busy doctor to do personal research on every drug that walks through his door in the salesman's bag. He is given samples of the newest drug to give away for free. Most doctors do not know the bottom line on the harm that drugs do. They were not taught much about it in med school and now they are busy. New drugs come out continuously. You **must study for yourself** and learn all you can about how the body works and what can be done to heal without drugs and their side effects. This will enable you to meet your own families' special needs in the way that is best for you. Always ask questions.

I suppose that this study came easier for me than some people since I had such fussy, sick babies and was trying desperately to find a way to help them. This, in turn, led me to a lot of really interesting information that I began to slowly process. The real climax came when I began to have my own health problems and the doctor was not able to help me. My journey intensified. To make it even more interesting, our family has had some unusual experiences with doctors. Some were downright scary, resulting in three near-death experiences. We need doctors, but they can and do make mistakes. These mistakes can mean very serious things when one is using drugs. They may mean the difference between life and death. We need to take responsibility when thinking about what medicines and treatments to take. Do your research carefully before taking any drugs at all.

Writing in the Journal of the American Medical Association (JAMA), one of the biggest medical magazines published in America, Dr. Barbara Starfield of the Johns Hopkins School of Hygiene and Public Health, says that 250,000 deaths per year are caused by medical errors, making this the third-largest cause of death in the U.S., following heart disease and cancer.

The American Medical Association (AMA) has studies to show how many times doctors have over-medicated, or given the wrong medication and have had serious results. They (the doctors) said that deaths resulting from the mistakes, treatments, or surgeries of doctors was the third leading cause of death in the USA. This was an amazing figure to me. They gave the figure at 250,000 deaths a year, higher than that of death by car accident! And standard medical pharmacology texts admit that relatively few doctors ever report adverse drug reactions to the FDA.

Gary Null PhD, Carolyn Dean MD ND, Martin Feldman MD, Debora Rasio MD, Dorothy Smith PhD wrote an interesting article entitled, The American Medical System Is The Leading Cause Of Death And Injury In The United States.

Here are a few of the things that they bring to our attention.

"A definitive review and close reading of medical peer-review journals, and government health statistics shows that American medicine frequently causes more harm than good. The number of people having in-hospital, adverse drug reactions (ADR) to prescribed medicine is 2.2 million. Dr. Richard Besser, of the CDC, in 1995, said the number of unnecessary antibiotics prescribed annually for viral infections was 20 million. Dr. Besser, in 2003, now refers to tens of millions of unnecessary antibiotics.

The number of unnecessary medical and surgical procedures performed annually is 7.5 million. The number of people exposed to unnecessary hospitalization annually is 8.9 million. The total number of iatrogenic [induced inadvertently by a physician or surgeon or by medical treatment or diagnostic procedures] deaths is 783,936.

The 2001 heart disease annual death rate is 699,697; the annual cancer death rate is 553,251.

It is evident that the American medical system is now the leading cause of death and injury in the United States. "Under-reporting of Iatrogenic Events - As few as 5 percent and only up to 20 percent of iatrogenic acts are ever reported. This implies that if medical errors were completely and accurately reported, we would have a much higher annual iatrogenic death rate than 783,936. Dr. Leape, in 1994, in a JAMA report, said his figure of 180,000 medical mistakes annually was equivalent to three jumbo-jet crashes every two days. Our report shows that six jumbo jets are falling out of the sky each and every day."

. . .Dr. Lucian L. Leape opened medicine's Pandora's box in his 1994 JAMA paper, Error in Medicine. He began the paper by reminiscing about Florence Nightingale's maxim – **"first do no harm."** But he found evidence of the opposite happening in medicine. He found that Schimmel reported in 1964 that 20 percent of hospital patients suffered iatrogenic injury, with a 20 percent fatality rate. Steel in 1981 reported that 36 percent of hospitalized patients experienced iatrogenesis with a 25 percent fatality rate and adverse drug reactions were involved in 50 percent of the injuries. Bedell in 1991 reported that **64 percent of acute heart attacks in one hospital were preventable and were mostly due to adverse drug reactions**."

Did you note here that the percentages are rising over the years rather than falling, even with our much advanced health care. Something is wrong with this system.

. . . in 1995, a report in JAMA said that: "Over a million patients are injured in U.S. hospitals each year, and approximately 280,000 die annually as a result of these injuries. Therefore, the iatrogenic death rate dwarfs the annual automobile accident mortality rate of 45,000 and accounts for more deaths than all other accidents combined." This admission, by their own pens, is alarming to any thinking person.

The Nutrition Institute of America reports that in 2003 iatrogenic deaths were tallied at 700,000. That number is just slightly higher than the 699,697 deaths by heart attack in 2001, and the 553,251 who died of cancer. That is a tremendous number of deaths that could have possibly been prevented."

And ponder this information: Medical imaging radiation isn't good for you, no matter what anyone tells you. Routine imaging is going to have disastrous results. Just one CT scan exposes you to as much radiation as 100 chest X-rays. Shockingly, many doctors don't know this! And they fail to take medical imaging radiation into account when prescribing these procedures for patients. The next time a doctor wants to subject you to medical imaging tests, ask WHY you need the test and WHAT the test might reveal that could be helpful to your physician. You might also ask if there's a safer alternative that could provide the same diagnostic information without the radiation shower. *See New England Journal of Medicine – Elements of Danger – The Case of Medical Imaging by Michael S. Lauer, M.D.

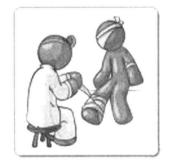

Ask yourself this: Why does **the doctor flee the immediate area** every time you get a chest X-ray, a mammogram, or a CT scan, and only returns after the imaging is done? The reason, of course, is because they're too intelligent to stay in the radiation zone and be exposed to the very same radiation they've ordered for you. Obviously they would get repeat doses since they work in this field, none-the-less, it is beginning to come to the attention of the medical world that the imaging that they are ordering is actually helping to raise the cancer rates.

We are glad for doctors. They are very helpful when we have a need. They are especially helpful in trauma, accidents, and emergencies. But Americans have been conditioned to use doctors without thinking to the detriment of their own health. Think with me, how many people over forty do you know who are not on any medication? This is not normal.

The reason I have given you this information is to get you to begin to think. Begin to ask questions. Begin to study. Do your own research before submitting to lots of tests or using drugs. Learn about your body and how it functions. Your body is a marvelous thing. God has created it to do all that you need to live and if you take care of it and feed it properly, it will work well for you but it is the only one that you will ever have. Care for it intelligently. Using many of the things that you have learned in this book, you will be able to cut down on the amount of drugs that you take and the amount of tests and doctor visits that you need. This should be beneficial to the health of your family.

Although I do not have a chapter on Immunizations in this book I really encourage you to study what is in them and what they are doing. If you have a computer go to Thinktwice.com and research the subject. There is a lot of thought provoking material out there to read.

Notes

Antibiotics –
America's Wonder Drugs!

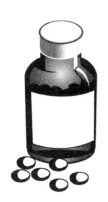

Antibiotics are the first line of defense for most doctors. When you take a child with the flu to the doctor you will almost always get an antibiotic.

Why should you be slow to use antibiotics? Following are some excerpts from medicine's own research. These are not health nut ideas!

"Almost half of patients with upper respiratory tract infections in the U.S. still receive antibiotics from their doctor. According to the CDC, 90% of upper respiratory infections are viral and **should not be treated with antibiotics.** *In Germany the prevalence for systemic antibiotic use in children aged 0-6 years was 42.9%. *Data indicates that on average, every child in America receives 1.22 antibiotic prescriptions annually.*

Group A beta-hemolytic streptococci is the only common cause of sore throat that requires antibiotics. Penicillin and erythromycin is the only recommended treatment. However, 90% of sore throats are viral. The authors of this study estimated there were 6.7 million adult annual visits for sore throat between 1989 and 1999 in the U.S. Antibiotics were used in 73% of visits. Furthermore, patients treated with antibiotics were given non-recommended broad-spectrum antibiotics in 68% of visits. The authors noted, that from 1989 to 1999, there was a significant increase in the newer, more expensive broad-spectrum antibiotics and a decrease in use of penicillin and erythromycin, which are the recommended antibiotics. "Orthomolecular Medicine News Service, Oct. 13, 08

Many health care practitioners advise that antibiotics should be reserved until absolutely necessary, because careless use can depress the immune system and lead to further illness. Certain portions of our gastrointestinal tract, including the mouth, small intestine and colon are populated by trillions of friendly bacteria. These friendly flora contribute to our health by increasing our immune competence and our ability to fight off disease. They help us eliminate wastes and provide many other helpful benefits. When antibiotics are used, they kill both the unfriendly and the friendly bacteria. Then harmful elements like candida (yeast) take over the space vacated by the friendly bacteria and cause many types of chronic illnesses and symptoms.

In addition, antibiotics can cause diarrhea and other disorders of the digestive system. They are also linked to asthma and many chronic illness and difficulties. When the immune system is thus comprised you get more and repeated illnesses.

My husband's sister had a routine tooth extraction that went well. No problem, except that the antibiotic that she was given was a problem! A few days later she had serious stomach ache and diarrhea. This escalated to a real problem that would not go away. Her husband, in talking to another nurse, learned that this type of reaction can be serious, cause a hospitalization, or even death. They immediately began to study what they could do to counteract the side effects of the drug that she had taken and heal her insides. She was so weak and ill that she just wanted to die. It took a long time before they were able to restore the health that she lost through one "harmless" antibiotic 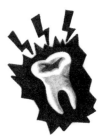 that was prescribed, "just in case," since there had been no infection at all when they gave it to her.

Many times when folks finally come to me for help, they have been to the doctor two or three times and been prescribed antibiotics but the problem has come back repeatedly. This is because overuse of antibiotics weakens the immune system.

There are medical studies that show that **women who have used antibiotics have a much higher incidence in cancer.** The authors of this JAMA study found that women who took antibiotics for more than five hundred days - or had more than twenty-five prescriptions - over an average period of seventeen years had more than twice the risk of breast cancer as women who had not taken any antibiotics. The risk was smaller for women who took antibiotics for fewer days. However, even women who had between one and twenty-five prescriptions over an average period of seventeen years had an increased risk; they were about 1.5 times more likely to be diagnosed with breast cancer than women who didn't take any antibiotics. The authors found an increased risk in all classes of antibiotics that they studied.

The study compared the antibiotic use of 2,266 women with breast cancer to similar information from 7,953 women without breast cancer. All the women in the study were age twenty and older, and the researchers examined a wide variety of the most frequently prescribed antibiotic medications.

The authors offer a few possible explanations for the observed association between antibiotic use and increased breast cancer risk. Antibiotics can affect bacteria in the intestine, which may impact how certain foods that might prevent cancer are broken down in the body. Another hypothesis focuses on antibiotics' effects on the body's immune response and response to inflammation, which could also be related to the development of cancer. It is also possible that the underlying conditions that led to the antibiotics prescriptions caused the increased risk, or that a weakened immune system - either alone, or in combination with the use of antibiotics - is the cause of this association. *Antibiotic Use in Relation to the Risk of Breast Cancer - Christine M. Velicer, Susan R. Heckbert, Johanna W. Lampe, John D. Potter, Carol A. Robertson, and Stephen H. Taplin JAMA. 2004;291(7):827-835.

This is not surprising when you understand that lowering the immune system, like antibiotics do, increases the risk of cancer. The overuse of drugs and the rise in cancer go hand-in-hand. To top it off, the treatments for cancer that America is spending billions on producing and using, are not working, and the doctors know that they are not. Sure, sometimes they help. But when they are really studied, they are proven to be majorly ineffective, not to mention that they have such terrible side effects that many people die from the side effects of the treatments.

America is involved in a wide-spread, overuse of drugs. Beside prescription drugs, there are antibiotics in our food and in the meats that we eat. This misuse has caused microbes to develop that are resistant to the present antibiotics, rendering many antibiotics potentially ineffective. It greatly contributes to today's medical crisis. Doctors are prescribing stronger and stronger antibiotics to control these resistant germs. These stronger drugs cause **more side effects** so they are **more dangerous and more expensive.** Many times the drugs, or combinations of the multiple drugs taken, combine to make the patient as sick or sicker than the disease that he was originally taking them for. We have had this happen numerous times in our family and in the families of our friends. It is a very real problem.

Another interesting thing about antibiotics is that they seem to work fairly well for bacterial infections but have very little positive effect on most viral infections. Many times your infections are viral in nature and medicine will have little or no effect on it, but will rather compromise your ability to get well. Thus, you are being given an ineffective medicine that will affect your health adversely later.

The American public is now living in a sort of terror about an epidemic of smallpox, or swine flu, or other potentially harmful sickness. The reality is that this could happen as a result of warfare or spread of a virus where the present antibiotics would be ineffective. With this in mind folks are discovering other ways to treat diseases. In France and Germany, doctors routinely treat diseases using plants and essential oils along with their traditional methods. You can actually go to a pharmacy there and purchase these treatments for your specific need. They are definitely ahead of America in their knowledge and ability in this area

Learn how to work with your body to fight sickness and disease so that you need to take very little antibiotics. Then when a serious illness comes along and you do need an antibiotic your body will be better able to deal with it. This kind of education is one of the missions of this book.

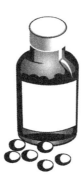

PART 3

PLANING AHEAD

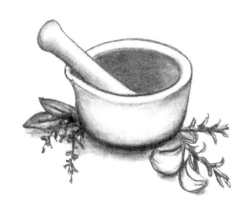

Making Medicine for Your Family

Teas, tinctures, and salves really help our family get through our hard times without needing the doctor. We try to keep our cupboard stocked so that we are prepared for any emergency, from strep throat to appendicitis or deep cuts and bad burns. It is really amazing that our family of 11 has used the doctor so little. We have had a cut sutured, a heart and thyroid condition checked out, and an appendix and a cyst removed. But we are usually, by God's grace, able to take care of our own needs and many of those in our church community around us. I will share some of my recipes with you so that you can be prepared to aid your family when the need arises.

How to Prepare Your Herbs

Tea

Tea that is made from leaves and stems is always made by bringing the water to a boil, turning off the heat, and then adding the herbs. Cover the kettle to keep in the valuable volatile oil in these herbs. Let the tea steep for 15 minutes. **Never boil leaves and stems! You will loose valuable nutrients.** Strain and sweeten.

You usually use a heaping teaspoon of tea to a cup of liquid. I use 2 tablespoons to a quart, and 1/2 cup of leaves for a gallon. Sometimes I double the amount of tea in the kettle and then ice it after it is sweetened to make 2 gallons. We all love to drink tea and it is a beverage that I do not mind if they have. The more I experiment with herbs, the more I think that if you made most any herb into a tea it would probably work almost as well as a tincture. So if you like drinking tea you might just like to make echinacea tea when you are coming down with a cold instead of taking the tasty echinacea tincture. It would be quick and easy! That applies to most herbs.

If you are using **bark or roots** you need to bring the water to a boil, add the roots or bark and simmer, covered, for a half hour. This will extract the medicinal properties from the harder material. Strain and sweeten.

Fomentation

To make a fomentation, dip a cloth in **double strength** tea and put it on the wound or sore place. Keep your fomentation warm by changing the cloth in the tea. I like to use a crock pot to keep the mixture warm. I put two old washcloths in the crock pot – use the one till it cools and then switch to the next one. In this way I can keep the area nicely warm and wet.

Hot and Cold Soaks.

This is a **very effective** way to speed healing for sprains, torn ligaments, rotor cuffs or muscles. Use double strength tea (like the fomentation) to make a hot soak and also prepare a bowl of ICE water. Have a few towels handy.

Soak the affected part in the hot solution for 4 minutes. This must be as hot as he can possibly tolerate it. You can keep it hot by adding hot water as your water cools.

Switch to the cold water. Immerse the area and keep it there until it becomes uncomfortable. This usually takes 45 seconds to a minute.

Plunge the area back into the hot soak. You have kept this warm by adding more hot if needed. Soak in the hot for 4 minutes. Then reverse to the cold soak for nearly a minute. Do this procedure for a half hour. You will have done the procedure six or seven times.

The reason that this speeds up the healing is that it dramatically increases the circulation to the area. Increasing circulation always speeds up healing.

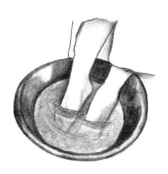

If the area is a knee or a place that does not soak well, use the fomentation method. Make sure your water is hot enough to really do the job and change washcloths often to keep the area really pink when doing the hot soak. Then use cold wash cloths from your ice water bowl. It can work marvels. Complete Tissue Herb is wonderful for this but plain hot water works too.

Poultices

A poultice is made by mixing powdered herb with warm water or oil until you have a spreadable mixture. Then spread it onto a cloth and apply it to the wound. Or you can heat water to boiling and crush a fresh leaf and dip it into the hot water until it is softened then apply the warm, wet leaf directly to the area that needs healing. Poultices can be kept warm with a hot water bottle or heating pad if needed. This is a very effective method of healing a wound or taking away pain.

Tinctures

Tinctures are a liquid way to take herbs. This is one of the easiest ways to get herbs into children besides tea. Tinctures are also stronger and easier to take wherever you go.

Dosages

Adults - 2 droppers. In sickness we take many herbs every hour or two without harm for a few days.

Children - 1 dropper; toddlers - 1/2 dropper

Infants - a few drops with every nursing.

The key to success in using herbs to make tinctures: Use **FRESH** herbs whenever possible to make your products. Take the herbs **IMMEDIATELY** when you begin to feel sick.

Take the herbs **OFTEN**, like every hour or two if needed until you begin to feel better. Then when you feel better, give your body a break so that it does not become accustomed to the herb, thus rendering the treatment of less effect.

Alcohol Tinctures

Use coarsely chopped fresh herbs or dried herbs.

Fill the jar **full** of chopped, **fresh** herb or ½ **full** of **dried** herbs.

Add alcohol (80 proof vodka) until it covers the herb and wets it completely with 1" of alcohol above the herb. Cap the jar tightly lining the lid with waxed paper so that the lid does not rust fast to the jar or use the plastic screw on lids.

Shake daily for two to four weeks. Strain out the liquid and wring out all you can from the wet herb. Bottle and label clearly. If you do not have a brown jar, store it in a cool, dark place so the light does not destroy your tincture.

Glycerin Tinctures

 # 1. Use coarsely chopped or ground fresh or dried herbs. Fill a pint jar full with the fresh herbs or ½ full of dried herbs. Add one-half cup of boiling water to moisten the herbs.

Add glycerin to cover the herb to 1 inch above the herb. Stir the mixture to mix well. Cap the jar tightly and let the jar stand for two or three weeks, shaking daily. Strain out the liquid and wring all you can from the wet herb. Bottle and label clearly. The ratio is 3 parts glycerine to 1 part water. Make sure your herb is not wet so that it does not get moldy.

Or **#2**. Fill your crock pot with water. Place a hot pad or folded dish cloth in the bottom of the crock pot. Set your jar(s) in the pot, making sure that water is as nearly up to the neck of the jar as possible. Turn the crock pot setting on low, making sure it will **not** boil. Add water as needed to keep the water level up to normal. Stir the liquid once a day, recapping tightly. At the end of two days remove from the water bath. Strain out the liquid and wring out all you can from the wet herb. Bottle and label clearly. If you do not have it in a brown jar store it in a cool, dark place.

Note: I like to make my alcohol and glycerin tinctures and then when they are finished I make a mix of half and half. This way you have the benefit of the strength of the alcohol and the sweetness of the glycerin. I find that most people take this mixture better than either the straight alcohol or glycerin. Do not give any alcohol to a small baby. Use glycerine tinctures for babies and young children.

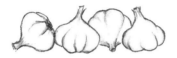

Tincture Recipes

Tasty Echinacea

> *2 parts fresh echinacea herb, chopped*
>
> *1 part fresh echinacea root chopped. (dried will work but it is much weaker in strength)*
>
> *1 part peppermint leaf chopped (for flavor)*

Make a mix of 75% glycerin and 25% water. Cover the herbs. Let stand two to four weeks shaking daily. Strain and bottle. Use liberally for children and adults alike.

Hot Echinacea

> *2 parts fresh echinacea herb, chopped*
>
> *1 part fresh echinacea root chopped*

1 part fresh garlic cloves

1 part cayenne (this one is hot and it is much more effective than Tasty Echinacea.)

Some folks put it in capsules to take since it is hot. This will not work quite as well, but it does keep your mouth from burning. Three capsules equal about 1 dropper. Cover the herbs with vodka. Let stand two to four weeks shaking daily. Strain and bottle.

Throat and Tonsil

To one pint of Hot echinacea add at least ½ cup fig syrup. Do not make it too sweet. *Then add ¼ teaspoon of peppermint oil.* Stir well and taste. You may want to add more peppermint to give it a cooling effect but add it drop by drop until it suits you. This coats and cools the throat for strep and other sore throats. Use hourly if needed.

Super Tonic

Use e*qual parts of freshly chopped or shredded onion – garlic – horseradish – ginger and cayenne (Use less if you do not want it too hot. You can use habanero or jalapeno peppers.)*

Fill quart jar with chopped mixture and cover with raw apple cider vinegar. Let stand for 2-4 weeks. Strain and bottle. Use liberally anywhere you would use an antibiotic. It works very well to ward off any cold or flu symptoms. It works best if you begin to use it at the first sign of illness or sniffles. I find that it will usually clear things up in a day if I start immediately at the first sign of sickness.

The Best "Dried" Echinacea Tincture

Buy 4 oz. good quality dried echinacea root. Grind the root (in a coffee grinder) and place it in a quart jar. Add the following to the jar:

☒ *2 handfuls grated ginger root*

☒ *4-6 orange slices*

☒ *2 handfuls freshly-chopped or dried peppermint*

Cover with 2 times more brandy (or vodka, brandy tastes nicer) than dry ingredients. You need the alcohol to extract the herb's qualities.

Cover the jar with plastic wrap and screw the lid on tightly. Shake the jar daily for two to four weeks. Strain the mixture through a cloth or a stocking and squeeze all of the liquid out of the "marc" (the herbal material).

Bottle the completed tincture in glass containers. Close tightly, label, and date it. Most alcohol-based tinctures keep indefinitely at room temperature in a dark cupboard.

Sleepy Time Tincture:

Mix together equal parts of

Lemon balm, catnip, chamomile, passionflower, oat straw, 1/4 part hops.

Cover with glycerin/water mix. See glycerin tincture recipe. Let stand for two to four weeks shaking daily.

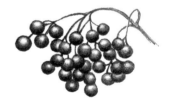

Sleepy time tincture is a combination of herbs that relax and calm. It contains the same herbs as the relaxing tea has. This tincture works well for both mamas and children. It quiets babies tummies when they have colic and calms older children and mothers. You can add ½ part valerian to the tincture for adults but **NOT for children.**

Elderberry Flu Tonic

Cover 1 pound of dried elderberries with 8 cups water. Bring to a boil and simmer on low for 10 minutes. Turn off heat and let set for 24 – 36 hours. Strain and wring out all juice through a cloth.

To 7 cups of juice add 6 or 7 cups of honey

*1 ½ cups of echinacea root glycerin tincture **without the peppermint***

Add vinegar to taste- about ¼ to ½ cup or more if desired. Vinegar will help to preserve and aid in chasing the flu but taste it as you add it so that you do not add more than you wish to taste. Vinegar does have a unique flavor.

Heat just enough to melt the honey and then bottle in dark bottles, or freeze. If you use fresh elderberries cover them with water and follow the recipe as directed above. This recipe is similar to Sambucol or Berry Well, works just as well and costs so much less. Berry Well has propolis in it. You can buy that and add 2-4 ounces to the above recipe if you wish.

Rose Hip Syrup

This syrup is an excellent source of vitamin C. It keeps well in the fridge.

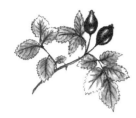

2 cups rose hips to 4 cups water. Bring to a boil and simmer for 20 minutes or until the water has been reduced by half. Cool slightly and strain through a cloth. Stir in 2 cups of honey to taste.

Use this as a syrup on pancakes or take by the spoonful for your daily dose of vitamin C.

Herbal Jello

A nice way for children or skeptics to take herbs.

1/4 box cherry jello (health food brand). Sugar will make it less effective medicine.

1/4 cup boiling water

1 oz. tincture

1 oz. cold water (2 tablespoons)

1. *Put the jello powder into a small loaf pan 2 1/2 x 6 1/2.*
2. *Dissolve with the boiling water, stirring well (make sure it is dissolved).*
2. *Add the tincture and stir well.*
4. *Add the cold water and stir well.*
5. *Pour into a loaf pan or similar container and chill.*
6. *Cut into 12 equal pieces and each piece will give about 2 ml of tincture, enough for a good dose of tincture.*

If you leave it uncovered in the fridge it will dry out and turn into a gummy!

When a child is really sick have him take a piece every half hour to forty-five minutes. This will give him the whole batch in about eight hours. You can do this with echineaca and you will see good results.

Helpful Herbal Teas

Pregnancy Tea

Mix:

3 parts - red raspberry leaf

1 part - alfalfa leaf

1 part – nettles

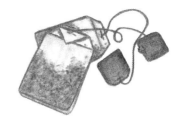

Drink one quart daily the last five months of your pregnancy. Use 1/4 cup of tea mix to 1 quart of boiling water. Let stand for fifteen minutes. Strain and sweeten. Add ice to make two quarts. This is enough for two days. Drinking this faithfully will really help to shorten your labor in most cases.

Flu Tea

We drink this tea when flu is going around the church. We make it by the gallon and chill it and drink it and it really helps. If someone does come down with the flu we drink it every hour.

3 parts - red raspberry leaf

1 part - alfalfa leaf

1 part – nettle leaf

1 part – peppermint leaf

¼ part –yarrow flower

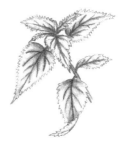

Pain ReliefTea

Boil 1 tablespoon of whole cloves in 3 cups of water for 20 minutes.

Add 2 bags of chamomile tea. Let steep 10 minutes. Strain and sweeten well.

Add plenty of warm milk. Drink this to help with pain or insomnia. Really relaxes the whole body!

Papaya Leaf Tea – (Lyme Tea)

Bring 1 quart of water to a boil. Turn off heat. Add 2 heaping tablespoons of dried papaya leaf and 2 heaping tablespoons of dried peppermint leaf – (use fresh when in season).Steep for 20 minutes. Sweeten, ice, and drink.

Relaxing Tea

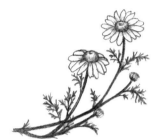

1 part chamomile

½ part peppermint

1 part passionflower

1 part oat straw

This is delicious and calming to the nerves and the body.

Combine and store in a glass gallon jar.

For **more serious** sleep or nerve difficulties add:

½ part valerian

½ part hops

DO NOT GIVE this second mixture to babies! It is too strong for them.

Respiratory Tea

Make a tea to clear out the respiratory system and help the immune system to work efficiently. Use:

2 parts – peppermint

1 part - oregano

1/2 part ea. – echinacea, mullein, comfrey leaf

Bring a half gallon of water to a boil. Turn off the heat. Do not continue to boil! Boiling makes the tea bitter and lessens the medicinal value, as the essential oils are evaporated into the atmosphere. Add one half cup of tea mixture to the water. Let it steep with the lid on, for twenty minutes. Strain and sweeten. Chill with ice and drink. This tastes nice enough to enjoy. Give them a cup every hour or oftener.

Herbal Salve Recipes

Plantain Salve for Bites and Stings

Pick plantain leaves, let leaves wilt for half a day then fill a small, clean jar. Fill the jar the second time with olive oil. Get out all the bubbles and cover all the plant material. Label the jar and let it sit for three weeks out of the direct sunlight. Shake every day. Set the jar on a paper towel since the oil will ooze a little. After four weeks pour off the oil and squeeze it out of the plants.

*To **every** ounce of oil add 1 tablespoon of grated beeswax and a capsule of vitamin E to prevent spoilage. Heat the oil stirring until the wax melts. This happens very quickly. Test by putting one spoonful of oil into the freezer. If it is too soft, add more wax. If it is too hard add more oil. Pour into jars and cool. A cup of oil makes a cup of salve.*

Skin Salve

For brush burns, wounds, infected sores, hang nails.

Follow the above directions using ½ chopped fresh comfrey and ½ comfrey root. Chop the root finely. Use olive or almond oil. Continue as above. Add enough lavender essential oil to make it smell nice. You could also mix the two and make just one salve. To **every** ounce of oil add 1 tablespoon of grated beeswax and a capsule of vitamin E to prevent spoilage. This salve works well for almost anything including chapped lips and diaper rash.

Chest Salve

Heat 1 ounce of olive oil   Add 1 capsule of vitamin E and 1 tablespoon grated beeswax.

When the wax is melted add 12 droppers of Deep Tissue Oil or use:

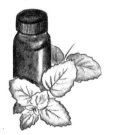

> *60 drops essential oil of eucalyptus*
>
> *20 drops essential oil of wintergreen*
>
> *10 drops essential oil of peppermint*
>
> *2 drop essential oil of thyme*

This is a great salve for chest congestion. Rub it on their back and chest and keep warm with a warm rice sock. Really helps quiet coughs.

Sleep Balm

Mix: 1/8 cup castor oil and 1/8 cup olive oil. Heat oil.

Add:

2 caps of vitamin E

2 tablespoon grated beeswax.

When the wax is melted add:

20 drops each of bergamot, ginger, rosemary, & balsam fir essential oil

40 drops of lavender

Stir and pour into jars.

Rub this on your temples and wrists if you are having trouble relaxing and falling asleep. It works very well for restless babies and children, too. I kept a tiny tin of it in my diaper bag to use for a restless baby when I needed it.

Comfrey Salve

Cut the comfrey leaves and shake them clean. Wilt leaves for half a day. Chop the leaves (and at least 6 inches of root) like you were going to make salad. Put them loosely into a wide-mouth quart jar. Cover with olive oil (or a mix of olive and almond oil). Heat to 100 degrees in your oven for one hour. Turn off heat and let set, covered with a cloth, on your counter for one to two weeks. Strain and squeeze out the leaves and you have a lovely, green oil.

Make your salve with this recipe.

2 cups of comfrey oil

1 ounce grated beeswax

1 tablespoon vitamin E oil

15 drops of lavender essential oil

Heat the oil mixture until the beeswax melts. Put a spoonful of the oil in your freezer and let it set for about 5 minutes. Is is thick enough for salve? If it is, pour it into jars. If not, grate a bit more wax and melt it and repeat the check until the salve consistency suits you.

Helpful Books

There are many, many book that you could read but do not go out and buy them all. Save money and use your local libraries whenever possible.

A Shot in the Dark – Coulter & Fisher - take an honest look at vaccines. Are they helpful?

Cancer- Step Outside the Box – Ty Bollinger – do not buy this book unless you want an alternative to the cut, poison and burn method of today's medicine. Unknown to many people, natural treatments work better than the normal medical route.

CharcoalRemedies.com – John Dinsley- you need this book to teach you more about charcoal.

Health Through God's Pharmacy – Maria Treben - great book to read and learn from

Dr. Mom's Healthy Living – Sandra Ellis

Doctor Yourself – Andrew Saul – Great reading and very helpful

Healing Lyme - Buhner - you need this if you need answers to Lyme!

Herbal Home Health Care – Dr. John Christopher - simple, basic information

How to Raise a Healthy Child in Spite of Your Doctor - Robert S. Mendelsohn – Great reading!

Natural Cures For Killer Germs – Dr. Cass Ingram - very interesting!

Mommy Diagnostics – Shonda Parker

Prescription for Nutritional Healing – James and Phyllis Balch

Smart Medicine for a Healthier Child – Janet Zand

Ten Essential Herbs – Lalitha Thomas - my first real exposure to using herbs - nice

The Green Smoothies Diet – Robyn Openshaw

Your Body's Many Cries For Water - Dr. Batmanghelidj - a must read!

What to Do When Antibiotics Don't Work – Dirk Van Gils

These books are just a place to begin. The way to learn is to read and study.

Supplies and Suppliers

Elysium Naturals – www.elysiumnaturals.com 616-965-1549

These suppliers make some of the strongest, most effective tinctures and salves that I know of, and their prices are really good. They carry Deep Tissue Oil, Complete Tissue Salve and bulk Complete Tissue Herbs for soaks. They supply Ladies Formula and Dental Formula. **Their specialty is a small first aid kit, ideal for in your car or kitchen cabinet, that includes 4 sample-sized salves, small containers of people's paste, deep tissue oil and arnica oil as well as charcoal and cayenne.** Check with them for less common things like yarrow tincture and salve, nettle tincture and others.

Natural Answers: 670 Phillips Rd, Millersburg, PA 17061   Ph: 717-692-5100.

Family owned and operated, they make and sell most of the good quality tinctures and supplies that I recommend. Their tinctures are stronger than most suppliers. They recently moved into a brand new manufacturing facility and are implementing GMPS (Good Manufacturing Practices). They make Deep Tissue Oil, salves and a large variety of tinctures. Call for a free catalog. **Mail order available.**

Nickle Mines Health Foods: 2123 Mine Rd. Paradise, PA 17562   Ph. 717-786-1426.

This family store carries most of the good quality tinctures and supplies that I recommend. They also carry glycerin tinctures without alcohol. Get Deep Tissue Oil, Comfrey Salve, Ladies Formula, Dental Formula, and lots more here. Leave a voice mail. Ask for price list. **Shipping available.**

Community Natural Foods - P.O. Box 578, New Holland, PA 17557   Ph: 717-355-0921

This store carries many of the **good quality tinctures and supplies that I recommend.** Get Deep Tissue Oil, Comfrey Salve, Ladies Formula, Echinacea Plus, Dental Formula, and lots more here. They also have American Botanical Pharmacy's (Dr. Schultz) line. Order Maximizer here. Shipping available. **Mail order available.**

Millers Natural Foods – 2888 Miller Lane, Bird-in-Hand, PA 17505   Ph: 717-768-7582

This family owned store carries most of the **good quality tinctures and other supplies that I recommend.** They specialize in burn supplies and B&W salve. Get Deep Tissue Oil, Comfrey Salve, Ladies Formula, Dental Formula, and lots more here. Carries American Botanical Pharmacy (Dr. Schultz) line. **Mail order available.**

Walnut Creek Botanicals: 2325 TR 444 Sugar Creek, OH 44681 Ph: 330-893-1095

This family business sells economical kits containing the supplies for you to make your own tinctures. Fun, easy to use and no wasted herbs. Kits make about a quart of finished product. Makes great gifts and so helpful to start you out in your tincturing adventure! Get Calcium tea, Dental Formula, Deep Tissue Oil and more. Ask for a price list. Shipping available.

Mountain Rose Herbs: PO Box 50220, Eugene, OR 97405   800-879-3337

This supplier carries almost any bulk herb and supply that you need for tinctures. The herbs are all wild-crafted or organic. They also have bottles for your tinctures, glycerin, essential oils and bees wax.

BuyActivatedCharcoal.com - PO Box 261Crawford, NE 69339   Ph: 308-665-1566

Natures Warehouse: 32654 Co Rte. 194, Theresa, NY 13691   Ph. 1-800-215-4372

This family based, Christian company provides supplements and books at reasonable prices. Their service is prompt and courteous and the shipping is low. Call for a catalog.

New Direction Aromatics – 1-800-246-7817

Order your Deep Tissue oils here; peppermint oil, wintergreen oil and   menthol crystals. These are not available at many other places.

Pacific Botanicals - 4840 Fish Hatchery Road, Grants Pass, OR 97527 Ph. 541- 479 - 7777

Use this company for your larger bulk orders. Order at least a pound at a time. Service and quality - excellent! Their herbs are fresh and not   chemically sprayed or irradiated. But remember that one pound is a lot of herb in most cases.

Wish Garden Herbs: 3100 Carbon Place, U. 103, Boulder, CO 80301   Ph. 303-516-1803

A supplier of good pregnancy and birthing related tinctures. Ask for their brochure. *Smooth Transitions* – ease labor contractions for the weary mother and give her a chance to regain some energy to birth the baby. *Womb Strings* – stops bleeding after birth. Blue Cohosh, Black Cohosh and Ginger tinctures are available here for midwives.

List of Supplies

Here is a list of things that I try not to be without. You will learn how to use them on the previous pages. Often an emergency comes on a weekend or in the evening after the store is closed. It pays to study and see what you feel comfortable with, and have that on hand. Most of these things are not expensive, at least not in light of a doctor visit.

- ☒ Ace bandages – a few of them
- ☒ Aloe vera gel or juice – keep in the fridge
- ☒ Band-aids
- ☒ Complete Tissue Salve
- ☒ Complete Tissue capsules
- ☒ Black salve – for drawing things out
- ☒ Brain Formula – 1- 800 – 437-2362 – for concussions, stroke or other brain issues
- ☒ Bulb syringe for children
- ☒ Natural CALM (Natural Vitality's magnesium powder)
- ☒ Cayenne pepper – powder & capsules - to stop bleeding and heart attacks
- ☒ Charcoal powder (at least 4 oz.) –for poisoning, and poultices
- ☒ Charcoal capsules – for diarrhea
- ☒ Clove buds & clove oil – tooth ache
- ☒ Coconut oil – for garlic salve
- ☒ Comfrey salve / tincture
- ☒ Comfrey root or BF&C (Bone Flesh and Cartilage) for soaking sprains
- ☒ Deep Tissue Oil – sprains, swollen glands
- ☒ Dental Formula – for cavities and toothache
- ☒ Digestive Tonic
- ☒ Echinacea – fresh root tincture (immune boost)
- ☒ Emergen-C vitamin C packets
- ☒ Enema kit for adults
- ☒ Epson salts
- ☒ Flax seed – 1 pound

- [x] Gauze rolls – at least 3 – 4″ rolls
- [x] Garlic bulbs
- [x] Ginger powder (4 oz.)
- [x] Kidney Bladder Formula
- [x] Hot water bottle
- [x] Ladies Formula/Hormone Health
- [x] Lavender oil
- [x] Lobelia tincture (for pain and seizures) - 1-800-215-4372
- [x] Maximizer (or any high quality protein digestive aid)
- [x] Male formula - 1- 800 – 437-2362 - helps with male hormone needs.
- [x] Nerve formula – 1- 800 – 437-2362 - really aides sleep and relaxes the nerves
- [x] Pantothenic acid
- [x] Peppermint oil
- [x] Sam splint (get this at a surgical supply store or from Mooremedical.com). You can construct great splints and casts from this stuff. It might even save you an emergency room trip!
- [x] Tiny sharp scissors
- [x] Slippery elm powder (at least 4 oz.)
- [x] Splinter remover
- [x] Super tonic (natural antibiotic)
- [x] Steri-strips for cuts that might need stitches. They work well!
- [x] Tape – for bandaging
- [x] Tea tree oil
- [x] Throat and Tonsil Formula –

Keep your supplies in a shallow, clear tote that has a lid on it. These totes can slide under a bed if needed. Put the wound care items together at one end. Put the tinctures together. Keep your herbal things together. Collect the supplies as you have time. It will save you many a doctor and emergency room visit. Can't find these? Check out the Suppliers list.

Quick Reference Emergency Chart

Copy and laminate these 2 pages and post in a prominent place to use in emergencies.

Appendicitis – see colon health chapter

Asthma attack - try 1 – 2 drops of unscented kerosene on a lump of brown sugar to dilate bronchial tubes and relieve spasms. Change diet – no dairy products or sugar till child is better. (See respiratory chap.)

Bee Sting – Rub with lavender

Bladder Infection - Drink 1 tsp baking soda in 8 oz. Water. Read Kidney Bladder Health.

Bleeding- Apply pressure at site – pack with bayberry or cayenne powder. **Internal Bleeding –** drink cayenne water 1 or more teaspoons to 8 ounce cup of warm water. Repeat in 5 minutes. Call 911 or transport to hospital yourself. You may have about 15 minutes before bleeding begins again. Repeat cayenne water during transport if needed.

Blood sugar drop – can result in migraine, serious headache, faintness and nausea. Occurs especially if meal is skipped or late. Give ½ cup orange juice followed by 1" square of cheese or some nuts.

Bruises – tape a bruised onion slice over area or rub with arnica oil

Burns – COOL in water with or aloe vera juice until pain subsides. Rub with lavender oil. For quick relief soak with vinegar water if the area is **not** open. (vinegar chap) Detailed directions in burn chapter.

Concussions – See emergency chapter for danger signs. Use brain formula for healing.

Coughs - wild cherry cough syrup for annoying sinus drainage cough. Garlic salve on chest and back for congestion and cough especially in babies and children.

Cramps - leg cramps – rub with deep tissue oil or soak feet in hot water with 1- 2 TBL of ginger powder. Tummy cramps – clove tea and heating pad or rice sock on stomach. Arm cramps – rub with deep tissue oil.

Croup – 1 – 2 drops of unscented kerosene on a lump of brown sugar to dilate bronchial tubes and relieve spasms. Change diet – no milk till child is better.

Diarrhea – take 8 oz. charcoal water after every run to the bathroom. (adult dose)

Give slippery elm gruel to babies and children. (slippery elm chap.)

Eye – to remove irritations use flax seed in tear duct area (flax chap.)

Fainting – Lay person down, loosen collar, open window or fan person. Apply cold to back of neck and forehead. Give sips of cayenne water till well revived.

Gas - Intestinal gas pain – Use 2-3 droppers digestive tonic in water or drink strong hot chamomile tea.

Heart Pain/Attack – drink 1 glass of warm water with 1 teaspoon of cayenne powder stirred into it. Repeat the dose in 5 minutes and again if needed.

Hiccoughs – Take 2 droppers of Digestive Tonic in a half glass of water. Startle the person!

High Blood Pressure – take 1 teaspoon of turmeric in glass of water to lower quickly. This is only an emergency measure. Treat with diet and exercise for further help.

Pain – cuts, wounds & breaks while healing – take Complete Tissue capsules 5-7 as often as needed. Drink clove tea to relax the area. Abdominal or back pain – use warm charcoal/flax poultice on area (flax chap.) Rub area with lobelia to relax muscles. Flax alone, will work too.

Poison – Drink charcoal water – 1 tablespoon in 1 8 oz. Glass of water. Repeat if needed. (charcoal chapter)

Seizures – drip lobelia in mouth, rub at base of skull and down spine. Or rub cayenne powder on gums to wake them up and bring them out of seizure.

Sinus congestion and pain - rub area frequently with deep tissue oil or sensei salve (not in eyes) Sniff salt water up nostrils and then blow – repeat every twenty minutes, as needed.

Stings – rub with lavender oil as needed. Does not work well for wasp stings. Use charcoal compress.

Stomach Ulcers – Stop solid food. Drink 8 oz. water hourly and 1 teaspoon cayenne in 8 oz. water hourly. (may burn but will soon soothe) read colon health chapter.

Sunburn – rub well with olive oil every half hour. For more cooling add a drop or two of peppermint oil to olive oil.

Tooth Abscess - Rinse mouth with salt water, take a clove of garlic and 2000 mg Vitamin C, hourly till resolved. Can tuck a garlic clove by sore spot in mouth.

Toothache – use clove tea to numb and sooth. Swish and swallow 2 droppers of Black Walnut hourly if needed for a day and then 4 x's daily till tooth heals.

Stroke - drink 1 glass of warm water with 1 teaspoon of cayenne powder stirred into it. Repeat the dose in 5 minutes and again if needed.

Alphabetical Index

Notes

Notes

Be Your Child's Pediatrician, is packed with valuable practical advice and personal stories. It is a refreshing change to use herbs, teas, and oils, instead of drugs, and with excellent results. Discover how to recognize childhood diseases, and deal with ADD, allergies, asthma, and much more. This full-color book makes being Dr. Mom much more doable. This is a companion book to *Be Your Own Doctor.* $24.95

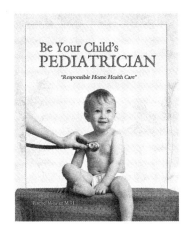

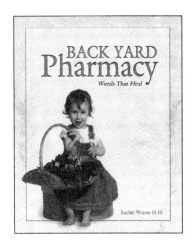

Backyard Pharmacy – Is filled with stories of how herbs, "weeds" from your backyard, may be the answer to some of your health needs. Again, it contains recipes of how to make medicine from these weeds, full color pictures of each plant discussed so that you can identify them yourself, and stories of folks who used them to heal their problems. Addresses and phone numbers of suppliers are included in each chapter as well as a list of people who market high quality salves and tinctures made from these "weeds".

Order these books online at www.drmomsherbs.com,

or call 717-435-4707, or send your order in the mail to:

Share-A-Care

240 Mohns Hill Road

Reinholds, PA 17569.